Understanding
Psychological
Assessment

PERSPECTIVES ON INDIVIDUAL DIFFERENCES

CECIL R. REYNOLDS, *Texas A&M University, College Station*
ROBERT T. BROWN, *University of North Carolina, Wilmington*

Understanding Psychological Assessment

Edited by

William I. Dorfman

Nova Southeastern University
Fort Lauderdale, Florida

and

Michel Hersen

Pacific University
Forest Grove, Oregon

Kluwer Academic / Plenum Publishers
New York • Boston • Dordrecht • London • Moscow

Library of Congress Cataloging-in-Publication Data

Understanding psychological assessment/edited by William I. Dorfman and Michel Hersen.
 p.   cm.—(Perspectives on individual differences)
 Includes bibliographical references and index.
 ISBN 0-306-46268-0
 1. Psychometrics. 2. Psychological tests. I. Dorfman, William I. II. Hersen, Michel.
III. Series.

BF39 .U54 2000
150'.287—dc21

00-033114

ISBN 0-306-46268-0

©2001 Kluwer Academic/Plenum Publishers
233 Spring Street, New York, N.Y. 10013

10 9 8 7 6 5 4 3 2 1

A C.I.P. record for this book is available from the Library of Congress.

Printed in the United States of America

To my parents Saul M. and Bettylou
                —WID

To my wife Vicki
                —MH

Contributors

Achilles N. Bardos, Division of Professional Psychology, University of Northern Colorado, Greeley, Colorado 80639

Yossef S. Ben-Porath, Department of Psychology, Kent State University, Kent, Ohio 44242

William J. Burns, Center for Psychological Studies, Nova Southeastern University, Fort Lauderdale, Florida 33314

Heather E. P. Cattell, Institute for Personality and Ability Testing, Inc., Walnut Creek, California 94595-2611

Adam Conklin, Austen Riggs Center, Stockbridge, Massachusetts 01262

Robert J. Craig, Bolingbrook, Illinois 60440-1214

William I. Dorfman, Center for Psychological Studies, Nova Southeastern University, Fort Lauderdale, Florida 33314

Sara Ehrich, Center for Psychological Studies, Nova Southeastern University, Fort Lauderdale, Florida 33314

Jan Faust, Center for Psychological Studies, Nova Southeastern University, Fort Lauderdale, Florida 33314

Johnathan David Forbey, Department of Psychology, Kent State University, Kent, Ohio 44242

Shawna M. Freshwater, Center for Psychological Studies, Nova Southeastern University, Fort Lauderdale, Florida 33314

Joseph J. Glutting, School of Education, University of Delaware, Newark, Delaware 19711

Charles J. Golden, Center for Psychological Studies, Nova Southeastern University, Fort Lauderdale, Florida 33314

Michael I. Lah, Middletown, Connecticut 06457-6215

Sean Leonard, Center for Psychological Studies, Nova Southeastern University, Fort Lauderdale, Florida 33314

Shane J. Lopez, Department of Psychology and Research in Education, University of Kansas, Lawrence, Kansas 66045

Jack A. Naglieri, George Mason University, Fairfax, Virginia 22030-4444

Shawn Powell, Division of Professional Psychology, University of Northern Colorado, Greeley, Colorado 80639

Bady Quintar, Center for Psychological Studies, Nova Southeastern University, Fort Lauderdale, Florida 33314

Gary J. Robertson, School of Education, University of Delaware, Newark, Delaware 19711

Joseph J. Ryan, Department of Psychology and Counselor Education, Central Missouri State University, Warrensburg, Missouri 64093

Barry A. Schneider, Center for Psychological Studies, Nova Southeastern University, Fort Lauderdale, Florida 33314

Alisa J. Snelbaker, School of Education, University of Delaware, Newark, Delaware 19711

Colby Sandoval Srsic, Department of Psychology, Ohio State University, Columbus, Ohio, 43210

Antonella P. Stimac, Department of Psychology, Ohio State University, Columbus, Ohio 43210

Scott W. Sumerall, Department of Psychology, William Jewell College, Liberty, Missouri 64048

W. Bruce Walsh, Department of Psychology, Ohio State University, Columbus, Ohio 43210

Drew Westen, Department of Psychology, Boston University, Boston, Massachusetts 02215

Gary S. Wilkinson, School of Education, University of Delaware, Newark, Delaware 19711

Christi Woolger, Kissimmee, Florida 34744

Preface

Introductory texts on psychological testing and evaluation historically are not in short supply. Typically, however, such texts have been relatively superficial in their discussion of clinical material and have focused primarily on the theoretical and psychometric properties of individual tests. More practical, clinically relevant presentations of psychological instruments have been confined to individual volumes with advanced and often very technical information geared to the more sophisticated user. Professors in introductory graduate courses are often forced to adopt several advanced texts to cover the material, at the same time helping students wade through unnecessary technical information in order to provide a basic working knowledge of each test.

Understanding Psychological Assessment is an attempt to address these concerns. It brings together into a single volume a broad sampling of the most respected instruments in the psychologist's armamentarium along with promising new tests of cognitive, vocational, and personality functioning. Additionally, it presents the most updated versions of these tests, all in a practical, clearly written format that covers the development, psychometrics, administrative considerations, and interpretive hypotheses for each instrument. Clinical case studies allow the reader to apply the interpretive guidelines to real clinical data, thereby reinforcing basic understanding of the instrument and helping to insure that both the student and practitioner can actually begin to use the test. *Understanding Psychological Assessment* includes cognitive and personality tests for adults, children, and adolescents, as well as chapters on the theory of psychological measurement and integrated report writing.

We think that this text will serve as a valuable introduction to graduate students in introductory testing and assessment courses, as well as to more seasoned practitioners needing a handy reference for a broad range of popular psychological tests.

Many individuals have contributed to the fruition of this textbook. First, we thank our eminent authors for taking time out from their busy schedules to write the chapters. Second, we thank Carole Londerée, Eleanor Gil, and Erika Qualls for their invaluable technical assistance. Finally, we acknowledge the goodwill of our editor, Eliot Werner, at Kluwer Academic/ Plenum Publishers.

WILLIAM I. DORFMAN
MICHEL HERSEN

Contents

II. CHILD/ADOLESCENT

III. INTEGRATION

1

Understanding Test Construction

Joseph J. Ryan, Shane J. Lopez,
and Scott W. Sumerall

Measurement typically involves the assignment of numerical values to objects or events. The attributes of persons that are generally assessed include, but are not limited to, career interests, intelligence, memory, and personality. A test may be designed to measure maximum performance as with intelligence scales and achievement tests, or usual performance as with questionnaires and inventories that assess feelings during the past week, personal attitudes, and vocational interests.

Psychological testing originated in China over 3000 years ago. By 200 B.C., the Chinese had developed a formal system of written, individually administered civil service examinations which were used until 1905. Within the West, the history of psychological testing can be traced to mid-19th-century Germany and Great Britain. Wundt, Weber, and others conducted studies that examined perception and motor speed. In so doing, they employed standardized data collection methods and set the tone for future work in the field. Sir Francis Galton examined differences among people and contributed to assessment by devising statistical methods for the analysis of relationships. In 1890, James Cattell initiated the term "mental testing" and developed norms to evaluate individual performance.

The methods by which attributes are assessed vary. They may involve direct observation of behavior, self-report, or some other approach. Direct observation is time consuming and often fails to identify the variable of interest. People sometimes alter their behavior patterns for personal reasons, or individuals may not be exposed to situations that elicit the desired behavior. Therefore, other methods of assessment are frequently utilized.

Basic self-report measures are employed for many clinical purposes. One can quickly gauge the presence and severity of a specific mood state such as depression. However, questionnaires and inventories that measure such constructs often are "transparent" and responses

Joseph J. Ryan • Department of Psychology and Counselor Education, Central Missouri State University, Warrensburg, Missouri 64093   Shane J. Lopez • Department of Psychology and Research in Education, University of Kansas, Lawrence, Kansas 66045.   Scott W. Sumerall • Department of Psychology, William Jewell College, Liberty, Missouri 64048

Understanding Psychological Assessment, edited by Dorfman and Hersen. Kluwer Academic/Plenum Publishers, New York, 2001.

are not always representative of an examinee's actual degree of emotional discomfort. In addition, there are some attributes that do not readily lend themselves to the self-report format. In many situations, tests that are less direct and do not convey an obvious purpose to the examinee, such as projective personality measures, may be used.

The present chapter is an introduction to test construction and item selection. First, the various techniques utilized to accomplish these tasks are presented and discussed. Next, a review of the empirical issues that pertain to validity and reliability of measures is provided. The chapter concludes with a discussion of test norms, test scores, and the rudimentary principles of score interpretation.

TEST CONSTRUCTION AND DEVELOPMENT

Typically, the first step in the development of a new measure is to determine its purpose and how individual scores will be interpreted. Will scores be used to make diagnoses, assist with vocational and career decisions, or identify high achievers or persons who need extra classroom assistance? Defining the purpose of a test is critical. For example, it would not be necessary to develop an academic measure with a very high ceiling if the goal of the assessment was to identify students who perform poorly in class and who would benefit from remedial intervention. Conversely, if the scores on a test were to be used for intelligence classification, the instrument should cover a wide range of performance that reflects both ends of the ability spectrum. A brief discussion of the three most widely used methods for constructing objective tests is given below.

Criterion-Keyed Approach

The criterion-keyed approach, or empirical method of test development, begins with an operational definition of the construct of interest. In most cases, groups of people who fall into specific categories (e.g., CPAs, social workers, persons with a diagnosis of schizophrenia or affective disorder) are selected as the operational expression of the construct. Next, test developers examine whether or not responses to a sample of items, thought to define the construct, differentiate the criterion groups. For example, if the task is to identify distinct interest patterns across selected professional occupations, a test might be administered to samples of C.P.A.'s, social workers, and persons in other job categories. If the individual samples respond in different ways to some or all of the items, it may be possible to arrange specific items into scales that more accurately characterize the response patterns of the target occupational groups. A problem with this approach is that it is not always apparent when an item truly differentiates the samples. Using a 5% level of significance to indicate that an item is specific to a certain group, assignment will occur five times out of 100 by chance alone. As a result, if some items are not strongly related to the construct or were incorrectly included in the test, interpretation of the results may be problematic. In addition, if more than one construct is reflected in a test or scale, examinees may earn the same set of scores but for distinctly different reasons.

Analytic Approach

The inductive/factor-analytic technique of test development begins with a group of items that, based on a theory, are thought to measure specific variables or factors. The items are given to a large sample, the data are subjected to factor analysis, and the results are interpreted according to the theory that guided item development. It is essential that the sample used in the factor analysis is representative of the persons to whom the test will be administered clinically. Replication studies also should be conducted to ensure the stability of the factor structure. This inductive approach has a number of drawbacks. For instance, in the absence of a strong theory to guide item selection and to explain the results, observed factors or traits may not have psychological meaning. Furthermore, statistical variables (e.g., the type of factor analysis and rotational method utilized and the portions of the sample that have strong intragroup positive correlations and significant intergroup differences on items) can influence the factors that are derived. These variables can alter the factor structure, the final version of the test, and the strategies used to interpret the results.

Rational/Deductive Method

The rational/deductive method of test construction combines the features of the empirical and analytic approaches. Items are generated on the basis of a theory and are then subjected to psychometric evaluation. Individual items and scales may be rejected if they do not meet or exceed minimal statistical standards or fail to demonstrate predicted empirical relationships. In the following pages, a brief overview of test construction using the rational/ deductive method is presented. This is the methodology most often employed by contemporary test developers.

Initial steps. Test construction begins with the selection of individual items that represent a specified domain. Assume that the test or scale will be used as a screening measure for depression. Based on a theoretical framework and the results of clinical and empirical research with the various depressive disorders, test items might be selected to cover psychological, behavioral, and biological factors. For example, unambiguous questions concerning suicidal ideation, crying spells, and disturbed sleep or loss of appetite might be selected and modified from available sources, or written specifically for the new scale. Another technique to examine a domain involves exploring the extremes of the construct. Thus, it may be important to define exactly what constitutes the strongest and the weakest expressions of the domain. Direct observation of persons with mild to severe depression will often be helpful in this regard. Once the items have been selected, experts may be asked to conduct a content analysis to insure that the domain of interest has been adequately sampled.

The item format must also be determined. Is the test or scale going to focus on dichotomous information and responses (i.e., true-false), use a Likert scale (i.e., the examinee indicates the degree of agreement or disagreement with statements on a five-point scale), follow a multiple choice format, or rely on open-ended questions or tasks? Test formats are typically driven by the purpose of the measure. Optimal performance tests, such as those that assess academic achievement often use multiple-choice or fill-in-the-blank questions. Objective personality tests or the depression scale discussed above frequently use true-false or Likert scaling. Projective measures are unique in that they often present novel stimuli (e.g., inkblots), ask the examinee to perform a specific task (e.g., draw a house, tree, person), or require an open-ended response (e.g., tell a story about a picture). The responses are then analyzed and interpreted in relation to a specific theory and a normative sample.

Once item selection and format problems have been resolved, a relatively large pool of items should be devised and subjected to expert review with regard to the appropriateness of content, cultural bias, and understandability. A trial or pilot study should be conducted in order to gain preliminary results so developers may further refine the test content and form. Next, the test is given to groups of carefully selected individuals who will serve as the normative sample. This provides data for reliability and validity studies as well as information to be used clinically so that comparisons can be made between the normative sample and individual examinees.

Item Analysis

Item analysis involves a review of test content and includes examination of item difficulty, item discrimination, and item response theory. Item difficulty levels are determined for measures of intelligence, aptitude, and achievement and indicate the number of persons who correctly respond to each item. Thus, .60 indicates that 60% of persons answering a question do so correctly. True-false questions on an aptitude measure that have difficulty values of .50 would be undesirable. The answers to these items can be obtained by guessing with a 50% probability of being correct. Likewise, in most situations, test developers do not want items with difficulty levels of 1.0 or 0.0. In both cases, the items do not differentiate among examinees. The first type is too easy and the latter is too hard. The difficulty of an item is best when it is centered between 1.0 and the likelihood of getting the item correct by chance. Thus, for a true-false aptitude test, the ideal item difficulty level would be .75, as differentiation among examinees is maximized. It is important to note that item difficulty levels will differ according to the purpose of the assessment. A screening test to select candidates for employment in a sheltered workshop should be composed of relatively easy items. Conversely, if a test is intended to identify candidates for advanced education in the basic sciences, it should be composed of relatively difficult items.

The relationship between responses to an item and overall performance on a test is referred to as discriminability. In most cases, if responses to an item are unrelated to the composite score, there is reason to suspect that the item failed to measure what it was intended to measure. To evaluate discriminability of items in a test that uses the true-false response format, a point-biserial correlation coefficient is appropriate because this statistic describes the relationship between a dichotomous variable (i.e., true-false) and a continuous variable (i.e., total test score). Other correlational procedures used for determining discriminability are the phi coefficient and the biserial coefficient. Another approach uses the discriminability index which is defined as: $D = P1 - P2$. Assume that $P1$ is the proportion of examinees in the upper 50%, based on the total score, who correctly answered the item, and $P2$ is the proportion of examinees in the lower 50%, based on the total score, who passed the item. Thus, the discriminability index is a measure of the difference between groups (i.e., persons who score very well on the test and those who do not) for each item. For example, if an item was answered correctly by 80% of persons in the upper half of the total-score distribution and by 35% of examinees in the lower half, this would yield an index of 45 (i.e., $80 - 35 = 45$). Conversely, if a given item was passed by 60% of persons in the top half of the total-score distribution and 40% of those in the lower half, the resulting index would equal 20. An index of 45 is better than one of 20, demonstrating that the item in the first example discriminated the groups more effectively than did the second item.

Item response theory provides information about item difficulty and item discrimination simultaneously, along with the probability of guessing correctly on any given item. It acknowledges the differences that sometimes are present when persons with varying degrees of the trait or ability of interest perform differently on a specific item. By the use of a mathematical model to predict performance at various trait/ability levels on an item, one can analyze the performance of examinees that have not responded to the same items. Item characteristic curves are plotted for each test question or task. This displays the likelihood of getting the item correct as a function of the magnitude of the presence of a single latent trait. Item response theory enhances test construction methodology because it renders tests more precise.

RELIABILITY AND VALIDITY

Reliability

Reliability reflects the extent to which a test measures a construct consistently. Adequate reliability is achieved when measurements are made in a way that reduces the impact of chance, although some degree of error will always be a part of the assessment process. Test scores are often influenced by sources of error related to inadequate test content, time intervals between assessments, failure to follow appropriate administration procedures, poor testing conditions, or examinee characteristics such as illness, fatigue, response bias, or poor test taking motivation. Different types of reliability coefficients are evaluated to assess the quality of a test (see Table 1.1). These statistics provide information about the amounts of true variance and error variance contained in a set of test scores. Some experts consider a coefficient of .80 the lower limit of acceptable reliability for tests used in clinical practice.

Internal Consistency Reliability

An internal consistency reliability estimate is obtained from a single administration of a test. It reflects content sampling and the degree to which items in the test "hang together" and measure the same construct. There are three primary methods for obtaining internal consistency estimates. The split-half technique divides a test into equivalent halves and correlates the two. Cronbach's coefficient alpha provides more information than the preceding method because it is the mean of all possible split-half correlations for the test. The split-half and alpha coefficients are designed for tests with items that have multiple possible answers. Finally, the Kuder-Richardson Formula 20 is a special modification of the alpha coefficient that is designed for tests that use the true-false or right-wrong answer format.

Test-Retest Reliability (Stability)

Administration of a test on two (or more) occasions to the same individuals allows for an estimation of test-retest stability. By correlating scores across two examinations, the extent to

Table 1.1. Types of Reliability

Type	Questions Addressed
Internal Consistency	Do comparable halves of the test reveal errors due to poor item sampling? To what degree do the test items measure the same construct?
Test-Retest	How stable are the test scores and how much random fluctuation occurs in scores from test to retest? To what extent can scores on retest be predicted by scores on initial testing?
Alternate Forms	Do parallel forms of the test produce similar results? Do the test items measure the construct of interest in a consistent manner?
Recording/Scoring Reliability	How accurately do examiners record the same response? How consistent are scoring judgments across different examiners?

which the results can be generalized from one situation to the next is determined. This methodology assumes that the characteristic being measured is a relatively stable trait such as general intelligence, vocational interests, or mechanical aptitudes. The test-retest intervals should be noted, as short periods between assessment probes increase the probability of practice effects (i.e., examinees remember items and successful problem solutions) on some tests (e.g., intelligence scales). Long intervals introduce confounds because of actual changes in the examinees caused by maturation, therapeutic interventions, educational attainments, or illness. The test-retest coefficient reflects the stability of scores for group data.

It is important to note that a high stability coefficient indicates only that the examinees ordered themselves in the same manner at both assessment points. This does not eliminate the possibility that individual scores change to a meaningful degree over time. If three examinees obtained IQ scores of 80, 90, and 100 during the first test session, and their IQs were 100, 110, and 120 at the second testing, this would yield a perfect stability coefficient. However, the level of intelligence suggested by each score would have changed significantly.

Alternate Forms Reliability

Content sampling, or the selection of items that occurs during the initial phases of test development, should be completed in a systematic manner so that the instrument is comprised of items that are representative of the attribute being measured. When a sufficient number of items have been developed, a second version of the test may be compiled. Administration of the two instruments, using a variety of test intervals (e.g., three hours and three weeks), provides an opportunity to assess alternate form reliability and the degree of variance associated with content sampling. If the correlation between alternate forms administered over a couple of weeks is low, and the correlation between the tests given on the same day is also low, this suggests that the two instruments have largely different content. If the correlation between the forms is high for the same day administration, but low for the two-week administration, the construct measured by the test is very likely a state variable (e.g., mood, anxiety level, etc.) that is unstable over time. If the two test forms yield high correlations (and similar means and standard deviations) regardless of the retest interval, the instruments appear to measure the same enduring trait. If there is minimal error in measurement, examinees will earn a highly similar score on both versions of the test.

Recording/Scoring Reliability

Interrater and interscorer reliability, although not typically measured by a correlation coefficient, should be carefully assessed when test scores depend, in any way, on examiner judgment or clerical accuracy. Variance in recording and scoring responses will directly affect the reliability and clinical utility of a test. Responses to some objective (e.g., Wechsler Adult Intelligence Scale-III Comprehension subtest) and most projective tests may challenge the scoring savvy of even highly experienced clinicians; so the extent to which different examiners arrive at similar scoring decisions needs to be evaluated. Error variance associated with recording and scoring errors quickly accumulates and can affect diagnostic impressions and treatment plans. According to formal studies on the scoring reliability of psychological tests, typical errors include the assigning of incorrect score values to individual responses, incorrectly recording responses, incorrectly converting raw scores to derived scores, and making calculation errors when obtaining raw and/or derived score totals. It is also noteworthy that, regardless of the examiner's level of experience with psychological testing, scoring errors occur frequently and detract from the accuracy of the assessment process.

Interpreting Reliability Coefficients

Qualifying terms such as *poor, appropriate, adequate, moderate,* and *high* are often used to describe the reliability of a test. The meaning of a coefficient is dependent on the type of construct measured and the method used to derive the reliability estimate. Reliability serves as a standard of test quality and informs the examiner of the amount of true and error variance in a set of test scores. Thus, a coefficient of .80 (which is a commonly accepted cut-off for clinical measures) reveals that 80% of the variance in a score is true and 20% represents random fluctuation or error. A coefficient of .70 (a commonly used cut-off for measures used in research) suggests that 70% of the score variance is "real" whereas 30% is "noise."

Another way to interpret reliability is to square it to obtain an estimate of predictability. Assume a test is given to a group of individuals on two occasions and the associated stability coefficient is .70. When this value is squared, it suggests that 49% of the variance in scores from the first administration is shared with scores from the second administration. In other words, scores on a readministration of the test are only 49% predictable and are 51% unpredictable based on results of the initial examination. Based on these findings one should not be overly confident in predicting future test results.

The correlation coefficient expresses the reliability of a test for a group of examinees. However, when working with a single client it is essential that reliability be evaluated in terms of individual scores. This is accomplished by using the standard error of measurement, which is defined as the standard deviation of the distribution of error scores. This statistic uses the obtained score and serves as a reminder that measurement error is inherent in all test results. The standard error of estimate, which is based on the estimated true score in place of the fallible obtained score, may also be employed. These statistics should be given in the test manual because they are needed to calculate confidence limits around obtained scores. Confidence limits reflect score precision by defining the upper and lower band of scores around the observed value in which a client's true score falls. Tests with large standard errors yield less precise scores than tests with small standard errors.

Validity

A test is valid if it does what it is intended to do. Validity is concerned with the usefulness of a test in both its applied and theoretical aspects. It relates to the ability of examiners to make inferences about people and environments from an examination of test scores. Evidence that supports the validity of a specific instrument comes from a variety of sources, relies heavily on empirical investigation, and is the result of an unending process.

Strictly speaking, one does not validate the test but instead validates the specific applications of a test. For instance, a test of musical talent may be valid for selecting applicants to a music school, but it would not necessarily be valid for other purposes, such as measuring general intelligence or identifying personality characteristics. The various types of validity are discussed below (see Table 1.2).

Face Validity

Face validity is not a psychometric concept, but it is important for many tests, such as those that measure general intelligence, aptitudes, and academic achievement. It refers to the extent to which the final version of a test looks like it measures what it purports to measure. Face validity is based on the subjective judgment of the examinee and may influence how one performs on the test. If an examinee feels a test is too simple, too hard, or unrelated to the

Table 1.2. Types of Validity

Type	Questions Addressed
Face Validity	Does the test appear to measure what it claims to measure?
Content Validity	Does the item content of the test adequately represent the domain of interest?
Criterion-Related Validity	
Concurrent Validity	Is performance on the test of interest highly associated with scores from other measures (e.g., tests and behavioral ratings) that are assumed to reflect the same construct and are obtained at about the same time?
Predictive Validity	Is performance on the test related to a future external measurement of the construct?
Construct Validity	What does the test measure? Does it measure the intended construct? How does the test measure the construct?

issue under investigation, a skeptical attitude or a reduced level of cooperation may result. In most situations, an unmotivated or disinterested examinee will produce scores that do not accurately reflect the abilities or other characteristics of interest.

Content Validity

The appropriateness of test content is relevant from the earliest stages of test construction. Content validity refers to whether the items composing a test adequately represent the domain or construct of interest. Items are selected to conform to a theoretical perspective (e.g., those that reflect state anxiety versus trait anxiety) or to cover a specific operationally defined skill level (e.g., arithmetic problems that tap the ability to perform basic addition and subtraction) or to do both. A proper balance of items in terms of content is achieved through careful consideration and formal reviews by qualified judges. Items may be reviewed during initial stages of test construction, as part of an item pilot-testing phase, and during standardization.

Criterion-Related Validity

Criterion-related validity reflects the extent to which test scores demonstrate an association with an external indicator or variable. Criterion-related validity is usually reported in two forms: concurrent and predictive. The former focuses on the extent to which test scores are related to some currently available measure of the criterion of interest collected at approximately the same time. Assume that a new intelligence test and an established measure of intelligence are given to the same sample of adults on the same day. If scores on the two tests are highly associated, the new intelligence test is said to have concurrent validity. Predictive validity reflects the relationship between a test and an external criterion, but unlike concurrent validity, there must be a meaningful time interval between test administration and performance on the criterion. For instance, an aptitude test might be administered to entering college freshman and later correlated with their four-year grade point averages. If scores on the aptitude test are highly correlated with grades, the test has demonstrated validity for predicting college success. The primary shortcoming of both approaches is that the usefulness of validity studies depends on the appropriateness of the criterion variables. In many situations this is problematic because there are no available criteria or those that are available suffer from various flaws.

Construct Validity

This type of validity focuses on how well a test measures a specific theoretical construct or trait and requires a three-stage process that involves (a) formulating an operational definition of the construct within a theoretical framework, (b) measuring the construct, and (c) determining the relationship between test scores and other variables hypothesized to be associated or unassociated with the latent trait. Studies that address the issues of concurrent validity and criterion-related validity also yield information about construct validity. However, unlike with these empirical approaches, it is not enough to know that a test correlates highly with other instruments that measure the same thing or that it accurately predicts future behavior. Instead, construct validation is aimed at determining why a test succeeds in predicting a criterion or why its results conform to theoretical expectations. Typical methods for evaluating construct validity include intercorrelations of multiple measures and factor analysis.

Interpreting Validity Coefficients

Validity refers to the various applications of a test and its determination is therefore an unending process. An instrument may have demonstrated validity for predicting an outcome such as school performance, but have little value for the identification of children with psychiatric or neurological problems. Thus, when a test is employed for a specific purpose, it is essential that the examiner be familiar with relevant validity studies that support the application. The association between a test and a criterion is typically reported in the form of a correlation coefficient. To evaluate a "validity coefficient," it must be squared (this yields the coefficient of determination) to determine the amount of shared variance between the test and the criterion. Thus, a correlation of .30 between an achievement test composite score and school grades indicates that the former variable accounts for only 9% of the variance in school performance. The remaining 91% of variation remains unexplained. It should be obvious that if the investigation that reported the coefficient of .30 was properly conducted (e.g., the sample did not show restriction of range of scores on either the predictor or the criterion), the achievement test cannot be used to predict school performance.

Some experts argue that the smallest acceptable validity coefficient should equal or exceed .60, but others feel that this is too liberal or too conservative. The most reasonable solution to this disagreement is to consider the purpose for which a test is being administered. If results will be used for important decisions such as IQ classification, diagnosis, or personal injury litigation, relatively high limits should be set. Keep in mind that the degree of predictability is determined by squaring the validity coefficient. If a test is used with a validity coefficient of .60, this accounts for only 36% of the variance between the test and the criterion. Thus, the test is a very poor predictor of the criterion.

Relationship between Reliability and Validity

Adequate reliability is a prerequisite for test validity. An instrument cannot be valid if it is unreliable. Only when a measure is accurate, consistent, and stable can the extent to which it measures what it purports to measure be ascertained. However, a reliable test may be invalid for a particular purpose. For example, a demographic questionnaire that requests information such as date of birth, race, sex, and the names of biological relatives will be perfectly reliable from test to retest. However, the questionnaire would be invalid if it were used to measure intelligence, mood, or vocational interests.

Reliability and Validity of Projective Tests

Projective tests are designed to gather information about personality and behavioral tendencies based on responses to ambiguous or novel stimuli. The most commonly used projective techniques include the Rorschach Inkblot Test, Thematic Apperception Test, Rotter Incomplete Sentences Blank, and House-Tree-Person Test. In terms of construction and application, projective techniques are theory driven. Historically, some clinicians have protested the application of traditional reliability and validity standards to these measures. The relevance of psychometric standards are questioned on the following grounds: (a) projective techniques are used for in-depth description of personality rather than formal measurement, (b) reliability indices that emphasize test-retest stability cannot account for the subjective and "state" experiences of respondents over time, nor can the tests be easily subjected to internal consistency analysis, (c) adequate criterion variables that are needed to conduct concurrent and predictive validity studies are often difficult to identify, and (d) available validation studies are inherently flawed due to administration variance and reliability issues. Despite these objections, practice standards dictate that tests used in clinical situations have adequate reliability, validity, and norms. Therefore, the proponents and opponents of projective techniques have produced a large body of research that should be carefully reviewed when the use of a projective test is being considered.

Test Bias

Those who use psychological instruments to assist with client placement, counseling, or classification should be familiar with the controversial issue of test bias. It represents inherent flaws within a test that result in discriminatory assessment because of an examinee's demographic (e.g., cultural and socioeconomic background), biological (e.g., gender and race) characteristics, or both. However, bias is not revealed by subjective opinion based on examination of individual test items, or even by significant mean differences between a minority sample and the majority population.

The specificity of item content may reflect varying degrees of cultural loading, a concept that is clearly different from cultural bias. The former is determined by subjective armchair analysis, while the latter is ascertained statistically by assessing a test's characteristics in terms of reliability and validity. For example, test questions that ask high school students from Los Angeles to name the capital cities of France, Italy, and Australia are more culturally loaded than items that ask the same students to name the capital cities of California, Arizona, and Nevada. However, these items may predict grades in geography equally well, irrespective of whether the answers are given by students from lower socioeconomic or middle-class backgrounds. Thus, culturally loaded items can demonstrate acceptable predictive validity. Moreover, if the items show similar difficulty levels, and internal analysis of the test shows the same degree of statistical properties across socioeconomic groups, evidence of cultural bias is lacking. The usual methods of internal analysis include the computation of internal consistency reliability coefficients and the use of exploratory and confirmatory factor analyses.

NORMS AND DERIVED SCORES

The raw score on a psychological or educational test, such as the number of items correctly completed, is not very meaningful when viewed in isolation. For instance, how might one interpret a score of 30 of 50 correct on a test of arithmetic computation? If the test is relatively easy, a score of 60% (30/50) correct might represent impaired performance. If the test is unusually difficult, a score of 60% might indicate superior achievement. To make sense out of a test score one must compare it with some type of relevant standard or norm. Basic normative data simply reflect the range and frequency of scores obtained by a sample of individuals who took the test.

To be relevant, norms must be representative. If the test is designed as a screening instrument for admission to a school of music, the normative sample might consist of students successfully completing the first semester of the program. If the test is to be administered to males and females, then the normative sample should include both sexes. However, if the test is intended as a more general measure of musical ability or talent, then a broader normative sample is necessary. In such cases, the purpose of testing might be to determine what constitutes typical performance among people in general on the specific musical tasks. The basic rule to follow is that the normative sample (also known as the standardization sample) should mirror the composition of those to whom the test will be applied. For people-in-general, one could use official census figures to select subjects to ensure proportional accuracy with respect to important demographic variables. If this goal is not met, the norms may yield inaccurate conclusions about the examinees.

The norms that accompany most published tests are collected during an official standardization process. After the items have been evaluated via pilot testing and tryout studies, a final or semifinal version of the instrument is administered to specific groups of people according to a carefully prepared plan that ensures a representative sample. Next, data are gathered by trained examiners under uniform conditions (e.g., lighting, ambient noise levels, and temperature in the examination rooms should all be uniform and items are administered in exactly the same manner to all examinees). Test responses are then scored according to specific criteria and all raw data are inspected, checked for accuracy, and eventually entered into a computer storage system. Based on the standardization sample, final statistics reflecting reliability, stability, validity, and potential test bias are generated.

To fully appreciate the appropriateness and adequacy of a normative or standardization sample, one must carefully read the test manual, or other relevant descriptive literature, or both. If the norms are not accompanied by a complete description of the people they represent, use them with caution, if at all. A good set of norms presents data that were recently collected under specified conditions (e.g., according to standardized test instructions and time limits). They should be stratified on demographic variables that are related to test performance or interpretation, such as age, sex, education, and occupation. The sample must also be large enough to yield stable estimates. A minimum of 30 to 50 subjects per cell is a reasonable rule of thumb when norms are intended for clinical use, although larger samples are always desirable. Finally, raw test scores must be equated with or transformed into percentiles, some standardized values or both to permit comparison of performance among various subjects or tests. The topic of transformed scores is discussed in the next section.

Norms usually are presented in the test manual in one or more tables giving corresponding values of raw scores and derived scores. The tabular information should be accompanied by descriptive statistics that include the average or mean score obtained by the standardization subjects along with measures of variability such as the range and standard deviation. These statistics allow one to compare an individual score with the expected scores of all participants in the normative sample. To illustrate the practical value of such data, assume that the mean score among standardization subjects on a music skills test is 100 and an advisor is providing academic counseling to a college freshman named Bob who has earned a score on the test of 115. Based on the norms, the advisor can tell the examinee that his score is above average. Now assume that the test manual also reports a standard deviation of 15. The advisor can now utilize knowledge of the normal curve to inform Bob that his obtained score equals or exceeds 84% of persons in the standardization sample.

The next interpretive conclusion depends on whether the norms consulted by the advisor represent a national sample of persons in general or a highly select group of individuals such as those admitted to a specific school of music. The latter data set is an example of local norms. Assume the comparative standard was a large stratified sample of high school graduates from all 50 states. Thus, Bob's score suggests that his musical ability and talents are above average for the general population of high school graduates. However, the manual also presents separate norms for applicants who have been admitted to the first year of music training at an institution comparable to the one that Bob attends. Suppose that the mean and standard deviation for the latter group were 130 and 15, respectively. Now Bob's score carries different implications since it is one standard deviation below the mean and equals or exceeds only 16% of persons in the normative group. If Bob was asking for advice about enrolling in an elective music appreciation class, more emphasis should be placed on the national norms. Conversely, if he was thinking about taking a major in musicology, the advisor would pay more attention to the local or special group norms. It should be obvious that the norms employed will influence test interpretation and that it is imperative to use the most appropriate norms for the individual examinee and the situation within which he or she is involved. Thus, no single set of norms can be used in all circumstances.

The importance of using an appropriate comparison standard cannot be overstated. However, there are occasions when one deliberately employs norms that appear to be unsuitable. For instance, suppose one is counseling a 65-year-old, unemployed carpenter who expresses an interest in returning to competitive employment. He retired three years ago following a stroke and has successfully completed a rehabilitation program. As part of the vocational evaluation, the Wechsler Adult Intelligence Scale-III (WAIS-III) is administered. In addition to examining the summary IQs, the results of the individual subtests are inspected. Suppose the client earned a raw score of 24 on Block Design, a subtest that requires the examinee to reproduce abstract designs using colored blocks. The test is thought to measure speed of performance and visuo-spatial and constructional ability. Now suppose the examiner is aware of empirical research that correlates performance on this subtest with success in general carpentry. As a result, the examiner feels that careful scrutiny of the Block Design score is in order. Using age-appropriate norms, it is found that a raw score of 24 converts to a percentile of 37. This represents average achievement for someone in the age range 65 to 69. However, the examiner knows that the typical carpenter is younger than the retired client. Therefore, his score is compared to the norms for the younger working population (age range 20 to 34) against whom he will compete, and it is found that a raw score of 24 converts to a percentile rank of nine. If only the age-appropriate score is considered, the client seems capable of working at his former occupation, but when he is compared to people in the general job market, his performance speed, visuo-perceptual ability, and constructional skills emerge as relative weaknesses. The client might be evaluated further by comparing his score to that of a group of local carpenters, if such a norm group was available. The process described here was intended to provide the client with important information about possible problems that might be encountered when he returns to competitive employment.

Derived Scores

As noted in the previous section, raw scores are usually transformed into derived scores. This procedure is followed so that the results of different tests can be put on the same scale to facilitate comparisons among the measures. The second reason for using derived scores is to enhance interpretation by defining an examinee's level and pattern of performance. There are many types of derived scores, but the most frequently utilized are percentiles, age-equivalents, grade-equivalents, and standard scores. Each of these scores has its own advantages and limitations.

Percentiles are derived scores that reflect an examinee's position relative to a normative standard. These scores are expressed in terms of the percentage of persons in the reference group who fall below a specified raw score. If 50% of the subjects fall below a given score, then that value is at the 50th percentile. An examinee who obtains a percentile rank of 50 on an aptitude test has performed as well as or better than 50 percent of the individuals in the normative group. To calculate percentile ranks one must first tabulate the raw scores of the normative sample into a frequency distribution. This is accomplished by grouping scores into class intervals and determining the number of cases in each interval. The size of the interval may vary from a single numerical value to a range of values (e.g., 50 to 54). A simple formula is than utilized to compute a percentile rank for each score in the normative sample. A good test manual will provide tables for converting raw scores to percentile ranks, and most elementary statistics books contain illustrations on how to calculate percentile ranks. There are obvious advantages to using this type of derived score. For instance, they are easily understood, can be utilized with a wide variety of tests, and work equally well with children and adults. The primary limitations of these scores are that they display a marked inequality of measurement units (i.e., differences between percentiles are smaller near the middle of the distribution than at the ends of the distribution) and are not readily amenable to statistical analysis.

Age-equivalent scores represent the mean raw scores obtained by a normative sample at each age level covered by the test. For instance, the raw score mean of all 5-year-olds in the standardization sample is at the 50th percentile and constitutes a mental age of five years. Age-equivalent scores are useful because they have popular appeal and provide an estimate of the examinee's repertoire of knowledge or absolute level of performance. However, the scores frequently do not represent equal units across age groups because mental growth is nonlinear. One year of mental growth from ages 4 to 5 is much larger than from ages 11 to 12. Finally, among persons with normal cognitive and adaptive functions, age-equivalent scores have little meaning for adults and older adolescents.

The results of educational achievement tests frequently are reported as grade-equivalents. These values reflect the mean raw score obtained by children at each grade level. For instance, if the average score on a spelling test given to third-graders is 25, then this raw score corresponds to a grade-equivalency of 3.0. These scores have considerable appeal within school settings, but they have numerous limitations. The scores frequently do not represent equal units for all groups because the content and emphasis of instruction varies across classrooms, schools, and grades. In addition, they are not applicable to most high school situations because skills such as basic reading and spelling reach their peaks at lower levels and are usually not taught in grades 10 through 12. Grade-equivalent scores also frequently lead to misinterpretation. It is incorrect to conclude that a third grader with an achievement test score at the fifth grade level in arithmetic has the same mastery of mathematical operations as the average child in the first month of fifth grade. Although a student may have correctly solved the same number of test problems as the average fifth grader, it is most likely that he or she did so because of superior mastery of third grade arithmetic.

Most ability, achievement, and personality tests provide tables that report the linear conversion of raw scores to standard scores. These linear transformations, which assume that one is working with a normal distribution, maintain the exact numerical relations of the original raw scores by subtracting a constant from each raw value and then dividing the result by another constant. The transformed scores express an individual's performance in terms of a specified mean and standard deviation. The latter statistic allows one to determine how far any obtained score lies from the mean of the standardization sample. There are many different types of standard scores including z-scores, T-scores, and deviation IQs.

The z statistic is the basic standard score since all other linear transformations may be established directly from it. To obtain a z-score, the group mean is subtracted from the specific raw score and then divided by the group standard deviation. The resulting z-scores have a mean of 0.0 and a standard deviation of 1.0. The typical range of standard deviations is from $+ 3.0$ to $- 3.0$. All z-scores above the mean carry a positive sign, while all scores below the mean carry a negative sign. This is a useful statistic for those conducting research with psychological and educational tests, but the z-score may cause confusion and inconvenience when used in clinical situations. Therefore, z-scores are usually converted into other standard scores in order to obtain smaller standard deviation units and to eliminate the decimal point and algebraic signs.

The T-score is probably the most widely employed linear transformation. Its rationale is identical to that of the z-score, except that it yields a mean of 50 and a standard deviation of 10. The typical standard deviation range is from a $T = 20$ to a $T = 80$. The formula for obtaining the standard score is $T = 10z + 50$. It is important to note that there is nothing sacred about a mean of 50 and a standard deviation of 10. One can create a system with any mean and standard deviation that is preferred. Simply multiply the z-score by the desired standard deviation and then add the number wanted as the mean of the new distribution. The deviation IQ employed with the many versions of the Wechsler scales of intelligence is an example of a widely used standard score. Unlike the typical T-score, the Wechsler scales use a mean of 100 and a standard deviation of 15 (i.e., deviation IQ $= 15z + 100$).

In some situations raw scores on a test are skewed and do not conform to a normal distribution. Under these conditions, it is often necessary to use a nonlinear transformation to change the shape of the original distribution into a normal curve. One well-known nonlinear transformation is the stanine scale. This system converts any set of scores into a distribution with a mean of 5, a standard deviation of 2, and a range from 1 to 9. The term stanine originated in the United States Army Air Force during World War II and refers to the fact that the scores run from 1 to 9. To transform a distribution into stanines, the mean and standard deviation of raw scores are used to convert each value to a z-score. Next, each z-score is converted to a percentile and the percentiles are converted to stanines. Table 1.3 gives the percentage of scores at each stanine.

SUMMARY

A test is an operational method of describing the extent to which examinees possess a specific trait, characteristic, or behavioral predisposition. There are multiple approaches to test development including those designated as criterion-keyed, analytic, or rational/deduc-

Table 1.3. Conversion of Percentiles into Stanines

Stanines	Percent of Cases in the Distribution	Percentiles
1	4	1–4
2	7	5–11
3	12	12–23
4	17	24–40
5	20	41–60
6	17	61–77
7	12	78–89
8	7	90–96
9	4	97–100

tive. The third approach is the most widely employed by contemporary test developers. Test publishers are ethically responsible for producing measures that are psychometrically sound. Nevertheless, it is the practitioner who must select the most appropriate instrument for a given application. This may be accomplished by evaluating a test in terms of its purpose, format, and psychometric characteristics. If two tests purport to measure the same construct or behavior and are equal in terms of ease of administration and scoring, then select the one with the highest reliability and validity coefficients, the smallest standard errors of measurement and/or estimation, and the most widely applicable set of norms. Also, one should look for norms on special groups, as no single set of norms is appropriate in all circumstances. Finally, it is important to examine the types of derived scores provided by a test publisher. At a minimum, there should be tables for converting raw scores to standard scores and percentile ranks.

SUGGESTED READINGS

Anastasi, A., & Urbina, S. (1997). *Psychological testing* (7th ed.). Upper Saddle River, NJ: Prentice Hall.

American Psychological Association. (1985). *Standards for educational and psychological testing*. Washington, DC: Author.

Crocker, L., & Algina, J. (1986). *Introduction to classical and modern test theory*. Fort Worth, TX: Holt, Rinehart, & Winston.

Golden, C. J., Sawicki, R. F., & Franzen, M. D. (1990). Test construction. In G. Goldstein and M. Hersen (Eds.), *Handbook of psychological assessment* (2nd ed.). New York: Pergamon.

Kaplan, R. M., & Saccuzzo, D. P. (1993). *Psychological testing: Principles, applications, and issues* (3rd ed.). Pacific Grove, CA: Brooks/Cole Publishing Company.

Reynolds, C. R., & Brown, R. T. (Eds.) (1984). *Perspectives on bias in mental testing*. New York: Plenum.

Sattler, J. M. (1988). *Assessment of children* (3rd ed.). San Diego: Author.

Walsh, W. B., & Betz, N. E. (1990). *Tests and assessment* (2nd ed.). Englewood Cliffs, NJ: Prentice Hall.

Wierzbicki, M. (1993). *Issues in clinical psychology: Subjective versus objective approaches*. Boston: Allyn and Bacon.

I

Adult

2

Wechsler Adult Intelligence Scale-III

Joseph J. Ryan and Shane J. Lopez

INTRODUCTION

The Wechsler Adult Intelligence Scale-III (WAIS-III) comes from a tradition of mental ability testing that began in 1939 with the publication of the Wechsler-Bellevue Intelligence Scale, Form I (W-B I). The W-B I, which was named after David Wechsler and the Bellevue Hospital where he was employed as chief psychologist, was considered a unique clinical instrument because it possessed good face validity with adolescents and adults, grouped items into subtests, and provided extensive assessment of both verbal and nonverbal abilities. The scale also utilized standard scores and deviation IQs instead of the mental age values and ratio IQs provided by contemporary tests such as the Stanford-Binet Intelligence Scale, Forms L and M.

David Wechsler was known for his pragmatic view of human intelligence. Early in his career as a test developer, he defined the construct of intelligence as "the aggregate or global capacity of the individual to act purposefully, to think rationally, and to deal effectively with his environment." This definition is not exclusively cognitive, but also includes affective (emotional) and conative (e.g., motivational) factors. Thus, Wechsler felt that intelligence was multifaceted, multidetermined, and a part of personality as a whole. To measure intelligence so defined, he selected items and procedures from ability tests already in use, such as the Army Alpha, Army Beta, Kohs Block Designs, Stanford-Binet, and Healy Picture Completion II. Some of the items were modified to increase their clinical potency, whereas others were retained in their original form. The resulting product consisted of six Verbal Scale subtests and five Performance Scale subtests. Wechsler considered the scales as different "languages" through which the underlying construct of general intelligence may be expressed. This format provided a separate Verbal IQ, Performance IQ, and overall composite score known as the Full Scale IQ. For ease of interpretation, these scores shared the same distributional characteristics (e.g., means and standard deviations) at all ages.

Joseph J. Ryan • Department of Psychology and Counselor Education, Central Missouri State University, Warrensburg, Missouri 64093   Shane J. Lopez • Department of Psychology and Research in Education, University of Kansas, Lawrence, Kansas 66045.

Understanding Psychological Assessment, edited by Dorfman and Hersen. Kluwer Academic/Plenum Publishers, New York, 2001.

The W-B I was a very popular instrument, but it had numerous structural shortcomings and an inadequate standardization sample. In 1955, these limitations were rectified with the publication of the Wechsler Adult Intelligence Scale (WAIS). This test was standardized on a large national sample of persons 16 to 75 years of age and measured a wider range of cognitive functions than its predecessor. Within a few years of its appearance, the WAIS was the most widely used psychological test in the United States. By the late 1970s, it was obvious that the WAIS needed to be modified, revised, and restandardized. This project was completed in 1981 with publication of the Wechsler Adult Intelligence Scale-Revised (WAIS-R).

TEST CONSTRUCTION AND DEVELOPMENT

A decade after publication of the WAIS-R, the test was in need of revision and restandardization. Psychologists and statisticians at The Psychological Corporation (TPC) recognized this fact and responded by assembling an in-house working group directed by Dr. David Tulsky to produce the WAIS-III. Tulsky and associates assembled an external panel of experts in the field of intellectual assessment to serve in an advisory capacity throughout the revision project. They also promulgated specific test development goals for the third edition which included: (a) retention of the basic structure of the previous editions, (b) updating the norms, (c) improving individual items, (d) enhancing clinical utility and strengthening the theoretical basis, and (e) providing extensive data on scale reliability and validity.

Structure of the WAIS-III

As with previous editions of the scale, the WAIS-III retains the 11 traditional subtests and yields Verbal, Performance, and Full Scale IQs. The revised Verbal Scale contains seven subtests. The Vocabulary, Similarities, Arithmetic, Digit Span, Information, and Comprehension subtests are combined to yield the Verbal IQ. The Letter-Number Sequencing subtest, which appears in a Wechsler Scale for the first time, is designated as a supplementary measure. It contributes to the Verbal IQ only when the Digit Span subtest has been spoiled (i.e., Digit Span administration is invalid due to an interruption in the test procedure or some other violation of standardization). Similarly, the Performance Scale consists of seven subtests where Picture Completion, Digit Symbol-Coding, Block Design, Matrix Reasoning, and Picture Arrangement are combined to yield the Performance IQ. The Symbol Search and Object Assembly subtests are designated as supplementary and optional tasks, respectively. The former may be substituted only for a spoiled Digit Symbol-Coding administration, whereas the latter may replace any spoiled Performance Scale subtest if the examinee is in the age range 16 to 74 years. The Matrix Reasoning and Symbol Search subtests are new to the third edition.

The six Verbal Scale and five Performance Scale subtests are combined to calculate the Full Scale IQ. After each subtest is scored, raw point totals are converted to scaled scores according to the examinee's age range in Table A.1 from the *WAIS-III Administration and Scoring Manual*. These scaled scores have a mean of 10 and a standard deviation of 3. Sums of scaled scores then are computed separately for the six Verbal Scale subtests, five Performance Scale subtests, and all 11 subtests which constitute the Full Scale. The sums are converted to deviation IQs using Tables A.3 through A.5 in the *WAIS-III Administration and Scoring Manual*. The IQs generated have a mean of 100 and a standard deviation of 15 at all age levels.

The WAIS-III introduces four new composites which have been designated as "index scores." They are based on a series of factor analyses performed on the standardization sample data.

The Verbal Comprehension Index is composed of the Vocabulary, Similarities, and Information subtests. The Perceptual Organization Index includes the Picture Completion, Block Design, and Matrix Reasoning subtests. A Working Memory Index is comprised of Arithmetic, Digit Span, and Letter-Number Sequencing. The fourth Index represents the construct of Processing Speed and contains two subtests, Digit Symbol-Coding and Symbol Search. The index scores are obtained by summing the scaled scores that constitute each of the composites and then converting the sums to deviation quotients using Tables A.6 through A.9 in the *WAIS-III Administration and Scoring Manual*. Each index score has a mean of 100 and a standard deviation of 15. Table 2.1 presents a brief description of the WAIS-III subtests, optional procedures, IQs, and indexes.

Table A.2 in the *WAIS-III Administration and Scoring Manual* provides optional norms that allow examiners to convert raw subtest scores to scaled scores relative to a group of 600 young adults 20–34 years of age. These scaled scores are not age-appropriate and are *never* used to compute the IQs and indexes. However, they can be consulted when a comparison of an older examinee's achievement levels with that of an optimally functioning group of young adults becomes relevant.

Updated Norms

The WAIS-III was normed on a stratified sample of 2450 individuals with negative histories for psychiatric conditions, medical conditions, or both that could potentially affect cognitive functioning. The stratification percentages for age, sex, race/ethnicity, educational level, and geographic region were based on the 1995 United States Bureau of the Census data. For each stratification variable, there was a very close match between the normative sample and the census figures. Table 2.2 summarizes the demographic characteristics of the WAIS-III standardization sample.

Item Development

The panel of experts assembled by TPC reviewed and critiqued the WAIS-III content and made suggestions for updating existing items, the creation of new items, and the addition of new subtests. Problematic items were identified and deleted from the Scale. With the assistance of the advisory panel, TPC conducted a series of pilot investigations and tryout studies. They assessed the psychometric characteristics of the modified Scale, determined item difficulty levels, and analyzed test content for potential bias. A variety of patient samples were tested in order to evaluate the clinical utility of new items, new subtests, and revised administration and scoring procedures.

Enhancing Clinical Utility/Strengthening the Theoretical Basis

The WAIS and the WAIS-R were often criticized because of their limited floors and ceilings. The IQs and subtest scores generated by these scales did not extend sufficiently downward to allow for discrimination among examinees with mild to moderate mental retardation or high enough to properly assess the intellectually gifted. To correct the former limitation, less difficult items were added to the third edition, the range of possible subtest scores was extended downward, and extrapolated IQs were generated at the lower end of the ability distribution. To address the second shortcoming, the ceiling of the WAIS-III was raised by five points. However, as the range of WAIS-III Full Scale IQs is only 45 to 155, the test is still

Table 2.1. WAIS-III Subtests, Optional Procedures, IQs, and Indexes

Subtest/IQ/Index	Description
Vocabulary	Contains 33 words arranged in order of increasing difficulty. The examinee defines each word aloud. It measures word knowledge, contributes to the Verbal Scale IQ and the Verbal Comprehension Index.
Similarities	Contains 19 pairs of words. The examinee is asked to identify similarities between each pair. The subtest appears to measure verbal concept formation and abstract thinking. It contributes to the Verbal Scale IQ and the Verbal Comprehension Index.
Arithmetic	Contains 20 arithmetic problems that require counting, addition, subtraction, multiplication, basic probability, or a combination of these. All items are timed, 3 use blocks with oral instructions, and 17 are word problems. The required skill level does not exceed 8th grade. The subtest always contributes to the Verbal Scale IQ and Working Memory Index.
Digit Span	Contains separate tasks of digits forward (series of numbers ranging from 2 to 9 digits in length) and digits backward (series of numbers ranging from 2 to 8 digits) and requires examinees to repeat digits in a prescribed order. Digits forward measures auditory attention and auditory sequencing. Digits backward appears to measure mental tracking, short term memory, and internal visual scanning. It contributes to the Verbal Scale IQ and the Working Memory Index.
Information	Contains 28 oral questions that assess general knowledge of objects, events, and places. It contributes to the Verbal Scale IQ and the Verbal Comprehension Index.
Comprehension	Contains 18 orally presented questions. Sixteen deal with everyday situations that assess knowledge of social conventionalities and common sense. The examinee is also asked to provide the meaning of two proverbs. It contributes to the Verbal Scale IQ.
Letter-Number Sequencing	Contains seven items that assess the ability to order random series of orally presented numbers and letters. The subtest measures auditory tracking, mental flexibility, and divided attention. It is a supplementary task that can substitute for Digit Span, if that subtest is spoiled. If substituted for Digit Span, it contributes to the Verbal Scale IQ. It always contributes to the Working Memory Index.
Picture Completion	Contains 25 drawings of people, animals, common objects, and scenes. Each drawing has a missing part that must be identified within 20 seconds. It measures the ability to differentiate essential from nonessential details and contributes to the Performance Scale IQ and the Perceptual Organization Index.
Digit Symbol-Coding	Contains a key with nine number-symbol pairs as well as 133 boxes with a number in the top portion and a blank space in the lower portion. The task requires drawing in the lower portion of each box the symbol that was paired with the number in the key. The subtest has a 120 second time limit and requires repeated visual scanning, visual tracking, handwriting speed, and paired-associate learning. It contributes to the Performance Scale IQ and the Processing Speed Index.
Block Design	Contains 14 items that require the reproduction of design patterns using colored blocks. All items are timed. It measures visuospatial problem solving, nonverbal concept formation, and constructional ability. It contributes the Performance Scale IQ and the Perceptual Organization Index.
Matrix Reasoning	Contains 26 nonverbal, multiple-choice items that involve pattern completion, serial reasoning, and/or classification. It has also been designated as a measure of fluid intelligence. It contributes to the Performance Scale IQ and the Perceptual Organization Index.
Picture Arrangement	Contains 11 individual sets of pictures. Each set is presented in a mixed-up order and needs to be put into a logical sequence within a specified time frame. It measures visual sequencing and the ability to plan and anticipate within a social context. It contributes to the Performance Scale IQ.

*Excellent Test mini Ravens Ravensis used worldwide.

Pretty non-biased – Culture free

Table 2.1. Continued

Subtest/IQ/Index	Description
Symbol Search	Contains 60 items that each present two symbols on the left side of a page and five on the right. Each requires a quick decision whether either symbol on the left is also presented on the right. The time limit is 120 seconds and the subtest measures perceptual discrimination, speed and accuracy, and sustained attention. It is a supplementary task that can substitute for Digit Symbol-Coding, if that subtest is spoiled. If substituted for Digit Symbol-Coding, it contributes to the Performance Scale IQ. It always contributes to the Processing Speed Index.
Object Assembly	Contains five jigsaw puzzles that must be solved within specified time limits. It measures visual organization, appreciation of part-whole relationships, and constructional ability. This is an optional task that may be administered for clinical reasons and may also be substituted for any spoiled Performance Scale subtest if the examinee is in the age range 16–74. If substituted for another subtest, it contributes the Performance Scale IQ.
Digit Symbol-Incidental Learning	Administered immediately after the Digit Symbol-Coding subtest. It evaluates memory for the associated number-symbol pairs and the individual symbols independent of the numbers. Thus, it is a measure of incidental learning of rehearsed material. This is an optional procedure that may assist with the interpretation of the Digit Symbol-Coding subtest.
Digit Symbol-Copy	Administered as the final component of a WAIS-III evaluation. It consists of the nine symbols used in the Digit Symbol-Coding subtest. Each item presents a symbol, with a blank space directly below. The examinee copies as many symbols as possible within 90 seconds. It measures perceptual and graphomotor speed. This is an optional procedure that may assist with the interpretation of the Digit Symbol-Coding subtest.
Verbal IQ	Comprised of the Vocabulary, Similarities, Arithmetic, Digit Span, Information, and Comprehension subtests. The Letter-Number Sequencing subtest is a designated supplementary measure. It contributes to the Verbal IQ only when the Digit Span subtest has been spoiled. This composite score reflects general verbal abilities including acquired knowledge, verbal reasoning, and attention to verbal information.
Performance IQ	Comprised of the Picture Completion, Digit Symbol-Coding, Block Design, Matrix Reasoning, and Picture Arrangement subtests. The Symbol Search and Object Assembly subtests are designated as supplementary and optional tasks, respectively. The former may be substituted only for a spoiled Digit Symbol-Coding administration, whereas the latter may replace any spoiled Performance Scale subtest if the examinee is in the age range 16 to 74 years. This composite score reflects perceptual organization, fluid reasoning, and attention to detail.
Full Scale IQ	Comprised of the 6 Verbal Scale and 5 Performance Scale subtests. This composite score serves as a global measure of intellectual functioning.
Verbal Comprehension Index	Comprised of the Vocabulary, Similarities, and Information subtests. It measures verbal knowledge and understanding and the ability to apply verbal skills across situations.
Perceptual Organization Index	Comprised of the Picture Completion, Block Design, and Matrix Reasoning subtests. It measures the ability to interpret and organize visually perceived material.
Working Memory Index	Comprised of Arithmetic, Digit Span, and Letter-Number Sequencing subtests. It measures auditory attention–concentration and verbal information processing capacity.
Processing Speed Index	Comprised of the Digit Symbol-Coding and Symbol Search subtests. It measures the ability to process visual information quickly.

Handwritten annotations:
- DERIVED SCORES
- 20-15 pts difference between these two is significant
- More gloss
- Similar to perceptual organization index.
- SUMMARY SCORE
- Pure measure of verbal
- measures - Focused - specific things

Table 2.2. Demographic Characteristics of the WAIS-III Standardization Sample

Variable	Description
Age	The 13 age groups were 16–17, 18–19, 20–24, 25–29, 30–34, 35–44, 45–54, 55–64, 65–69, 70–74, 75–79, 80–84, 85–89 years.
Sex	For all age groups between 16–17 years and 55–64 years, there were 100 males and 100 females. There were 90 males and 110 females in the age range 65–69 years and 88 males and 112 females for those 70–74 years. For individuals in the age ranges 75–79 years, 80–84 years, and 85–89 years, the male-female numbers were, respectively, 83 and 117, 54 and 96, and 32 and 68.
Race/Ethnicity	There were 1,925 whites, 279 African Americans, 181 Hispanics, and 65 individuals from other racial/ethnic groups.
Educational Level	Five educational categories were represented. The groups were $\leq$8 years (n = 284), 9–11 years (n = 289), 12 years (n = 853), 13–15 years (n = 579), and $\geq$16 years (n = 445). Individuals 16–19 years of age were classified according to years of parental education.
Geographic Region	The U.S. was divided into four regions consisting of nine northeastern states, 12 north central states, 17 southern states, and 12 western states. Individuals were recruited from each of these areas.

inappropriate for the assessment of examinees with moderate to severe mental retardation or persons identified as extremely gifted.

To increase the clinical information provided by the WAIS-III, a new measure of incidental learning was added. Following administration of Digit Symbol-Coding, there now is an optional procedure for evaluating an examinee's recall of the nine number-symbol pairs that constitute the subtest. A second optional procedure requires the examinee to copy symbols as quickly as possible without the need to form number-symbol associations. By comparing the results of these optional tasks, it is often possible to ascertain the reasons for poor performance (e.g., symbol recall inaccuracy or copying difficulties) on the Digit Symbol-Coding subtest.

The WAIS-III was co-normed with the Wechsler Memory Scale-III (WAIS-III) for all age groups in the standardization sample and linked with the Wechsler Individual Achievement Test (WIAT) for persons 16–19 years of age. Co-norming involved the administration of both the WAIS-III and WMS-III in counterbalanced order to 1,250 individuals in the WAIS-III standardization sample. Because of the relatively high correlation between intellectual ability and memory functions, this procedure allows the clinician to determine if an examinee's memory skills are commensurate with his or her level of intelligence. The linking process was based on administration of both the WAIS-III and WIAT to a supplementary sample of 142 individuals in the age range 16 to 19 years. This provides a method of comparing an examinee's intellectual ability to his or her academic proficiency, a frequently important piece of information when there is a need to identify the presence of a specific learning disability.

To strengthen the theoretical basis of the third edition, TPC made a number of changes. First, a subtest that purportedly measures fluid intelligence was added to the scale. The Matrix Reasoning subtest provides information that should assist examiners who wish to interpret WAIS-III scores according to the Horn-Cattell theory of fluid and crystallized intelligence. Also, by the addition of two supplementary subtests, Letter-Number Sequencing and Symbol Search, examiners now have the option to regroup the various subtests and calculate theory-based summary values that appear to measure the constructs of Working Memory and Processing Speed. These dimensions are important for understanding cognitive functions since they are thought to contribute to information acquisition and problem solving. Despite these changes, the WAIS-III remains theoretically grounded in David Wechsler's pragmatic view of intelligence.

Extensive Reliability and Validity Data

Internal Consistency

A series of studies conducted on the WAIS-III standardization sample indicated that it has exemplary internal consistency. This type of reliability measures consistency with regard to content sampling, as it is derived from a single administration of the test. For IQs and indexes, it is derived by a formula for determining the reliability of a composite group of tests; for the subtests, it is calculated by the split-half technique. The Full Scale reliability coefficients are .97 or above across the entire age range in the standardization sample; Verbal Scale coefficients are .96 or higher; Performance Scale coefficients are .93 or higher. For the Verbal Comprehension, Perceptual Organization, Working Memory, and Processing Speed indexes, the reliabilities are at least .94, .90, .91, and .86, respectively. Of the 14 subtests, Vocabulary has the highest reliabilities (ranging from .90 to .95), whereas Object Assembly has the lowest (ranging from .50 to .78). The Verbal Scale subtests are generally more reliable than the Performance Scale subtests.

Standard Error of Measurement

Standard Error of Measurement (SEM) statistic reflects the reliability of the individual score. It is the standard deviation of the distribution of error scores and is expressed in terms of confidence limits that are placed around the obtained composite score or individual subtest score. The larger the SEM, the larger is the band of error and the less precise the score. The SEM is obtained by taking the square root of one minus the reliability coefficient and then multiplying by the standard deviation of the test (i.e., $SD \sqrt{1-r_{xx}}$). The average SEM for the Full Scale IQ across all age groups is 2.30. The average SEM is larger for the Performance IQ (3.67) than for the Verbal IQ (2.55). Because the indexes are based on fewer subtests than the traditional IQs, they yield scores that have slightly lower reliabilities and are somewhat less precise. The average SEM is 3.01 for the Verbal Comprehension Index, 3.95 for the Perceptual Organization Index, 3.84 for the Working Memory Index, and 5.13 for the Processing Speed Index. Of the seven Verbal Scale subtests, Vocabulary (0.79) has the smallest average SEM, whereas Letter-Number Sequencing (1.30) has the largest. Within the Performance Scale, the smallest average SEM is on the Matrix Reasoning subtest (0.97) and the largest is on the Object Assembly subtest (1.66).

Test-Retest Stability

The WAIS-III has excellent temporal stability which was demonstrated by evaluating 394 individuals on two occasions with an average test-retest interval of thirty-five days. Uncorrected stability coefficients for the Verbal, Performance, and Full Scale IQs were, respectively, .91, .83, and .91 for persons in the age range 16–29 years; .95, .88, and .96 for 30–54 years; .97, .91, and .96 for those 55–74 years; and .95, .93, and .96 for 75-89 years. Uncorrected stability coefficients for the Verbal Comprehension, Perceptual Organization, Working Memory, and Processing Speed indexes were, respectively, .89, .79, .82, and .83 for persons in the age range 16-29 years; .95, .86, .90, and .87 for 30–54 years; .96, .89, .90, and .89 for 55-74 years; and .93, .89, .85, and .92 for 75–89 years. Of the seven Verbal Scale subtests, Information (.94) is, on the average, the most stable, whereas Letter-Number Sequencing (.75) is the least stable. Within the Performance Scale, the Digit Symbol-Coding subtest (.86) demonstrated the highest stability. The poorest stability was noted on the Picture Arrangement subtest (.69).

The *WAIS-III–WMS-III Technical Manual* reports changes in test scores by individuals in the four age groups who were tested on two different occasions. The average Verbal IQ increased by 3.2, 2.0, 2.1, and 2.4 points, respectively, for individuals in the age ranges 16–29 years, 30–54 years, 55–74 years, and 75-89 years. The average Performance IQ gains for each of the four age groups were 8.2, 8.3, 5.7, and 3.7 points. On the Full Scale IQ, increases from test to retest averaged 5.7, 5.1 3.9, and 3.2 points. These retest changes, which are greater on the Performance Scale than on the Verbal Scale, are likely the result of practice effects. However, the trend for retest gains on the Performance and Full Scale IQs to decrease in magnitude as one moves from the youngest to the oldest groups is noteworthy. Perhaps they reflect age-related cognitive changes in visual-spatial problem solving or incidental learning or both. Retest changes on the four indexes are similar to those associated with the IQs. The average practice effects across the four age groups was 2.4 points for the Verbal Comprehension Index, 5.4 points for the Perceptual Organization Index, 2.4 points for the Working Memory Index, and 3.9 points for the Processing Speed Index. The largest increases from test to retest were on the Perceptual Organization and Processing Speed indexes. Of the seven Verbal Scale subtests, the Vocabulary and Comprehension subtests demonstrated the smallest average retest gains across the four age groups (0.23 points), whereas Information had the largest mean retest gain (0.58 points). Within the Performance Scale, the smallest retest gain was on the Symbol Search Subtest (0.45) and the largest retest gain was on the Picture Completion Subtest (1.80).

Content Validity

A test that purports to measure intelligence must demonstrate appropriate content coverage and content relevance. To meet these requirements, test developers conducted extensive literature reviews to identify any problems with items on previous editions of the scale. Next, experts in the field of intellectual assessment reviewed potential WAIS-III items, designed new ones, and helped update others. Data from item tryout and pilot studies were also reviewed. Based on these efforts, TPC felt that the third edition had achieved an appropriate level of content validity.

Concurrent Validity

High correlations have been found between the WAIS-III and other measures of intelligence, achievement, and memory. These findings support concurrent validity because the WAIS-III and other tests were administered at approximately the same time. Concurrent validity studies reported in the *WAIS-III–WMS-III Technical Manual* indicate that the WAIS-III Full Scale IQ correlates .93 with the WAIS-R Full Scale IQ, .88 with the Wechsler Intelligence Scale for Children-III Full Scale IQ, and .88 with the Stanford-Binet Intelligence Scale-IV Composite Score. Correlations between the WIAT composites for Reading, Mathematics, Language, and Writing and the WAIS-III Full Scale IQ are high and range from .68 to .81. The magnitude of these associations allows for the prediction of achievement test performance of an examinee based on knowledge of his or her WAIS-III scores. Another example of concurrent validity is the relationship between various scores from the WMS-III and the WAIS-III. Correlations between the eight memory scores and the Full Scale IQ are moderately high and range from .36 to .68. These findings indicate that the WAIS-III and WMS-III, although significantly related, are measures of different constructs.

Construct Validity

The pattern of intercorrelations among the WAIS-III subtests conform with expectations based on practical knowledge and psychological theory. For example, the Verbal Scale subtests intercorrelate more highly with each other than they do with the Performance Scale subtests, whereas the Performance Scale subtests tend to intercorrelate more highly among themselves than they do with the Verbal Scale subtests. Also, the 14 subtests are intercorrelated to a statistically significant degree. This observation supports the premise that a pervasive, general intelligence factor underlies the WAIS-III.

Exploratory factor-analytic studies of the WAIS-III standardization sample at five age ranges (16–19, 20–34, 35–54, 55–74, and 75–89) using 13 subtests (Object Assembly was excluded) were reported in the WAIS-III–WMS-III Technical Manual. These procedures identified four factors, as mentioned previously: Verbal Comprehension, Perceptual Organization, Working Memory, and Processing Speed. These factors were supported by a confirmatory factor analysis of data from the same five age groups in the standardization sample. A separate exploratory factor analysis using a diagnostically heterogeneous patient sample (n = 152) was conducted by the present authors. Using the same 13 subtests and identical statistical methodology, highly similar results emerged. However, the Working Memory factor was composed of only Digit Span and Letter-Number Sequencing. For the patient sample, the Arithmetic subtest could not be uniquely allocated to any of the factors. Finally, a series of exploratory factor analyses was conducted on the standardization sample separately for the total group and each of the 13 age groups by Sattler and Ryan (1999). All 14 subtests (Object Assembly was added) were used in the analyses. A four-factor solution characterized the WAIS-III, but the subtests that contributed to each factor varied somewhat across age ranges.

The Verbal Comprehension and Perceptual Organization factors bear a close resemblance to the Verbal and Performance scales. This provides construct validity support for interpretation of the Verbal and Performance IQs as meaningful cognitive dimensions. The significant intercorrelations among the 14 subtests and the magnitude of the subtest loadings on the first unrotated factor reported by Sattler and Ryan support the construct validity of the Full Scale IQ. Overall, 50% of the variance in the WAIS-III may be attributed to the construct of general intelligence.

Another way to assess construct validity is to ascertain whether scores on the WAIS-III conform to the expectations of a credible theory of intelligence. For example, the Horn-Cattell theory postulates that general intelligence can be divided into two separate components that represent fluid and crystallized ability. The former involves the capacity to solve novel problems and think abstractly, whereas the latter involves the retrieval of previously learned and stored verbal information. Fluid ability tends to decline with advancing age and is disrupted by damage to the central nervous system. Crystallized ability is relatively resistant to age-related deterioration and, in the absence of aphasia, severe brain dysfunction, or both, shows less decline secondary to brain damage than do fluid abilities.

If the WAIS-III is viewed within the Horn-Cattell framework, the majority of Verbal Scale subtests may be considered measures of crystallized intelligence, whereas most of the Performance Scale subtests may be designated as measures of fluid intelligence. Inspection of the WAIS-III norms indicates that there are few differences between the older and younger standardization participants in verbal ability. Thus, on subtests such as Vocabulary and Information, it takes about the same number of raw score points to earn a scaled score of 10 (50th percentile) regardless of age. The situation is dramatically different for older and younger standardization participants on the Performance Scale subtests, as the norm tables indicate that older individuals have less adequate fluid abilities than do younger persons. This is clearly demonstrated by the observation that, in the age range 20–34 years, it takes 76 raw score points on the Digit Symbol-Coding Subtest to earn a scaled score of 10. However, in the age range 85–89 years, it takes only 33 raw score points to earn the same scaled score. Likewise, on the Symbol Search subtest, persons in the age range 20–34 need at least 33 raw score points to earn a scaled score of 10, whereas individuals in the age range 85–89 years need to earn only 14 raw score points to obtain a scaled score of 10.

ADMINISTRATION

Applications of the WAIS-III

The WAIS-III is a standardized instrument developed for use with persons in the age range 16–89 years. Examinees must have adequate vision and motor functions to permit a valid administration of the Performance Scale subtests and should also be fluent in English and possess adequate hearing to permit a valid administration of the Verbal Scale subtests. However, administration and interpretation of the measure to English-speaking persons from countries other than the United States should be done cautiously. In such cases, the examiner must be alert to the possibility that failure on certain test items (e.g., Information subtest items 10 and 11) reflects cultural loading, not an intellectual limitation. Interpretation of performance data of individuals over 89 years of age should be done cautiously as norms are not available. The use of the WAIS-III with elderly Hispanics and members of ethnic groups such as Asian Americans and Native Americans should be carefully considered given that minimal data were collected from these subgroups of the population.

As a measure of intellectual functioning, the WAIS-III can be used with individuals described above. General applications of the measure include obtaining IQ estimates for both adolescents with above-average functioning and adults, for determining examinees' cognitive strengths and weaknesses, and for examining the influence of psychiatric difficulties on cognitive functioning. Specific uses of the WAIS-III include diagnosing giftedness and mental retardation and determining the extent of neuropsychological impairments and cognitive decline due to age-related and non-age-related factors.

Test User Qualifications

Examiners should have training and experience in the administration of standardized psychological instruments. Formal graduate courses in psychometrics and clinical assessment (e.g., interviewing, mental status examination) are highly desirable. The examiner must be thoroughly familiar with the instructions and procedures contained in the *WAIS-III Administration and Scoring Manual*, including the proper sequence of subtest administration, subtest starting points and discontinuance rules, and the specific time limits required for administration of individual items. The last requirement is significant because some of the WAIS-III subtests emphasize speed of performance and require precise timing to insure valid administration. The examiner should also know when to utilize the supplementary and optional subtests.

Finally, some of the subtests are complex and require the examiner to simultaneously manipulate the test manual, stimulus materials, and a stopwatch. Therefore, it is imperative that examiners practice scale administration numerous times prior to using the WAIS-III with a client or patient. The Sattler and Ryan (1999) *Administrative Checklist for the WAIS-III* provides a useful guide for judging the adequacy of an examiner's administrative performance.

Establishing and Maintaining Rapport

It is important for the examiner to establish and maintain rapport throughout each testing session. Characteristics of empathy, genuineness, and warmth help communicate a desire that each examinee perform at his or her best. The rapport-developing process includes an appropriate greeting of the examinee and explanation of the reason for the assessment and the nature of the testing procedures. Next, rapport building involves the establishment of a conversational manner, an interactive relationship, and a non-threatening environment. The skilled examiner will encourage the client to work efficiently, will respond to his or her questions, and will attend to obvious needs for encouragement, redirection, or a break. Verbal and nonverbal reinforcement should be given freely to maintain a high degree of effort on the part of the examinee, but reinforcement should *not* be contingent on whether a response is correct or incorrect. The *WAIS-III Administration and Scoring Manual* provides additional hints for establishing and maintaining rapport with individual examinees.

Standardized Administration

Reliability and validity of test scores are directly affected by test administration techniques. The *WAIS-III Administration and Scoring Manual* provides the detailed instructions for administration which should be read verbatim. Order of administration along with starting, reverse, and discontinuation rules should be followed carefully. The manual also provides information about some of the nuances of administration that are described below.

Repetition of Items

Repetition of subtest instructions is allowed. Use judgment when deciding to repeat items from Verbal subtests. *Digit Span and Letter-Number Sequencing items cannot be repeated as that would invalidate the test.* Repetition or practice of Performance subtest items should only be done when indicated by the standardized instructions. Excessive requests for repetition of items should be discussed and a reevaluation of the examinee's physical ability to complete the WAIS-III should be considered.

Querying Responses

During scale administration, the use of some probing questions or queries is necessary to help clarify vague or incomplete responses. The decision to query a response is made by the examiner, but the *WAIS-III Administration and Scoring Manual* provides examples and guidelines concerning when to initiate the process. During a typical WAIS-III administration, the Vocabulary, Comprehension, and Similarities subtests require the most frequent queries.

Administration Time

Wechsler (1997) reported that administration of the 11 standard subtests required to yield the three IQs takes 75 minutes (range from 60 to 90 minutes), whereas administration time for the 11 subtests that produce the four indexes is approximately 60 minutes (range from 45 to 75 minutes). Measurement of both the IQs and Indexes requires administration of 13 subtests and takes 80 minutes (range from 65 to 95 minutes).

These estimates reflect the time needed to administer the WAIS-III to healthy individuals. Assessment of persons with physical, cognitive, psychiatric, or a combination of these disabilities is more time consuming and individual examiners must be aware of this fact so that they can plan their testing sessions accordingly. For instance, the present authors tested 62 patients with a variety of medical and psychiatric conditions and found that average administration time for the 11 standard subtests exceeded 90 minutes and for 13 subtests was almost 100 minutes.

Testing of Limits

Testing of limits is a term that describes the practice of going beyond standard testing procedures to gather additional performance data from the examinee. Limits testing should only be conducted after the entire test has been administered via standard procedures. Then, additional procedures could be utilized to determine if an examinee's abilities surpass the ceiling established by standard administration of the test or if elimination of time limits improves performance. Additionally, probing questions could be used to establish the methods by which examinees reach solutions. This extension of the standard testing procedure generates qualitative information that could shape clinical impressions of an examinee's abilities.

Scoring the WAIS-III

Scoring the WAIS-III subtests, scales, indexes and optional procedures is no simple matter. The literature indicates that graduate students, and even experienced psychologists, sometimes convert scores incorrectly, give inappropriate credit to individual items, and make mistakes when adding raw score points and scaled scores. On occasion, credit may be assigned incorrectly to the number-symbol pairs on the Digit Symbol-Coding subtest and on optional procedures. These scoring errors can result in misleading and inaccurate results. Examiners need to be particularly cautious when scoring the Comprehension, Similarities, and Vocabulary subtests. Personal experience indicates that examiners sometimes fail to credit responses that appear in the test manual or do give credit to spoiled responses (i.e., examinee's elaboration reveals a misconception of the item). To guard against error, examiners need to have a full appreciation of the scoring criteria, scoring guidelines, and scoring examples in the *WAIS-III Administration and Scoring Manual*.

INTERPRETATIVE GUIDELINES

Extracting the meaning of WAIS-III results can be a difficult task for clinicians of all experience levels. Thus, rules of thumb for interpreting quantitative and qualitative performance data are provided. The rules should be applied within the framework of a hypothesis-driven interpretive approach, which will be outlined and discussed below.

Analysis of WAIS-III Results

Examining Quantitative Data: Analyzing IQs and Index Scores

The analysis of WAIS-III results begins by assessing the degree of intersubtest scatter (i.e., variability between the subtests) in the profile. This is done to determine whether the various composites (e.g., IQs and indexes) hang together and provide adequate reflections of the constructs under consideration. For example, it is appropriate to interpret the Verbal IQ as a measure of verbal comprehension and expression and the Performance IQ as a measure of perceptual organization and nonverbal problem solving when the component subtests of the scales cluster around their respective scaled score means. It is inappropriate to interpret the constructs if marked variability is present in one or both scales.

It is important to note that a considerable degree of intersubtest scatter characterizes the WAIS-III. For the standardization sample, the median and mean scatter ranges were both 7 scaled score points when 13 subtests were administered. Therefore, the present authors question whether a composite group of subtests provides a meaningful dimension of ability whenever the degree of scatter within the composite equals or exceeds that for 95% of standardization participants. If the magnitude of scatter is below that of 95% of the standardization sample, the composite is usually accepted as a unitary reflection of mental ability.

Table 2.3 provides an illustrative example of a WAIS-III protocol in which all the standard composites hang together according to the rule of thumb provided above. On the Verbal Scale, the largest deviation from the mean ($M = 10$) is 2.0 points. By consulting Table B.3 in the *WAIS-III Administration and Scoring Manual,* it can be seen that when seven subtests are administered from the Verbal Scale, deviations greater than or equal to those found in 95% of persons in the standardization sample range from 3.00 points on Vocabulary to 4.43 points on Digit Span. On the Performance scale, when six subtests are administered the largest deviation from the mean ($M = 8.2$) is 3.8 points. From Table 2.4 it is apparent that when six subtests are administered, deviations from the mean that equal or exceed those of 95% of the standardization participants range from 3.57 points on Symbol Search to 4.14 points on Digit Symbol-Coding. None of the subtests scores deviate meaningfully from the mean. Even the large deviation noted for the Picture Arrangement subtest is not considered meaningful because a difference of 4.03 points is required to equal or exceed 95% of the standardization sample.

Base rate tables that report cumulative scatter values for the indexes within the standardization sample are not yet available. However, the authors' preliminary calculations suggest that the reasonable threshold (i.e., scatter that equals or exceeds that of 95% of the standardization sample) for questioning whether a subtest composite reflects a meaningful dimension of ability is when one or more of its component subtests deviates from the mean by three or more points. As demonstrated in Table 2.3, each of the Indexes provides a unitary estimate of the construct it purportedly measures.

In the present example, none of the subtest scores deviate meaningfully from their respective scale or index means. Therefore, it is feasible to interpret the various WAIS-III composites. From Table 3.3 it is apparent that the Verbal and Performance IQs differ by 11 points. By consulting Table B.1 in the *WAIS-III Administration and Scoring Manual,* it can be seen that a difference of this magnitude is reliable at the 95% level. Thus, it probably is not the result of measurement error and likely reflects a real difference in how the examinee expresses his or her intelligence. However, inspection of Table D.3 in the *WAIS-III Technical Manual* indicates that a difference of 11 points occurred in approximately 32% of persons in the standardization sample whose Full Scale IQ fell within the ability range 90–109 when the direction of the discrepancy is ignored. The frequency is 16% when the direction of the difference is consid-

Table 2.3. Illustrative WAIS-III Results

Subtests, Scales, and Indexes	Scaled Score	Scale Mean[a]	Difference	
Verbal Scale				
Vocabulary	10	10	0.0	
Similarities	9	10	−1.0	
Arithmetic	10	10	0.0	
Digit Span	11	10	1.0	Verbal IQ = 101
Information	10	10	0.0	
Comprehension	12	10	2.0	
Letter-Number Sequencing	8	10	−2.0	
Performance Scale				
Picture Completion	8	8.2	−0.2	
Digit Symbol-Coding	7	8.2	−1.2	
Block Design	6	8.2	−2.2	
Matrix Reasoning	10	8.2	−1.8	Performance IQ = 90
Picture Arrangement	12	8.2	3.8	
Symbol Search	6	8.2	−2.2	
				Full Scale IQ = 97
Verbal Comprehension				
Information	10	9.7	0.3	
Vocabulary	10	9.7	0.3	Index = 98
Similarities	9	9.7	−0.7	
Perceptual Organization				
Picture Completion	8	8.0	0.0	
Block Design	6	8.0	−2.0	Index = 88
Matrix Reasoning	10	8.0	2.0	
Working Memory				
Arithmetic	10	9.7	0.3	
Digit Span	11	9.7	1.3	Index = 97
Letter-Number Sequencing	8	9.7	−1.7	
Processing Speed				
Digit Symbol Coding	7	6.5	0.5	Index = 81
Symbol Search	6	6.5	−0.5	

[a]Scale means are the average respectively of the seven verbal subtests and six performance subtests. Index means are composed of only the subtests that contribute to the composite scores that contribute to the Scale/Index.

ered (divide the cumulative percentage from Table D.3 in half). This indicates that the 11-point Verbal IQ–Performance IQ discrepancy is not unusual (the authors consider a difference to be unusual if it occurred in 5% or fewer of the standardization participants) and that the Full Scale IQ provides a reasonable explanation of the examinee's cognitive functioning.

Once the decision has been made to interpret the Full Scale IQ, it is necessary to convert the score to an ability level using Table 2.2 in the *WAIS-III Administration and Scoring Manual*. Next, the IQ is assigned a percentile rank and banded by either the 90% or 95% confidence limits. Tables A.3 through A.5 in the *WAIS-III Administration and Scoring Manual* list the percentile ranks and confidence limits for the Verbal, Performance, and Full Scale IQs. These

Table 2.4. Deviations from the Mean of Six Performance Scale Subtests that Occurred in $\leq$ 5% of the Standardization Sample[a]

Subtest	Deviation from the Mean
Picture Completion	3.93
Digit Symbol-Coding	4.14
Block Design	3.65
Matrix Reasoning	3.79
Picture Arrangement	4.03
Symbol Search	3.57

[a]Adopted from LoBello et al. (1998)

confidence limits are based on the standard error of estimation (SEE), not the SEM discussed previously and presented in Table 3.4 of the *WAIS-III–WMS-III Technical Manual*. Confidence limits based on the SEM for all age groups in the standardization sample are provided in Table 0-1 of Sattler and Ryan (1999). The SEE and the SEM are interpreted in exactly the same manner and yield highly similar confidence limits for IQs within the middle portion of the ability distribution. However, at the extremes of the distribution the SEE provides confidence limits that are asymmetrical around the obtained score. The SEM provides symmetrical confidence limits at all intelligence levels. The reason for this difference is that the SEE takes into consideration the phenomenon of regression to the mean and assumes that examinees with high IQs benefit from positive chance error and those with low IQs are compromised by negative chance error.

As mentioned above, the present example has an 11-point difference which is statistically significant and therefore reliable, but not unusual because a Verbal-Performance IQ discrepancy of this magnitude occurred in 16% of the standardization sample. Also, because the subtest scores within the Verbal Scale do not differ meaningfully from their mean, evidence that the Verbal IQ reflects the unitary dimension of verbal comprehension and expression is provided. Similarly, the absence of meaningful scatter within the Performance Scale indicates that the IQ may be interpreted as a unitary measure of the perceptual organization and clerical speed construct.

The next step in the interpretative process is to examine the relationships between and among the index scores by consulting Table B.1 in the *WAIS-III Administration and Scoring Manual*. It can be seen that the Verbal Comprehension Index is significantly larger than both the Perceptual Organization and Processing Speed Indexes, whereas the Working Memory index is superior to the Processing Speed Index. On the other hand, the Working Memory Index does not differ from either the Verbal Comprehension or Perceptual Organization indexes. Finally, the Perceptual Organization and Processing Speed indexes are essentially the same.

The Verbal Scale of the WAIS-III reflects two major abilities, the first associated with the Verbal Comprehension Index and the second with the Working Memory Index. In the present example, these composites are comparable and indicate that the Verbal IQ provides an effective measure of the global construct of interest. The Performance Scale subtests measure two principal abilities, with Perceptual Organization corresponding to the first and Processing Speed to the second. For the current example, these composites are comparable and indicate that the Performance IQ likely provides a valid measure of the major construct of interest.

Examining Qualitative Information: Detecting Errors

Numerical scores are not always sufficient for detecting and understanding a client's problems. Qualitative information, such as that gained by behavioral observations, may provide important insights into an examinee's cultural background, cognitive deficits, thought processes, psychiatric status, or some combination of these. Likewise, it is often helpful to document the nature and effectiveness of the strategies that an examinee employs enroute to either passing or failing individual items. Table 2.5 provides examples of qualitative errors on selected WAIS-III subtests that, if encountered during a WAIS-III administration, should not be overlooked.

Hypothesis-Driven Approach to Interpreting the WAIS-III

To fully utilize the quantitative and qualitative information provided by a WAIS-III examination, an organized approach that attempts to integrate historical information, behavioral observations, and test results should be followed. The approach used in this chapter is summarized in Table 2.6. It begins with a thorough review of available information from the client's medical, educational, and social histories, the reason for referral, and the behavioral observations made during test administration. Prior to calculating the WAIS-III scores, the examiner formulates a few hypotheses and expectations about the test results.

Table 2.5. Examples of Qualitative Errors Associated with Selected WAIS-III Subtests

Subtest	Errors and Hypothesized Interpretations
Similarities	*"Not alike" response*: May reflect concrete thinking, low IQ, or a psychological characteristic such as negativism.
	Stimulus bound response: Provides common associations to the word pairs, not similarities. For example, in response to item 8, the examinee states, "Ear you hear out of and eye you see out of." Sometimes given by concrete thinkers, persons with low IQ, or patients with brain damage.
Digit Span	*Incorrect sequencing*: The examinee recalls all the elements, but fails to maintain the order of presentation. Sometimes associated with a learning disability and occasionally noted in the records of individuals with significant depression or anxiety.
	Initial errors: Incorrectly recalls the first or second digit in a sequence containing five or fewer digits. When made by an examinee who is fully alert, it is likely that he or she deliberately failed the item
Block Design	*Broken gestalts:* Failure to maintain the 2x2 or 3x3 configuration of one or more designs. Seen occasionally in the records of persons with documented brain damage. Reflects a marked impairment of visuospatial ability.
	Stacking: Blocks piled one on top of the other. An unusual error that suggests the presence of brain dysfunction.
Digit Symbol-Coding	*Shape completion:* Symbols are converted into perceptually similar forms. For instance, the symbol ∧ is converted into an "A." Seen occasionally in the records of patients with brain damage.
	Associating wrong symbol with a number: Suggests failure to comprehend instructions, inattention, or visual scanning problems.

Table 2.6. Hypothesis-Driven Approach to Interpreting the WAIS-III[a]

Phase I: Generating Hypotheses

1. Prior to calculation of the WAIS-III scores, gather data about the client's background information (e.g., medical, educational, and social histories) and review the behavioral observations made during test administration. Formulate *a priori* expectations or hypotheses about the examinee's test performance.
2. Translate *a priori* expectations or hypotheses into specific test results using a sequential process as follows:
   a. Full Scale IQ
   b. Verbal and Performance IQs
   c. Index Scores
   d. Subtest Scores
   e. Individual Item Responses

Phase II: Profile Analysis and Hypothesis Testing

3. Evaluate the degree of intersubtest scatter in the Profile and determine the feasibility of interpreting the various WAIS-III composites.
4. Test *a priori* expectations or hypotheses against the obtained scores.
5. If *a priori* expectations and hypotheses do not account for the data, formulate *a posteriori* explanations and hypotheses for the findings.

Phase III: Gathering More Data and Drawing Conclusions

6. Collect additional data to test or support the *a priori* and *a posteriori* explanations and hypotheses.
7. Draw conclusions, but place an emphasis on explanations and hypotheses that are supported by at least two pieces of evidence.

[a]When implementing this framework, clinicians should employ clinical decision-making strategies that minimize bias and misuse of heuristics.

CASE EXAMPLE

Hypothesis-Driven Interpretive Approach

This section describes the WAIS-III results of F.M., a 23-year-old woman with a high school diploma who attended junior college for approximately two years. She had recently transferred to a small, four-year liberal arts college in hope of obtaining a bachelor's degree in political science. Her career goal was to become "...a paralegal and maybe even a trial lawyer."

Phase I. She is socially active and well liked by fellow students, but she has experienced difficulty with most of her courses. The teaching faculty have given her extra attention during class and also have provided one-on-one tutoring in mathematics and science. Because F.M. has not benefited academically from these interventions, she was referred by her academic advisor for an evaluation of cognitive, academic, and general adaptive capacities.

F.M. denies the presence of medical or psychiatric problems and takes no prescription medications. However, the history is positive for multiple head injuries. The first occurred when she was three years old and was associated with a brief loss of consciousness. A second head injury was sustained in a motor vehicle accident when she was 18 years old. She remembers hitting her head on the windshield and receiving one or more lacerations that required stitches. This trauma was not associated with loss of consciousness, although she was confused for a brief period and then fell asleep shortly after the injury. According to F.M., during the second grade she was identified as having a learning disability, but she is unable to provide further details. This problem was again identified during attendance at junior college, where she received special assistance. (Please note that there is no way of knowing if the head injury as a toddler caused the learning problems. A cause-and-effect relationship cannot be inferred.) After two years of judicious course selection, her grade point average was sufficient for transfer to a four-year college.

F.M. was seen for evaluation at 9:00 a.m. and was then administered an extensive battery of tests. However, the present discussion will focus exclusively on the WAIS-III. Behavioral observation revealed a friendly, talkative, and cooperative young lady. Affect was stable and mood was mildly anxious, but generally appropriate to the situation. There was no evidence of formal thought disorder or unusual thought content, but she was somewhat unsure of herself and giggled excessively. The latter behavior seemed immature for a 23-year-old woman, but it may have been her way of handling test-related anxiety. Although the session took over five hours, she worked without evidencing significant fatigue and her approach to the tasks was slow and deliberate. Finally, she was frequently aware of her failures, but appeared discouraged and frustrated on only one occasion. She was visibly uncomfortable and tense during a task that required the solution of basic arithmetic problems without the aid of pencil and paper. During this task she commented, "I've always been dumb in math, just don't get it!"

As Table 2.6 recommends, available background information and behavioral observation data were reviewed and reasonable *a priori* expectations about F.M.'s WAIS-III performance were generated. Listed below are some expectations and hypotheses presented in a sequential manner starting with the most global score:

1. The history of head injuries and possible learning disability suggests that her general cognitive functions (i.e., Full Scale IQ) may be lower than expected, even through she has completed high school and two years of junior college.
2. Comparable achievement is expected on the Verbal and Performance IQs. Persons who have fully recovered from a closed head injury do not usually exhibit marked IQ discrepancies. Also, data on groups with either traumatic brain injury or learning disabilities reported in the *WAIS-III–WMS-III Technical Manual* did not produce large Verbal–Performance IQ differences.
3. The Working Memory and Processing Speed indexes may reveal selective weaknesses. Data in the *WAIS-III–WMS-III Technical Manual* indicate that learning-disabled individuals score poorly on the former index. Also, it was readily apparent during the examination that she was unable to deal effectively with basic arithmetic calculations, a component of the Working Memory Index. The *WAIS-III–WMS-III Technical Manual* also indicates that persons with a history of traumatic brain injury demonstrate a relative weakness on the Processing Speed Index.
4. F.M. had received tutoring in mathematics and during administration of the Arithmetic subtest she was unable to cope with task requirements. Therefore, her scaled score on the Arithmetic subtest should emerge as a relative weakness in the overall profile. Memory problems sometimes contribute to poor academic performance. Thus, it is reasonable to expect F.M. to experience some difficulty on the supplementary Digit Symbol-Incidental Learning procedure.
5. The history of learning disability suggests that auditory sequencing problems may be seen on the Digit Span items and that answers to the Arithmetic items may reveal specific types of errors (e.g., difficulty in carrying or borrowing).

All of the hypotheses offered in this example may not be supported by the calculated WAIS-III scores. However, they constitute an attempt to integrate external information with the test results and force the examiner to consider the complete array of information provided by the WAIS-III.

Phase II. The next step in WAIS-III interpretation is to evaluate the degree of intersubtest scatter in the profile and thereby determine whether the summary scores represent valid estimates of their respective constructs. Table 2.7 summarizes the quantitative and qualitative information gleaned from F.M.'s evaluation. Analysis begins with an examination of the values provided in the "Difference" column of Table 2.7. For the Verbal subtests, the numbers are compared to the values in Table B.3 of the *WAIS-III Administration and Scoring Manual.* As can be seen, the Vocabulary (4.3 points) and Arithmetic (–6.7 points) scores deviate meaningfully from the Verbal Scale mean. These are considered meaningful deviations because only 5% of the WAIS-III standardization sample had scores that equaled or exceeded 3.00 points on Vocabulary and 3.57 points on Arithmetic. These findings suggest that the Verbal IQ does not provide a unitary estimate of the verbal comprehension construct and that a comparison of this value with the Performance IQ will yield misleading information.

Examination of scatter within the Performance Scale is accomplished by comparing the deviation scores under the "Difference" column in Table 2.7 with the values provided in Table 2.4. This indicates that none of the subtest scores deviate meaningfully (i.e., equal or exceed that of 95% of the standardization sample) from the mean. Therefore, the Performance subtests represent a unitary construct and the resulting IQ may be interpreted as a valid estimate of F.M.'s processing speed and perceptual organization abilities.

Next, the cohesiveness of the four indexes is evaluated using the rule of thumb presented previously. That is, an index is considered cohesive if none of its component subtests deviate from the mean by 3.0 or more points. As can be gleaned from Table 2.7, the subtests that comprise the Verbal Comprehension, Perceptual Organization, and Processing Speed indexes demonstrate minimal scatter from their respective means and appear to represent unitary abilities. On the other hand, F.M. performed inconsistently on subtests comprising the Working Memory Index. Two of the three subtest scores deviate from the mean by 3.0 or more points, indicating that this composite is not unitary in what it measures.

The fourth step in WAIS-III interpretation involves testing the a priori expectations and hypotheses against the obtained scores. As can be seen from Table 2.7, the Verbal, Performance, and Full Scale IQs are significantly below expectations for someone with 14 years of education, which confirms the first hypothesis. Based on F.M.'s demographic characteristics (e.g., age, sex, education, race, social economic status, and urban vs. rural residence) it is reasonable to expect average to above average IQs. The second hypothesis is also confirmed since there is no Verbal-Performance IQ discrepancy.

To address the third hypothesis, it is necessary to consult Table B.1 in the *WAIS-III Administration and Scoring Manual.* By reading down the appropriate columns in the table, one can see that the Working Memory Index is significantly lower than each of the other indexes. By following the same procedure, it is can be seen that the Processing Speed Index is significantly below the Verbal Comprehension Index, but statistically equivalent to the Perceptual Organization Index. These findings confirm the third hypothesis since the Working Memory and Processing Speed indexes represent weaknesses in F.M.'s WAIS-III profile.

The Arithmetic scaled score emerges as the single most prominent weakness in the profile. Examination of the Digit Symbol-Incidental Learning scores indicates that F.M. freely recalled six of the nine individual symbols and six of the associated number-symbol pairs. These scores are below the 10th percentile and suggest that F.M. may experience learning and memory problems. These findings confirm the hypothesis that addressed individual subtest performance.

Finally, examination of item responses reveals errors on the Digit Span subtest that are suggestive of a deficit in auditory sequencing. Analysis of F.M.'s answers to items on the

Table 2.7. F.M.'s WAIS-III Results

IQs		Indexes	
Verbal	86	Verbal Comprehension (VC)	101
Performance	86	Perceptual Organization (PO)	80
Full Scale	85	Working Memory (WM)	69
		Processing Speed (PS)	88

Verbal Subtests	Scaled Score		Mean		Difference
Vocabulary	12	–	7.7	=	4.3
Similarities	9	–	7.7	=	1.3
Arithmetic	1	–	7.7	=	–6.7
Digit Span	6	–	7.7	=	–1.7
Information	10	–	7.7	=	2.3
Comprehension	8	–	7.7	=	0.3
Letter-Number Sequencing	8	–	7.7	=	0.3
Performance Subtest					
Picture Completion	8	–	7.8	=	0.2
Digit Symbol-Coding	9	–	7.8	=	1.2
Block Design	7	–	7.8	=	–0.8
Matrix Reasoning	5	–	7.8	=	–2.8
Picture Arrangement	11	–	7.8	=	3.2
Symbol Search	7	–	7.8	=	–0.8
VC Subtests					
Vocabulary	12	–	10.3	=	1.7
Similarities	9	–	10.3	=	–1.3
Information	10	–	10.3	=	–1.7
PO Subtests					
Picture Completion	8	–	6.7	=	1.3
Block Design	7	–	6.7	=	0.3
Matrix Reasoning	5	–	6.7	=	–1.7
WM Subtests					
Arithmetic	1	–	5.0	=	–4.0
Digit Span	6	–	5.0	=	1.0
Letter-Number Sequencing	8	–	5.0	=	3.0
PS Subtests					
Digit Symbol-Coding	9	–	8.0	=	1.0
Symbol Search	7	–	8.0	=	1.0

Digit Symbol-Coding, Optional Procedures
Incidental Learning - Pairing   6
Incidental Learning - Recall   6

Qualitative Features
Digit Span (Forward)
    –4-2-7-3-1   repeated as "4-3-2-7-1"
    –6-1-9-4-7-3   repeated as "6-9-1-4-7-3"
    –5-9-1-7-4-2-8   repeated as "5-9-7-4-2-1-8"
Digit Span (Backward)
    –6-2-9   repeated as "9-6-2"
Arithmetic - careless errors such as $4.00 plus $5.00 = "$8.00"
        - apparently lacks mastery of basic multiplication and division

Arithmetic subtest suggest that she lacks mastery of basic mathematical operations and concepts. These findings confirm the last two *a priori* hypotheses.

F.M.'s WAIS-III protocol contains one result that was not predicted. The Verbal Comprehension Index is 21 points higher than the Perceptual Organization Index. The practical implication of this finding is that F.M. demonstrates her intelligence more effectively via the expression of previously learned and stored verbal information than by perceptual organization and nonverbal problem solving. Obviously, it would be incorrect to interpret the absence of a Verbal-Performance IQ difference as evidence of similar verbal and nonverbal cognitive functioning. To explain this fact, it is necessary to formulate an *a posteriori* hypothesis. For instance, it is reasonable to assume that F.M.'s fund of information, word knowledge, and understanding of verbal relationships has been artificially increased beyond the expected baseline because of her almost three-years exposure to college courses and associated educational experiences.

Phase III. The sixth and seventh interpretative steps listed in Table 2.6 address the need to collect additional data to support the interpretative hypotheses. To accomplish this goal, F.M. was administered a battery of tests that included measures of language, memory, academic proficiency, executive functions, and constructional ability. When the battery results are considered in conjunction with the history of two head injuries and learning problems, it appears reasonable to assume that F.M. experiences a mild cerebral dysfunction and that this factor is responsible, at least in part, for her lower than expected IQs and the various problems related to academic achievement (please note that this is only an inference, cannot be proven, and should not appear in a formal report). These conclusions are further reinforced by the presence of subtle problems on tasks involving language (e.g., naming difficulties) and mental flexibility. Memory evaluation indicates that she is significantly better at retaining information presented via the auditory modality than through the visual modality, a finding that makes sense in light of the superiority of the Verbal Comprehension Index over the Perceptual Organization Index. She also displayed a significant retrieval deficit during a word list memorization task. Academic proficiencies are low average in reading and factual knowledge, whereas marked deficits are noted in writing and mathematics.

Preparing the WAIS-III Report

The WAIS-III was administered to help answer the referral question and to provide insights into F.M.'s cognitive and adaptive abilities. However, the scores have little meaning in and of themselves and must be translated so that F.M. and the referral source can utilize the information. This requires drawing conclusions and the preparation of a formal report. The following paragraphs attempt to demonstrate this process with respect to the WAIS-III results:

Reporting the IQs

On the WAIS-III, F.M. achieved a Verbal IQ of 86, a Performance IQ of 86, and a Full Scale IQ of 85. The chances that the range of scores from 81-89 includes her true Full Scale IQ are about 95 out of a 100. Her overall achievement is classified in the low average range and is ranked at the 16th percentile. These results appear to be reliable and valid.

Comment. It is often important to provide the sophisticated reader with traditional IQs. F.M. was referred by her academic advisor and there was a clear expectation that such information would be forthcoming. Also, it is recognized that the Verbal IQ does not constitute an accurate measure of the verbal comprehension construct and that the Verbal-Performance IQ discrepancy is misleading. However, for practical reasons this information is presented in another section of the report. The goal of this paragraph is to communicate information concerning F.M.'s general intellectual level. Finally, the results appear valid and reliable because F.M. was cooperative, and motivated to perform and because most of the *a priori* hypotheses and expectations were addressed by reviewing data from multiple sources external to the WAIS-III (e.g., history, behavioral observations, other test results).

Subtest Analysis (Verbal Scale)

Analysis of the Verbal Scale subtests revealed average achievement on measures of verbal comprehension and expression (53rd percentile). She effectively handled tasks that require the ability to orally define words, recall facts about common events, people, and places, and identify similarities between word pairs that describe objects and concepts. She also demonstrated an average understanding and appreciation of social conventionalities and performed adequately on a test of auditory tracking and information processing. With respect to the latter observation, she listened to a series of random letters and numbers and then repeated the numbers in ascending order and the letters in alphabetical order. However, when asked to repeat strings of orally presented digits, her score fell within the low average to borderline range (9th percentile). This was not the result of an attention problem since behavioral evidence of distractibility or fluctuating motivation was absent during task administration. Instead, it appeared to reflect auditory sequencing problems since F.M.'s repetition was limited to five digits forward in the prescribed order. F.M.'s most impaired score emerged during mental arithmetic calculations (1st percentile) when she became frustrated and tense and made errors on basic problems that involved addition ($4.00 + $5.00 = "$8.00"), subtraction ($10.00 – $6.00 = "$5.00"), and multiplication (25 x 6 = "70").

Comment. This paragraph describes F.M.'s achievement levels and, where appropriate, attempts to integrate behavioral observations and subjective impressions gleaned from item analysis and the various subtest scores. It should also be apparent that whenever possible the emphasis is put on the composite index (Verbal Comprehension Index) over single subtest scores. However, is this case the Working Memory Index was not unitary and it was necessary to focus on results from the individual subtests to adequately describe F. M.'s performance. Also, the Comprehension subtest is not officially a part of the Verbal Comprehension Index, leaving the examiner to decide whether to ignore it, report it, or subsume it under the Verbal Comprehension Index (The latter option is justified by factor analytic research.)

Subtest Analysis (Performance Scale)

Analysis of the Performance Scale subtests revealed a high average capacity to plan and anticipate within a social context. When confronted with sets of pictures in mixed-up order, she quickly and efficiently rearranged them into logical stories. Low average achievement was evidenced on measures of visual processing speed and clerical efficiency (21st percentile). She was able to work under time pressures, visually scan arrays of numbers and symbols, and rapidly copy stimuli or place marks in designated places on the protocol. Low average scores were also obtained on tests of perceptual organization and nonverbal problem solving (9th percentile) since she demonstrated an adequate capacity to identify omitted parts in pictures of common objects and settings, reproduce abstract patterns using colored blocks, and recognize missing elements in a series of gridded patterns. On a measure of incidental learning for rehearsed material, her scores were again low average. Thus, she repeatedly copied 9 number symbol pairs for 120 seconds and later remembered 6 individual symbols and 6 associated pairs when a surprise recall trial was conducted.

Comment. This paragraph describes F.M.'s achievement levels and puts emphasis on the Processing Speed and Perceptual Organization Indexes. However, specific interpretations are made for the Picture Arrangement subtest and the Digit Symbol-Incidental Learning procedure. These single subtest interpretations are necessary because neither measure contributes to the composite index scores within the Performance Scale.

Overall Conclusions

Overall, F.M. performed within the low average range of intelligence as evidenced by a Full Scale IQ of 85 (16th percentile). Equal functioning on the Verbal and Performance Scales was suggested, but analysis of subtest scores lead to a different conclusion. Specifically, scores on measures of verbal comprehension and expression (53rd percentile) were superior to those on tasks of processing speed and clerical efficiency (21st percentile) as well as those that reflect perceptual organization and nonverbal problem solving (9th percentile).

F.M. displayed a satisfactory appreciation of social conventionalities and her ability to plan and anticipate within a social context was solidly average. She also demonstrated normal attention-concentration and auditory tracking skills. However, difficulty with number processing was noted during a digit repetition task when she displayed sequencing errors. Problems were also documented on a test of mental arithmetic when she became tense and frustrated by an apparent inability to successfully carry out even the most basic calculations. Finally, on tests of incidental learning of rehearsed material, her scores fell within the low average range.

Comment. These paragraphs summarize the WAIS-III results and provide a clarification statement concerning the misleading Verbal-Performance IQ relationship. Many implications could be drawn from F.M.'s results, but the fact that her general intelligence is in the low average range should not be overlooked. F.M. is attempting to succeed at a competitive college among students whose average entrance examination score suggests at least high average intelligence. As a transfer student, F.M. was not required to take an entrance examination. Moreover, because of her normal verbal skills and appreciation of social conventionalities, it is postulated that she was able to present a facade of adequacy during required pre-enrollment and orientation activities. Apparently her problems went undetected until she was well into her first semester of academic courses.

In most assessment situations, as with the present case, the WAIS-III is administered as part of an extensive test battery. The findings for F.M. were presented orally and in writing to involved faculty, the student, and her significant others. It was decided that F.M. would leave college at the end of the semester and in the interim she would be referred for therapeutic and vocational counseling. Every effort was made to insure that F.M. had a smooth transition from the traditional college program to a more appropriate educational setting that emphasized job skill acquisition. Tutoring in college level courses was terminated and remediation efforts were focused on the development of proficiencies in basic, everyday mathematics.

SUMMARY

The WAIS-III is a psychometrically sound measure of general intelligence for individuals who are 16 to 89 years of age. Updated norms and enhanced clinical utility make the measure appropriate for use in a wide range of clinical situations.

Improvements in the stimulus material and test protocol make the measure more user-friendly for both the examinee and the examiner. However, a strong foundation in psychological assessment remains a prerequisite for test use and examiner precision and accuracy are necessary for proper administration and scoring.

As suggested in this chapter, interpreting the WAIS-III is a challenging task given the volume of client data generated. Nevertheless, with implementation of the hypothesis-driven interpretive framework, meaningful information that *is* or *is not* consistent with other client characteristics can be extracted.

SUGGESTED READINGS

Kamphaus, R. W. (1993). *Clinical assessment of children's intelligence: A handbook for professional practice.* Boston: Allyn and Bacon.

LoBello, S. G., Thompson, A. P., & Evani. V. (1998). Supplementary WAIS-III tables for determining subtest strengths and weaknesses. *Journal of Psychoeducational Assessment, 16*, 196–200.

Sattler, J. M., & Ryan, J. J. (1999). *Assessment of children, revised and updated third edition: WAIS-III supplement.* San Diego, CA: Sattler.

The Psychological Corporation. (1997). *WAIS-III–WMS-III technical manual.* San Antonio, TX: Author.

Wechsler, D. (1997). *WAIS-III Administration and scoring manual.* San Antonio, TX: The Psychological Association.

3

General Ability Measure for Adults (GAMA)

Achilles N. Bardos

INTRODUCTION

The measurement of intellectual ability is an important component of many psychological assessments conducted by mental health professionals. Psychologists often face the challenge of assessing the cognitive ability of individuals who, for a variety of reasons, are either limited in their ability to understand directions (and therefore the requirements of a test) or have verbal expression difficulties. For example, recent demographics in the United States suggest that the percentage of individuals of diverse ethnic backgrounds, language backgrounds, or both is on the rise. Mental health professionals searching for ways to measure the cognitive ability of children and adults have used ability tests typically referred to as nonverbal. These tests assess a person's intellectual ability using minimal verbal requirements. For example, they include very short verbal directions and minimal-to-nonexistent English language verbal expression skills. These characteristics have made nonverbal intelligence tests very popular among psychologists who need to employ fair assessment techniques in their evaluations. The General Ability Measure for Adults (GAMA), is a nonverbal test that shares many of the above features. By reducing the effects of item verbal content, the GAMA is free of the confounding requirements for expressive language skills and overall academic achievement. This assessment approach offers the advantage of providing an instrument that is accessible to a wide variety of persons with different linguistic and cultural backgrounds, to those with limited educational experiences or verbal skills, to those with difficulties with verbal communication, and to those who are deaf or hearing impaired. In addition, the GAMA can be administered in a variety of settings. These may include high schools, community mental health centers, hospitals, and private practice offices using a paper and pencil format and in the near future, online, using a personal computer.

Achilles N. Bardos • Division of Professional Psychology, University of Northern Colorado, Greeley, Colorado 80639

Understanding Psychological Assessment, edited by Dorfman and Hersen. Kluwer Academic/Plenum Publishers, New York, 2001.

TEST CONSTRUCTION AND DEVELOPMENT

Theoretical Structure and Goals

Many theorists refer to the concept of "g" as a person's overall ability to apply knowledge and reasoning skills in solving problems. Problems can present themselves in various formats and varieties of content and can include tasks that require verbal reasoning, quantitative reasoning, short-term and long-term memory and visual abstract reasoning. These constructs are included in individually administered intelligence tests such as the Wechsler intelligence scales (Wechsler, 1981). For example, the Wechsler tests utilize several tasks that are organized into global scores to provide an assessment of general cognitive ability. Many of these tasks, however, can pose difficulties in the evaluation process of a person's overall ability. For example, many tasks require verbal comprehension and verbal expression skills and others require the manipulation of objects, while optimal performance on some tasks might be compromised by the required time limits at the item level.

The primary goal in the development of the GAMA was to design a brief test of general ability using a variety of tasks that require visual abstract reasoning. This was accomplished by developing a test that:

- is normed on a recent and large standardization sample of individuals 18 to 96 years old. There were a total of 2,360 individuals who were included in the final standardization sample.
- is a measure on which a person's performance is not influenced by the motor requirements of its tasks since the test includes no manipulatives. All test items are designs printed on the stimulus booklet.
- provides a fair estimate of intellectual ability for persons from diverse backgrounds by requiring minimal verbal comprehension and no verbal expression skills.
- has minimal administrative instructions, while feedback from sample items introduced prior to the administration of the test facilitate the understanding of the task requirements.
- where appropriate, can be self-administered individually or in groups with minimal examiner involvement.
- uses colorful designs that help to maintain interest. The colors used in the designs are those that are least problematic for those with color-impaired vision.
- provides an overall score with a mean of 100 and a standard deviation of 15 and subscale scores with a mean of 10 and standard deviations of 3. This metric allows comparisons with a majority of intelligence and achievement tests.

Description of the GAMA

The GAMA is designed to measure nonverbal intellectual ability using a variety of tasks. It includes 66 items organized into four item types. The four item types are organized with a mean of 10 and a standard deviation of 3. The four item type subtests contribute to the overall GAMA total score, which is organized with a mean of 100 and a standard deviation of 15. The structure of the GAMA is presented in Figure 3.1. Samples of the four item types will also be presented and described.

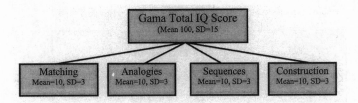

Figure 3.1. The structure of the General Ability Measure for Adults.

Matching

"Matching" items consist of a stimulus presented at the left side of a rectangle followed by six options to the right (see Figure 3.2). These items require the person to perceive various shapes and visually differentiate among shape and color combinations while inspecting each of the characteristics of the stimuli in each of the options to detect the same exact features. Performance on this task requires the ability to delay the impulse to respond until an exact match is found. Both the shapes as well as the colors of the designs contribute to their complexity.

This book has four kinds of problems for you to solve. Samples of the problems are shown on the next few pages. Read the directions above each sample and then solve the problem. The correct answer is given below each sample. Be sure to solve each sample carefully. Look at the sample below.

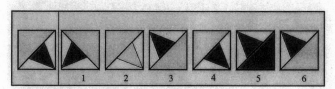

The Matching subtest requires the recognition of the spatial orientation of the designs and identification of the option with the same arrangement of shapes.

Figure 3.2. Sample Matching item.

Analogies

With this item type called "Analogies," the examinee must inspect the relationship between and analyze the shapes and designs of the first pair of geometric designs and determine the analogy for the second pair (see Figure 3.3).

Sample : Which answer (1, 2, 3, 4, 5, or 6) goes on the question mark?

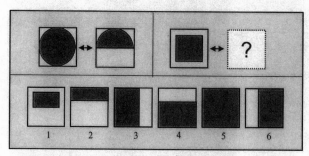

Analogies require the recognition of the relationship(s)
between the figures in the sample and identification of
the option with the same conceptual relationship.

Figure 3.3. Sample Analogies item.

Sequences

With "Sequences" the examinee is shown a sequence of events represented by figural designs. The examinee must follow the temporal relationship of the various shape and color combinations and recognize their progressive relationship (see Figure 3.4).

Sample : Which answer (1, 2, 3, 4, 5, or 6) goes on the question
mark to complete the pattern?

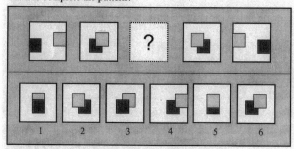

Sequencing requires the recognition of the pattern of
change in the sample and identification of the option
with the same sequential pattern.

Figure 3.4. Sample Sequences item.

Construction

The final item type, "constructions," requires the examinee to decide how various shapes can be combined to produce one of the two-dimensional designs (see Figure 3.5) which in turn requires the analysis and breakdown of each design into its parts, examination of their relationship, mental rotation of shapes, and synthesis of the individual parts into the original design.

Sample : Which answer (1, 2, 3, 4, 5, or 6) can be made with the shapes in the top box?

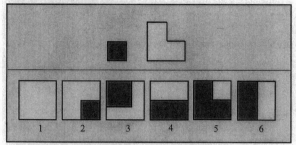

Construction requires analysis and syntheses of the spatial characteristics of the shapes to mentally construct one of the options.

Figure 3.5. Sample Construction item.

Uses of the GAMA

The GAMA might be the appropriate instrument of choice in a variety of situations when a general estimate of cognitive ability is desired. For example, the test can be part of a comprehensive evaluation and it can be used either as the primary instrument to assess a person's ability or to test hypotheses generated followed the administration of a comprehensive individually administered battery. For example, if the examiner suspects that a client might have had difficulty manipulating objects in a subtest on the Wechsler scale due to impaired motor skills, the GAMA can provide an additional measure to verify this hypothesis. The variety of GAMA's administrative forms, especially self-administration, will minimize the amount of time the psychologist must spend on this part of the evaluation. In other cases, an examination of a person's intellectual ability might begin with the GAMA, and if needed, be followed by a comprehensive individually administered test.

In counseling settings, the GAMA can be used in inpatient or outpatient settings when an estimate of intellectual ability is needed prior to counseling or as part of a diagnostic personality evaluation. The evaluation of a client's intellectual ability is warranted when there is no current data on overall intellectual ability and such knowledge would facilitate the mode of therapy. For example, such knowledge can assist the therapist in the selection of the most appropriate therapeutic method (e.g., behavior modification, rational emotive therapy, or insight therapy) or allow the therapist to plan interventions that are consistent with the client's intellectual ability and problem-solving skills.

Similarly, the GAMA can be used in career counseling since intelligence tests have consistently demonstrated their ability to predict educational performance. The relationship of intelligence tests to occupational level attainment has been documented in the literature.

In business and industry settings, the GAMA can be a viable addition to or alternative for tests such as the Wonderlic Personnel Test, especially when testing individuals with limited English skills. In these settings, the GAMA can be especially helpful when large groups need to be tested (e.g., training programs, prisons, the military).

In addition, the GAMA can be used in public schools, especially with mentally retarded students to whom the schools are required by law to offer services up to the age of 21. For example, in many instances when psychologists participate in the evaluation of a client's transition from a public school to another setting, a comprehensive intelligence test might not be warranted. Instead, an update of a student's overall intellectual ability might be required. In other cases, the GAMA might be appropriate with students with learning disabilities who are planning to pursue studies in a community college or four-year college. An update of the student's record should include at least some recent measure of cognitive ability. This is a desirable, if not necessary, component of a student's record prior to the determination of services that will be offered by the respective college.

PSYCHOMETRIC PROPERTIES

Earlier in this chapter we have made certain claims about the GAMA's goals and identified numerous possible applications for the test. In this section, we will present evidence to support these claims. All of the evidence presented relates to the test's validity, that is, the quality of inferences that can be made by the GAMA IQ score.

Standardization Sample

A sound standardization sample is critical in the development of a normative test. Following pilot studies of approximately 200 test items in an initial item pool, the final test was selected on the basis of a series of psychometric studies. These studies included examining mean scores by age and gender, examining biased items, computing the internal consistency coefficients for each item type and computing item difficulty and item discrimination values. The national standardization sample for the GAMA consisted of a sample of 2,360 people who ranged in age from 18 to 96 years. The sample was selected using a stratified random sampling plan so that the sample would closely match the United States population according to the 1990 census. The standardization sample was comprised of nine age groups of approximately equal numbers of people: 18–19, 20–24, 25–34, 35–44, 45–54, 55–64, 65–69, 70–74, and 75–96 years. Each age group was stratified by gender, race or ethnic group (African American, American Indian, Asian or Pacific Islander, Hispanic, or white), educational level (less than 9 years completed, grade 9-12 without high school graduation, high school diploma or GED, some college including vocational programs and 2-year college degrees, and bachelors degree or more), and geographic region (Northeast, South, Midwest, and West).

Reliability

The GAMA's reliability was examined using two methods. Internal consistency was determined by the split-half method while stability of scores over time was determined through a test-retest study. The GAMA IQ score average reliability across the 11 age groups was .90 and ranged from .79 for the 80 and older group to .94 for the 35–44 year olds (see Table 3.1).

The stability of the test scores was also examined in a study with 86 individuals who were readministered the GAMA within a 2 to 6 week interval (the mean test-retest interval was 25 days with a SD of 7.7). The mean performance of the test-retest administrations of the GAMA scores are shown in Table 3.2. The similarity of the test-retest means suggest that the scores remained stable over the time interval. Practice effects are indicated by the small gain in scores; they are standard score points for the overall score and less than one standard score point for the subtests. The test-retest coefficient of .67 was statistically significant, an additional indicator of the GAMA IQ score stability across time.

Table 3.1. Split-Half Internal Consistency Reliability Coefficients[a]

Age group	Sample Size	Reliability coefficient	Standard Error of Measurement
18–19	265	0.91	4.78
20–24	271	0.91	4.69
25–34	310	0.90	4.29
35–44	300	0.94	4.10
45–54	274	0.92	4.46
55–59	153	0.92	4.36
60–64	104	0.88	4.88
65–69	238	0.91	4.72
70–74	219	0.86	4.72
75–79	135	0.85	5.20
80 +	91	0.79	5.77
All ages	2,360	0.90	4.76

[a]The reliability for the GAMA IQ score was calculated on the basis of a lineaar composite of the subtest split-half coefficients (Nunnally & Bernstein, 1995). The standard errors of measurement (SEM) for the GAMA IQ and subtests were obtained from the reliability coefficients using the following formula: $SEM = SD \times \sqrt{1 - r_{yy}}$.

Validity

The GAMA was designed as a measure of overall cognitive ability. In this respect, the validity of the GAMA was demonstrated by examining: a) mean scores across the 11 age groups, b) correlations with other comprehensive (WAIS-R) and brief intelligence tests of general cognitive ability, c) correlations with achievement tests and d) performance of a variety of groups such as individuals with learning disabilities, the deaf, elderly nursing home residents, individuals with traumatic brain injuries, and individuals with mental retardation. In all studies, the GAMA and the other criterion tests were administered in counterbalanced order. Where appropriate, a control matched sample was derived from the standardization sample to demonstrate group mean score differences. These studies are presented in Appendix A and demonstrate the validity of the GAMA as a measure of general cognitive ability. For a continuous update on research regarding the GAMA, the reader is encouraged to visit the author's home page http://www. edtech.unco.edu/abardos/.

ADMINISTRATION AND SCORING

It is important to recognize that administration and interpretation of the GAMA demand different levels of expertise. Interpretation of GAMA scores should always be made by indi-

Table 3.2. Stability of Test Score Performance

| Subtest | Test | | Retest | | | |
	M	SD	M	SD	Gain	r
Matching 10.15	3.0	10.07	3.3	.08	.55*	
Analogies 9.71	3.0	10.56	3.4	.85	.65*	
Sequences	9.73	3.4	10.72	3.8	.99	.74*
Construction	9.71	3.1	10.57	3.5	.86	.38*
Total score	99.2	15.6	103.2	17.6	4.0	.67*

viduals with formal training in psychological testing and assessment and in consultation with the local licensing boards and regulatory agencies regarding test administration and appropriate test use and supervisory arrangements.

The administration and scoring procedures for the GAMA are simple and straightforward. Thus, with proper supervision and training, examiners who may not be qualified to administer comprehensive batteries such as the Wechsler scales can obtain valid scores. Since any psychological test can be misused, it is the responsibility of the test user to ensure that all the methods and procedures described in the manual are followed.

Test Materials

The test is comprised of the manual, the test booklet, and two types of response forms. The examiner's manual provides general information about the test, guidelines for administration and scoring, test psychometric properties, and information on the interpretation of results. The test booklet includes the test directions, sample items, and the 66 test items. Directions are printed in English. A separate booklet with directions printed in Spanish is also available. There are two response forms, a self-scoring record form and a scannable answer sheet. The *Self-Scoring Record Form* gives the examiner the ability to immediately score the test using the guidelines presented on the form and without having to refer to the examiner's manual. The scannable answer sheet is a two-page form that can be scanned and processed using the Microtest-Q software. This scoring program generates a report for each test administration. Microtest-Q is the software developed by National Computer Systems (NCS) and can be used to score the GAMA and other tests, such as the MMPI-2, the Millon, career-related inventories, and all other products published by NCS.

Administration

One of four sets of directions for the administration of the GAMA is used, depending on the setting (individual or group) and the type of form used (scannable or self-scoring). People with a second-grade reading level should be able to read and understand the instructions. Nevertheless, the examiner should read the test directions out loud while the examinee(s) follows along in the test booklet. For those subjects who are unable to read in either English or Spanish, the examiner can pantomime the test directions. The examiner should monitor the examinee as the four sample items are completed. Once the samples are completed and the task is understood, the examinee may begin the test. The examiner should begin timing when Item 1 is exposed.

Scoring

The scoring requirements for the GAMA vary according to the administration form that is used. For example, if the scannable form is used, all scoring is completed through the Microtest-Q software. The Microtest-Q software can be installed in the user's personal computer or the form can be mailed to the publisher for scoring. The program generates a report for each client. For an illustration using the self-scoring form, the reader is encouraged to follow the various steps described below as part of a case study.

CASE EXAMPLE

Nicolette referred herself for an evaluation to the career services office at a local university. She is a 24-year-old single female who has decided to pursue her education in the local community college (see Figure 3.6). Nicolette was concerned about her ability to handle the coursework requirements. Following an interview, a counselor administered a career interest inventory, a brief academic achievement test and the GAMA.

Nicolette B.
Name

201-38-4671
Identification Number

12/30/99   *9/24/75*
Test Date   **Birth Date**

Gender ☐ Male
        ☒ Female

FOR OFFICE USE ONLY

	Year	Month	Day
Test Date	99	12	30
Birth Date	75	9	24
Age	24	3	6

LEVEL OF EDUCATION (check only one)
- ☐ Grade 8 or less
- ☐ Grade 9 to 12 (without graduation)
- ☒ High school graduate or GED
- ☐ Some college
- ☐ Associate degree (2-year degree)
- ☐ Vocational/technical school certificate/diploma
- ☐ Bachelor's degree or more

EMPLOYMENT STATUS (check all that apply)
- ☐ Employed full-time
- ☒ Employed part-time
- ☐ Homemaker
- ☐ Retired
- ☐ Student
- ☐ Unemployed
- ☐ Other (please specify)
  _____

SETTING (check only one)
- ☐ (Inpatient/Outpatient) Mental Health Center
- ☐ General Medical
- ☐ College Counseling
- ☐ Correctional
- ☒ Career/Vocational Counseling
- ☐ Human Resources
- ☐ Other (please specify)
  _____

LANGUAGE
1. What language do you speak in your home?
   - ☒ English
   - ☐ Other (please specify)
     _____

2. What language do you speak outside of your home?
   - ☒ English
   - ☐ Other (please specify)
     _____

RACE/ETHNIC GROUP (check only one)
- ☒ White
- ☐ African American (Black)
- ☐ Hispanic/Latino
- ☐ Asian
- ☐ American Indian (Native American)
- ☐ Pacific Islander
- ☐ Other (please specify)
  _____

3. How well do you speak English?
   - ☐ Not well
   - ☐ Well
   - ☒ Very well

Figure 3.6. Self-Scoring Record Form, age grid and demographics.

Figures 3.6–3.10 represent sections of the GAMA self-scoring record form with Nicolette's responses. The four GAMA subtest's scaled scores are obtained from the sum of the raw scores for Matching, Analogies, Sequences, and Construction. The GAMA IQ score is derived from the sum of the four subtest's scaled scores.

After the client provides answers for the various items, the examiner tears open the perforations at the bottom and sides of the self-scoring form and scores each item. The correct answer for each item appears in blue on the record form. The examiner marks a one (1) in the box to the right of each item if the response is correct. A zero (0) is marked if the correct answer was not selected, there was no response to the item, or more than one answer was marked. The examiner then performs the following steps.

- The examiner adds the numbers correct recorded in the boxes next to each item on page 7 of the record form and records the column sums in the diamonds below each column (see Figure 3.7).
- The examiner adds the column sums in the two diamonds that correspond to each subtest and records the subtest raw score in the appropriate oval. The various shapes (diamonds, ovals) and colors assist in this process. In Nicolette's case, she earned scores of 9, 14, 8 and 13 for the four respective item types.
- The examiner then transfers each subtest raw score from this page to the Subtest Raw Score column in the GAMA RESULTS summary section (see Figure 3.8).
- Using the examinee's age (see Figure 3.6) the examiner locates the appropriate raw-score-to-scale-scores-transformation table and records the scale scores. There are 11 tables printed on the record form (but only four are shown) representing the subtest raw score to scale score conversions needed. The norm tables were placed on the record form to expedite the scoring process. In this case Nicolette's scale scores were 10 for Matching, 13 for Analogies, 9 for Sequences, and 15 for Construction.

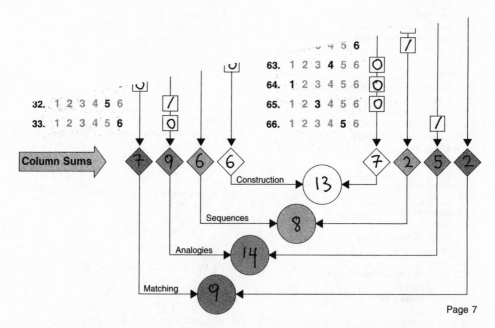

Page 7

Figure 3.7. Calculations of subtest raw scores using the Self-Scoring Record Form. Part of the record form has deleted to protect the test security. Diamonds and circles are color coded on the actual form to facilitate the scoring.

GAMA RESULTS

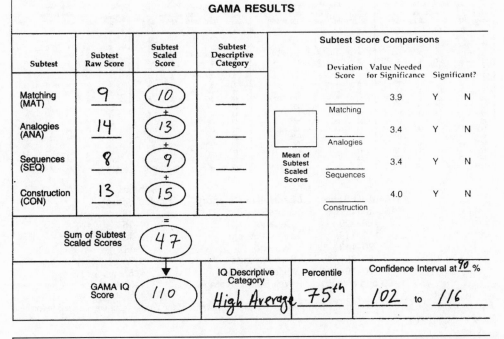

Subtest	Subtest Raw Score	Subtest Scaled Score	Subtest Descriptive Category
Matching (MAT)	9	(10)	____
Analogies (ANA)	14	(13)	____
Sequences (SEQ)	8	(9)	____
Construction (CON)	13	(15)	____

Sum of Subtest Scaled Scores = (47)

Subtest Score Comparisons

	Deviation Score	Value Needed for Significance	Significant?	
Matching	____	3.9	Y	N
Analogies	____	3.4	Y	N
Sequences	____	3.4	Y	N
Construction	____	4.0	Y	N

Mean of Subtest Scaled Scores

GAMA IQ Score (110)

IQ Descriptive Category: High Average Percentile: 75ᵗʰ Confidence Interval at 90 %: 102 to 116

GAMA IQ Score Graph

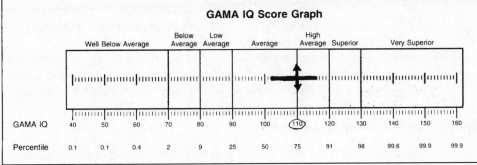

GAMA IQ	40	50	60	70	80	90	100	(110)	120	130	140	150	160
Percentile	0.1	0.1	0.4	2	9	25	50	75	91	98	99.6	99.9	99.9

Well Below Average | Below Average | Low Average | Average | High Average | Superior | Very Superior

Comments/Observations:

_____

_____

_____

_____

Figure 3.8. Self-Scoring Record Form, GAMA Results Section.

- Next, the examiner obtains the sum of the subtest scale scores (Nicolette's score = 47) and using the conversion table (see Figure 3.10) also printed on the record form finds her GAMA IQ score of 110 and records it in the appropriate oval in the GAMA RESULTS section of the form (see Figure 3.8). Similarly, the examiner records the corresponding percentile value, the 90% confidence interval values, and the overall classification range of ability.

Scaled Score	Age Group: 18–19 Raw Scores				Scaled Score	Age Group: 20–24 Raw Scores				Scaled Score	Age Group: 25–34 Raw Scores				Scaled Score	Age Group: 35–44 Raw Scores			
	MAT	ANA	SEQ	CON		MAT	ANA	SEQ	CON		MAT	ANA	SEQ	CON		MAT	ANA	SEQ	CON
1	0-1	0	—	0	1	0-1	0	—	0	1	0-1	0	—	0	1	0	—	—	—
2	2-3	1	0	1	2	2	1	0	1	2	2	1	—	1	2	1	0	—	0
3	4	2-3	1-2	2-3	3	3	2	1	2	3	3	2	0	2	3	2	1	0	1
4	5	4-5	3	—	4	4	3-4	2	3	4	4	3-4	1-2	3	4	3	2-3	1	2
5	—	6-7	4	4	5	5	5-6	3-4	4	5	5	5	3	4	5	4-5	4	2	3
6	6	8	5	5	6	6	7-8	5	5	6	6	6-7	4-5	5	6	6	5-6	3	4
7	7	9	6	6	7	7	9	6	6	7	7	8	6	—	7	—	7-8	4	5
8	8	10	7	7	8	8	10	7	7	8	8	9	—	6	8	7	—	5	6
9	—	11	8	—	9	—	11	8	—	9	—	10	7	7	9	8	9-10	6	—
10	9	12	9	8	10	9	12	9	8	10	9	11	8	8	10	9	11	7	7
11	—	13	10	9	11	—	13	10	—	11	—	12-13	9-10	—	11	—	12	8-9	8
12	10	—	11	10	12	—	—	11	9	12	—	—	11	9	12	—	13	10	—
13	—	14	12-13	11	13	10	14	12	10	13	10	14	12	10	13	10	—	11	9
14	11	—	14	12	14	11	—	13	11-12	14	11	—	13	11-12	14	11	14	12	10
15	—	15	15	13	15	—	15	14-15	13	15	—	15	14	13	15	—	—	13-14	11
16	—	16	16	—	16	—	—	16	—	16	—	—	15	—	16	—	—	15	12
17	—	—	17	14	17	—	16	17	14	17	—	16	16	14	17	—	15	16	13
18	—	17	18	15	18	—	17	18	15	18	—	17	17	15	18	—	16	17	14
19	—	—	19-20	16-18	19	—	—	19-20	16-18	19	—	—	18-20	16-18	19	—	17	18-20	15-18

GAMA IQ Score	Descriptive Category	Subtest Scaled Score
130 and above	Very Superior	16–19
120–129	Superior	14–15
110–119	High Average	12–13
90–109	Average	8–11
80–89	Low Average	6–7
70–79	Below Average	4–5
69 and below	Well Below Average	1–3

Figure 3.9. Norm tables printed in the Self-Scoring Record Form (part of the record form was deleted to protect the test's security).

- Finally, the examiner completes the GAMA IQ score graph (see Figure 3.8). This graph will be used to share with Nicolette her test results.
- The examiner might complete the optional subtest score comparison (profile analysis) to determine whether her performance was consistent through all item types or whether she demonstrated any strengths or weaknesses relative to her own overall performance.

Optional Subtest Score Comparisons

To accomplish this analysis, strictly for hypothesis testing purposes only, the examiner performs the following steps.

1. Divides the sum of the subtest scaled scores by 4 to obtain the mean of the subtest scaled scores rounded to one decimal place. Records the result in the appropriate box.
2. Subtracts the mean of the subtest scaled scores from each of the subtest scaled scores to obtain the deviation score for each subtest. Records the results in the appropriate place in the deviation score column.
3. Compares each deviation score with the corresponding value needed for significance. If the deviation score is equal to or greater than the value needed for significance, the examiner circles the Y (yes). Otherwise, the N (no) is circled.

Interpretation

There are several steps in the interpretation of the GAMA. Decisions about a client's overall ability should rely only on the GAMA IQ score. It is the most reliable score and represents the performance on all four subtests. The GAMA IQ score is organized with a mean of 100 and a standard deviation of 15, a common metric for intelligence tests. Further meaning for the

Appendix B—GAMA IQ Score
Conversion Table (from manual)

Sum of Subtest Scaled Scores	GAMA IQ Score	Percentile	90% Confidence Interval	95% Confidence Interval
1	43	0.1%	42–56	40–57
2	45	0.1%	44–58	42–59
3	46	0.1%	44–59	43–60
4	48	0.1%	46–60	45–62
5	49	0.1%	47–61	46–63
6	51	0.1%	49–63	48–65
7	52	0.1%	50–64	48–65
8	54	0.1%	52–66	50–67
9	55	0.1%	53–67	51–68
10	56	0.2%	53–68	52–69
11	58	0.3%	55–69	54–71
12	59	0.3%	56–70	55–72
13	60	0.4%	57–71	56–73
14	61	0.5%	58–72	57–74
15	63	0.7%	60–74	58–75
16	65	1%	62–76	60–77
17	66	1%	62–77	61–78
18	68	2%	64–78	63–80
19	69	2%	65–79	64–81
20	71	3%	67–81	66–82
21	73	4%	69–83	67–84
22	75	5%	70–85	69–86
23	76	5%	71–86	70–87
24	77	6%	72–87	71–88
25	79	8%	74–88	73–90
26	80	9%	75–89	74–91
27	81	10%	76–90	75–91
28	83	13%	78–92	76–93
29	84	14%	79–93	77–94
30	86	18%	80–95	79–96
31	87	19%	81–96	80–97
32	89	23%	83–97	82–99
33	90	25%	84–98	83–100
34	91	27%	85–99	83–100
35	93	32%	87–101	85–102
36	94	34%	88–102	86–103
37	95	37%	88–103	87–104
38	97	42%	90–104	89–106
39	98	45%	91–105	90–107
40	100	50%	93–107	92–109
41	101	53%	94–108	92–109
42	102	55%	95–109	93–110
43	104	61%	97–111	95–112
44	106	66%	98–113	97–114
45	107	68%	99–113	98–115
46	109	73%	101–115	100–117

Figure 3.10. Obtaining the gama Total IG score (portion of the table has been removed for test security purposes).

GAMA IQ score should be obtained through the use of percentile scores, confidence intervals around the obtained score, and descriptive categories for the GAMA IQ score (see Figure 3.9).

Intra-individual comparisons allow the examiner to explore possible strengths or weaknesses for the individual. The four subtests were not designed to represent separate abilities but rather different means of assessing general ability. When this optional intra-individual performance comparison is conducted, it is important to note the levels of performance indicated by the subtest scores that are to discussed as strengths or weaknesses. For example, an Analogies scale score of 12 might be a weakness for an individual with an overall mean of 16. However, it is a relative weakness since the person is still performing in the high average range of ability when compared to others of the same age in the general population. In another scenario, a weakness represented by a scale score of 6 might be both a weakness relative to the individual's overall performance as well as a cognitive weakness when compared to individuals of the same age in the general population. To supplement this subtest analysis, we also calculated the frequency of occurrence of specific intra-individual differences. Therefore, the meaning attached to a particular strength or weakness should be examined in light of the commonality or rarity of the subtest difference in the general population as well as the referral question.

Finally, GAMA IQ scores can be obtained for an individual at two points in time to monitor changes associated with neurological conditions or the course of treatment. Specific tables were developed that allow the examiner to determine whether a change from one administration to the second is reliable. When GAMA is first administered, a range of scores is established that allows the determination of significant improvement or deterioration. For example, in our case study, if Nicolette was undergoing some type of therapy or her overall cognitive ability functioning was being monitored, we could say that a change has occurred in her overall ability if in the second administration her scores were outside the expected range of 98 to 120 at the 90 % confidence level. Depending on the nature of the treatment and the rationale for the administration of the second GAMA, a higher or lower score might take on a different meaning for the client and his or her care provider.

Integrating the GAMA in the Psychological Report

Results from the GAMA can be described in a psychological report within the paragraph that describes the person's overall cognitive ability. If additional tests of nonverbal ability have been included along with the GAMA, the data should be integrated. In our case, Nicolette's performance could be presented as follows.

> Nicolette's general cognitive ability was measured using a nonverbal test that required her to apply her reasoning and problem solving abilities. On this measure she earned a GAMA IQ score of 110, which falls in the high average category of mental ability. There is a 90% chance that her true GAMA IQ score falls between 102 (average) to 116 (superior) range of cognitive ability. Her overall score is ranked at the 75th percentile which indicates that her performance exceeded that of 75% of individuals her age in the general population. Her performance throughout the various tasks administered was consistent. (A concluding sentence in this paragraph should present implications of the obtained scores in view of the referral question and her performance on other instruments (e.g., achievement, career inventory, or other relevant information).

SUMMARY

The GAMA was designed as a self-administered test of general cognitive ability. It has minimal language requirements, which makes it an attractive alternative when an assessment of ability is desired for individuals who might have difficulties with the English language for a variety of reasons. In this chapter we provided information about the test development, reliability and validity studies and illustrated its use with a case study. The findings of all studies conducted support the validity of the GAMA as a measure of general intellectual ability in adults.

REFERENCES

Lidenmann, J. E., & Matarazzo, J. D. (1990). Assessment of adult intelligence. In G. Goldstein & M. Hersen, *Handbook of psychological assessment* (2nd ed., pp. 79–101). New York: Pergamon Press.

Naglieri, J. A., & Bardos, A. N. (1997). *General Ability Measure for Adults (GAMA)*. Minneapolis, MN: National Computer Systems.

Wechsler, D. (1981). *WAIS-R (Wechsler Adult Intelligence Scale-Revised) manual*. San Antonio, TX: The Psychological Corporation.

Wonderlic Personnel Test, Inc. (1992). *Wonderlic Personnel Test and Scholastic Level Exam user's manual*. (1992). Libertyville, IL: Author.

Zachary, R. A. (1991). *Shipley Institute of Living Scale revised manual*. Los Angeles: Western Psychological Services.

APPENDIX
VALIDITY STUDIES OF THE GENERAL ABILITY MEASURE FOR ADULTS

VALIDITY EVIDENCE FOR THE GAMA

- ✦ TEST DEVELOPMENT
- ✦ MEAN RAW SCORE PERFORMANCE
- ✦ RELATIONSHIP TO OTHER TESTS
- ✦ PERFORMANCE OF SPECIAL POPULATIONS
    - ✦ For additional validity studies visit: http://www.edtech.unco.edu/abardos

TEST DEVELOPMENT

- ✦Items were developed and pilot studies were performed, along with external experts reviews.
- ✦Tryout studies determined the final item selection.
- ✦An excellent standardization sample was selected.

MEAN RAW SCORES ACROSS AGE

Age	N	Mean	
18-19	265	37.5	
20-24	271	37.6	
25-34	310	36.2	Age trends were similar to those
35-44	300	33.7	reported with other intelligence
45-54	274	30.1	tests
55-59	153	28.9	
60-64	104	25.1	Kaufman , Reynolds, MckLean
65-69	238	23.8	(1989).
70-74	219	21.6	
75-79	135	19.4	
80 +	91	15.7	

RELATIONSHIP TO OTHER TESTS

- ✦Correlations with other ability tests.
    - ✦WAIS-R and K-BIT
    - ✦WONDERLIC and SHIPLEY
- ✦Correlations with Achievement
    - ✦NELSON- DENNY TOTAL READING TEST .52 (P<.01)

GAMA, WAIS-R & K-BIT

	Total sample			
	Mean	SD	N	Correlations
GAMA IQ	104.5	13.8	194	
WAIS-R PIQ	106.7	15.9	194	.74
WAIS-R VIQ	104.6	13.5	194	.65
WAIS-R FSIQ	105.9	14.9	194	.75
K-BIT Matrices	106.7	10.9	189	.72
K-BIT Vocabulary	104.9	11.5	189	.54
K-BIT IQ	106.4	11.1	189	.70

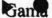

GAMA, WONDERLIC & SHIPLEY

	Mean	SD	Correl.
Wonderlic	103.8	16.3	.70
Shipley Vocabulary	97.2	14.1	.56
Shipley Abstraction	109.1	12.8	.73
Shipley Total	104.4	13.7	.72
GAMA IQ	104.7	15.0	----

Note: Wonderlic scores converted to a mean of 100 and Sd=15.

PERFORMANCE OF SPECIAL POPULATIONS

✦ Learning disabilities
✦ Deaf
✦ Elderly nursing home residents
✦ TBI
✦ Mental retardation

Adults with Learning Disabilities

	r	Clinical (LD) Mean SD	Control Mean SD
GAMA IQ		97.1 19.4	99.5 16.2
WAIS-R VIQ	.52*	96.7 11.6	
WAIS-R PIQ	.66*	99.6 14.5	
WAIS-R FSIQ	.65*	97.6 12.0	

Deaf adults (n=49)

	Clinical Mean SD	Control Mean SD
GAMA IQ	101.5 14.9	103.8 14.9

Elderly nursing home residents (n=43)

	Nursing home Mean SD	Control Mean SD
GAMA IQ	93.6 9.4	100.9 13.4
K-BIT Vocabulary	98.7 10.0	
K-BIT Matrices	96.6 7.3	
K-BIT Composite	97.3 8.3	

Adults with Traumatic Brain Injuries (n=50)

	TBI sample Mean SD	Control group Mean SD
GAMA IQ	83.6 13.4	101.4 15.3
K-BIT Vocabulary	87.1 12.3	
K-BIT Matrices	89.3 16.1	
K-BIT Composite	87.0 13.1	

Adults with mental retardation (n=41)

	Mean SD	r
GAMA IQ	66.2 6.7	
WAIS-R VIQ	64.4 7.1	ns
WAIS-R PIQ	63.1 7.8	.39*
WAIS-R FSIQ	62.1 5.7	.36*

4

Luria-Nebraska
Neuropsychological Battery

Charles J. Golden and Shawna M. Freshwater

INTRODUCTION

The Luria-Nebraska Neuropsychological Battery (LNNB) is a method which integrates the qualitative information generated by the techniques of A. R. Luria with traditional American psychometric procedures. This hybrid approach takes elements from both significant traditions.

Since its official publication in 1978, the LNNB has generated many reactions, both positive and negative. Opponents have criticized the test for evaluating specific functions (such as motor skills) with a variety of types of items rather than the repetition of one procedure or item type many times to insure reliability of the scores. Opponents less psychometrically oriented have criticized the test for being too psychometric and "tainting" qualitative procedures with quantitative scoring and rules.

However, proponents have found the test to offer both a strong psychometric base and an opportunity to make numerous valuable qualitative observations and discriminations of specific problems in clients which cannot be made easily with traditional psychometric instruments. The test battery provides a brief but comprehensive evaluation in less than three hours which makes it very practical with an impaired client.

This chapter begins with a description of the test protocol and organization unique to the LNNB, then describes the test content and scoring procedures, and concludes with clinical interpretive strategies.

TEST CONSTRUCTION AND DEVELOPMENT

Traditionally, the major goal of neuropsychological tests has been classification of individuals as "brain damaged" or "normal." Extensive literature throughout the twentieth century has

Charles J. Golden and Shawna M. Freshwater • Center for Psychological Studies, Nova Southeastern University, Fort Lauderdale, Florida 33314

Understanding Psychological Assessment, edited by Dorfman and Hersen. Kluwer Academic/Plenum Publishers, New York, 2001.

attempted to validate individual tests or batteries of tests for the purpose of this basic identification. While this designation remains a goal of neuropsychological testing, its importance
has diminished with introduction of computerized tomography (CT), magnetic resonance
imaging (MRI), and measures of brain metabolism including regional cerebral blood flow
(rCBF), positron emission tomography (PET), and single photon excitement computed tomography (SPECT). These neuroradiological techniques have increased our ability to diagnose
the presence of brain injury, although certain disorders still manage to evade detection by
these techniques.

As neuroradiological techniques have improved, neuropsychological testing has increasingly focused on the sequelae of brain injuries rather than on the presence of a brain injury.
The goals of that testing can range from localizing an injury to detailed description of the
strengths and weaknesses of the client.

Luria's qualitative procedures were ideally suited for a detailed evaluation of the client's
strengths and weaknesses. However, their application to clients was difficult because the examination lacked consistently employed content, was devoid of a scoring system other than
the examiner's impressions, and lacked a systematic interpretive strategy which could be evaluated for its accuracy and usefulness in different populations. Traditional neuropsychological
techniques, alternatively, were psychometrically sound but lacked the ability to provide the
rich clinical interpretive information which could be gained from Luria's work.

The LNNB provides a framework for Luria's evaluative style by adding an objective scoring system and standard administration procedures. This structuring provides a foundation of
items which can be given to all clients, scored in an objective and reliable manner, and evaluated for systematic effectiveness across different populations. At the same time, Luria's qualitative and flexible administration is retained around this framework, yielding an instrument
which can be studied psychometrically while at the same time used in a purely clinical and
impressionistic manner.

ADMINISTRATION

In order to reach these dual goals, it was necessary to carefully modify administration of
the test so that it was reproducible but also accounted for the client's individuality and allowed the clinician adequate flexibility to investigate qualitative behavior. To achieve this
adaptability, several changes were made in test administration.

First, instructions for items were made flexible so that the clinician could be assured that
the client understood the instructions. In the case of many "standardized" instructions, clients
make errors because they do not understand the task requirements. The LNNB permits para-
phrasing and repeating instructions, answering client questions, and the offering of examples
to insure that the client understands what is required. Simultaneously, client information is
garnered in this communicative process. For example, if the client learns only from examples,
or rapidly forgets instructions and needs frequent repetition, information directly relevant to
the client's condition and learning style is gained. Attention to this communicative process
throughout the test can lead to an accurate diagnosis and description of the client.

Second, "testing of the limit" procedures is encouraged throughout the evaluation. While
such procedures are built into the items themselves, the test's organization allows the clinician
to add these procedures without affecting the validity of the standard scores. An important
aspect of this flexibility is the emphasis on identifying the process underlying client's perfor-

mance. Any item on any test, regardless of its simplicity, can be failed for a variety of reasons. A full understanding of the client's condition can be achieved only by understanding why the client failed.

Further, qualitative observations are encouraged throughout the test. These observations not only focus on the question of "why" an item was failed, but on behavior between items and during the test. For example, a person with attention problems who is otherwise intact may receive normal scores on the test if sufficiently redirected to the questions. The need and nature of such redirection, while not scored in any item, becomes a significant part of the evaluation. In traditional tests, client errors are often misinterpreted in terms of item content rather than the attentional process. Through clinician involvement in the testing process, the LNNB separates the issues of item content from consideration such as the clients' arousal, attention, concentration, emotionality, frustration, motivation, and fatigue.

Finally, the emphasis of the LNNB is obtaining optimal client performance. Many traditional tests encourage suboptimal performance in brain-injured clients through minimal feedback, excessive testing times, misunderstood instructions, and other similar features. Such procedures maximize differences between the brain-injured clients and normals, increasing "hit rates" but decreasing individual differences among brain-injured clients. Indeed, the goal for many tests is to maximize the manifestation of client impairment.

The LNNB emphasizes that only clients with a deficit in an area should fail a specific item by optimizing performance. It is believed that optimal performance tells us more about how the *brain* functions, although the individual may not perform at such levels due to various potential psychiatric and environmental reasons. By understanding which problems arise from brain injury and which from other sources, we again maximize our understanding of the individual. For example, on the motor speed items of any test, clients may become distracted, forget what they are doing, lose interest, or perform at an inappropriate rate, resulting performances below their capabilities. The LNNB accounts for this problem qualitatively and diagnostically. An item is readministered so that the final standard score is not affected by extraneous factor. This method has the effect of making individual items and scales less "sensitive" to brain injury but more specific to the underlying cause of impaired performance.

DESCRIPTION OF THE TEST CONTENT

The LNNB, Form II, consists of 279 items organized into 12 basic scales. Since many of the items have more than one subpart, the actual number of procedures in the test is approximately 1000. The LNNB scales are nontraditional because the same procedure or question is not asked repeatedly at different levels of difficulty. The purpose of the LNNB is not to stratify individuals as "average" or "superior" but rather to address basic functions which underlie all complex behavior. Each scale is organized to test different aspects of behavior within each area evaluated. While the items differ from one another in a variety of ways, they all have a common theme such as "memory functions" or "language functions." Below is a description of the content of each of the 12 scales.

The 51-item *Motor scale* begins with four items measuring the motor speed of the left and right hands. Speed is measured on one simple item (opening and closing a hand) and one complex item (touching each finger in sequence with the thumb). This is followed by four items which examine the role of muscle feedback in performance of simple motor behaviors, and 10 items which examine the ability to perform simple bilateral motor movements by imitation. Two items examine the ability to perform simple items by command. Three items examine bilateral speeded coordination. Perseverative and fine motor skills are examined with an item which requires the copying of a repetitive figure (alternating m's and n's).

The ability to perform complex motor movements by verbal instruction and without "props" is measured by four items such as, "Show me how you would open up a can with a can opener." This evaluation is followed by nine items evaluating the ability to perform simple and speeded oral motor movements, and 13 items looking at the speed and quality of work when making simple drawings by command and by copying. The final four items request contradictory behavior under verbal control, such as, "If I tap once, you tap twice." These latter items examine the ability of the client to inhibit imitation and to control behavior through inner speech, or endophasy.

The 12-item *Rhythm scale* evaluates the ability to hear rhythmic patterns and musical tones, to evaluate these stimuli, and to reproduce them. Items include identifying similarity among patterns or tones and reproducing patterns, tones, and musical sequences.

The 22-item *Tactic scale* uses a series of 11 measures on both the right and left sides of the body each independently. These tasks include indicating where the person is touched, whether a touch is hard or soft, whether a touch is sharp or dull, how many points are touching the person, the direction of movement of a touch, which letters or numbers are written on the wrist, copying gross motor movements by muscle feedback, and identifying simple objects placed in the hand.

The 14-item *Visual scale* examines visual and visual-spatial skills which do not require motor movements. While some of the items involve verbal feedback, clients do not need to name objects accurately but must indicate they recognize the object's purpose or use. The items include simple identification, identification when parts of the item are missing, and identification of overlapping items. Spatial items include completing visual patterns (similar to Raven's Matrices), telling time on an analog clock, identifying directions, imagining items in three dimensions, and rotating items into new configurations.

The 33-item *Receptive Language scale* evaluates comprehension of speech including basic phonemes and complex sentences. Eight items examine phonemic comprehension and six items examine word comprehension, while the remainder evaluate the comprehension of sentences at various levels of complexity.

The 42-item *Expressive Language scale* evaluates speech utilizing simple sounds and complex sentences under a variety of conditions. The first 10 items look at repetition of sounds and words, while the next 11 involve reading similar sounds and words (with the diagnostic emphasis on the fluency of pronunciation rather than accuracy of reading). Three items involve repetition of sentences. Three items examine naming skills, while five items evaluate automatic naming (such as counting or the days of the week). The remainder of the items concern complex and less structured speech, such as responding to a question, describing a picture, speaking about the weather, using specific words in a sentence, and reorganizing words into a sentence.

The 12-item *Writing scale* scores both for motor writing errors (the motor performance of forming letters and words) and spelling. The items range from single letters to sentences. One composition sample is included as well. The scale measures basic writing and spelling skills up to a seventh-grade level.

The 13-item *Reading scale* involves the reading of items ranging from single letters to paragraphs. Two items look at the ability to hear letters and articulate them into sounds and words. Unlike the reading items on the Expressive Language scale, the items are scored for reading accuracy, not expressive fluency. As with the Writing scale, the test measures basic abilities up to a seventh-grade level.

The 22-item *Arithmetic scale* evaluates the reading and writing of numbers as well as simple computational skills. Nine items examine number recognition and writing at various levels of complexity. Two items involve simple number comparison, while nine items look at basic computational skills up through a seventh-grade level. The final two items involve serial sevens and serial thirteens. Items are designed to examine the spatial nature of numbers as well as more basic number recognition.

The 13-item *Memory scale* evaluates verbal and nonverbal immediate memory with and without interference. The scale begins with the learning of a seven-item word list, followed by picture memory with and without delays. Immediate rhythmic and tactile-visual memory are assessed, as is verbal-visual memory. These appraisals are followed by simple list learning with interference and sentence learning with interference. One item involves recall of a paragraph, while the last item examines visually cued verbal memory using a seven-item paired list.

The 34-item *Intelligence scale* yields an estimate of general IQ, employing many types of items traditionally used in intelligence evaluations. Four items involve picture interpretations, while an additional two involve picture sequencing. Verbal items include interpretations of stories and proverbs, vocabulary, similarity items, difference items, the ability to generalize from the specific to the general, the ability to specify from the general to the specific, and categorization skills. The final 12 items involve simple mathematical word problems.

The *Delayed Memory scale* tests delayed memory of items (initially required to be memorized in the Memory scale section) as well as recognition and retention of material in the remainder of the test. This procedure usually involves delays ranging from 30 minutes to 2 hours. Both verbal and nonverbal items are included.

Scoring Procedures

Scoring of the LNNB occurs on several different levels, including scoring of specific items, scoring of the scales, and qualitative scoring.

Item Scoring

All items on the LNNB are scored as either a 0 (indicating normal performance), 1 (borderline performance), or 2 (impaired performance). For items which are only scorable as right or wrong, a 0 represents right and a 2 represents wrong. For those items (such as motor speed items) which involve counting of responses, the raw score is translated into a 0, 1, 2 score using norms given on the test form. Use of this common scoring procedure allows for statistical and clinical inter-item comparisons.

Scale Scoring

Each scale is scored by adding up the 0, 1, and 2 scores from each of the items. A total raw score is generated which is converted into a T-score using the table in the test form. The T-scores have a mean of 50 and a standard deviation of 10. Higher scores reflect poorer performance. These scores are classified as normal or impaired by reference to a cutoff score which is individually determined by the client's age and education using a table in the test form.

Scores above the cutoff are considered impaired. The average cutoff is 60, but may vary from 50 to over 70 depending on the client.

In addition to these basic scales, the LNNB items may be rearranged into scales for specific purposes. Three of these scales are used frequently. The Left Hemisphere scale consists of all items related to the right side of the body, while the Right Hemisphere scale consists of all items related to the left side of the body. The Pathognomonic scale consists of a series of items which are sensitive to the severity and acuity of the cognitive dysfunction.

Additional scales also include the factor scales, which represent factors extracted from individual scales as well as the overall test. All of these additional scales are scored in the same way as the original scales, adding up the scale scores on each item. These scales represent such subfactors as motor speed, drawing, basic language, spatial skills, repetition, verbal memory, verbal arithmetic, general intelligence, simple tactile, complex tactile, naming, verbal-spatial skills, phonemic skills, complex expressive language, basic reading, and so on. Other scales have been developed for specific uses. There is no limit to the range and type of scales which can be developed from the basic data.

Qualitative Scoring

In addition to the item and scale scoring, the LNNB includes 60 qualitative scoring categories which can be scored at any time during the test including in between items. It is not within the scope of this chapter to review all of these indices, but a sample can be discussed to show their usefulness. In general, qualitative indices represent recording of observations by the tester during the scope of the examination. These reports generally fall into the categories of: (a) problems related to inadequate client comprehension of procedures, (b) observations which tell why the client fails an item, (c) unusual behaviors between items which impact the testing, and (d) problems displayed during an item performance but not related to the objective scoring of the test.

Problematic client comprehension generally involves confusion, insufficient vocabulary, attention deficits, arousal problems, fatigue, and motivation. Observations made during the item which clarify errors differ depending on the scale but will include paralysis, motor slowness, motor awkwardness, hearing difficulties, attentional problems, tactile sensation loss, visual difficulties, visual agnosia, inability to comprehend speech, naming problems, slowness in comprehension, inability to attend to the left side of stimuli, dysarthria, slowness of speech, word substitutions in speech, sound substitutions in speech, syllable substitution in words, inability to progress from one sound to another, perseveration, concreteness, dyslexia, failure to recognize letters, failure to recognize sounds, failure to recognize number, visual-motor problems, memory problems, fatigue, and so on.

Unusual behaviors may include distractibility, the inability to recall the instructions, the examination's purpose, or even the examiner, inappropriate emotional reactions, excessive fatigue, hyperactivity, lack of cooperation, poor arousal, seizures, and other related problems. The final category can include any problems seen when the person responds correctly but still shows a problem. For example, an individual may correctly describe an object but fail to name it correctly, thus demonstrating dysnomia. An individual may be literate, but only in a dysfluent manner, suggesting expressive speech problems such as dysarthria.

The qualitative indices are not limited to those discussed here and in the test manual, but rather reflect any behaviors which help further understand the client. Any observations of behaviors which do not make sense or seem normal should be recorded even if the examiner does not know what they mean or their etiology.

Clinical Interpretive Strategies

With the LNNB, there are many levels of client classification ranging from normal/abnormal to sophisticated analysis of the precise deficits and precise neurological causes of a given deficit. The first and most basic classification concerns quantifying profiles as normal or abnormal. The second classification involves a more detailed pattern analysis using the quantitative scores. The third classification involves a detailed item analysis yielding a description of what the client can and cannot do without any inferences about neurological causes. The fourth classification involves an analysis of the qualitative data and its integration with the quantitative data. The fifth classification brings the client's history into the analysis. The final classification involves the integration of psychometric, qualitative, historical, and medical findings to form a definitive picture of the client's problems, their causes, their interaction with the environment, the role of the client's personal and medical history, and the implications of this data for rehabilitation and prognosis in general.

Identifying Brain Damage

The LNNB provides several independent methods to identify the possible presence of a brain injury. The first involves a comparison of the 12 basic skills along with the pathognomonic scale to the critical level (CL) discussed in the scoring section. More than three scores above the CL is indicative of brain injury. The probability of this occurrence in a normal individual is less than 1 in 100. If none or one scale is elevated, the profile is considered to be normal. If two scales are elevated (which is likely to happen in 1 of 25 normals), the profile is a borderline case.

Since the CL is dependent on age and education, the accuracy of this rule depends on the accuracy of the information. While age is rarely misstated in a significant fashion, education can be much more difficult to quantify. For example, the CL will overestimate the premorbid abilities of a client who has simply attended school for 12 years but was impaired due to retardation or brain injury. In such a case, the choice of a specific level of education for the formula often depends on the question being asked. If we simply wish to know how the person is performing in relation to other people with 12 years of education, then using 12 is appropriate. If we wish to ask if the person had a recent brain injury (since the end of school), then using the client's actual achievement level may be more appropriate. In addition, the test manual includes a formula for calculating the critical level from premorbid IQ levels.

A second method for the identification of brain injury is to consider the difference between the lowest and highest T-score. Normal individuals typically show less than a 20-point spread between the lowest and highest scores, with a few normals showing up to a 25-point difference (with the highest scores often being on Arithmetic or Writing (because of spelling) in such cases. Brain-injured clients typically show greater variability. Using this information, score differences exceeding 30 points are considered clearly indicative of brain dysfunction. Score differences of 21 to 30 are considered borderline, while ranges 20 and under are considered normal. It should be emphasized that the absence of a wide range does not itself make a profile normal.

Pattern Analysis Using the Quantitative Scores

The basic quantitative scales of the LNNB yield profiles much like the Minnesota Multiphasic Personality Inventory (MMPI) and other similar tests. These profiles suggest which scales represent the highest elevations and are most likely to show the general areas where the client has the most difficulty. Two-point codes (the highest two scales) and three-point codes (the highest three scales) can be determined to generate statistical descriptions of the client's most likely problems. This information can be generated without reference to the full complexity of the profile, often yielding a valuable starting point for profile classification.

Most work has been done on the interpretation of the two-point profiles with some work on three-point profiles. Before interpretation, a distinct profile classification must be determined. A clear-cut, two-point profile is one in which both of the two highest scales are at least ten points higher than the third highest scale among the 12 basic scales plus the Pathognomonic, Right Hemisphere, and Left Hemisphere scales or in which the two scales are the only scores elevated over the critical level. A clear-cut, three-point profile is one in which all three of the three highest scales are at least ten points higher than the fourth highest scale or in which the three scales are the only scales higher than the critical level. Four-point and five-point code types may be defined in a similar manner. A scale is generally not included in a high point profile if it does not exceed the critical level. Interpretive suggestions given in research or in the test manual are generally more accurate when the profile is "clear-cut."

While the test manual provides more extensive descriptions of the many possible high point codes, several examples which involve the Motor scale can be given here to clarify the process. A common two-point code is the elevation of the Motor and Tactile scales. This combination is often seen in clients where there is lateralized impairment, often caused by a cerebral vascular accident of some kind. In general, these occurrences are cortical strokes, and the affected side can be reliably determined by the comparison of the Left and Right Hemisphere scales. These strokes are generally accompanied by severe cognitive deficits, the nature of which depends on lateralization of injury. In general, the scales representing those cognitive areas (e.g., Expressive Language) will show secondary elevations.

Two-point elevations on the Motor and Visual scales are most often associated with anterior right hemisphere injuries. The client shows intact basic visual skills, but has trouble with more abstractive and visual reasoning tasks. Motor impairment is generally greatest on the left side of the body. Impairment on the Rhythm scale may be seen as well, producing a Motor-Visual-Rhythm three-point code. When the two-point code is Motor/Rhythm, the lesion is generally more anterior than when the two-point code is Motor/Visual. The Motor/Rhythm combination is generally associated with attentional problems, difficulties in emotional control or emotional recognition, poor insight, poor social skills (especially if the lesion is long-standing), and difficulties in following the relationships between sequences of events. This profile may also be seen in many subcortical injuries, including mild to moderate head injury.

The two-point Motor/Receptive Language combination is rare and occurs most often after injuries to the anterior left hemisphere and the subcortical left hemisphere. Such individuals generally have problems with bilateral coordination and difficulty following complex verbal commands, especially those which require an action that differs from the one the client is viewing, such as, "When I tap once, you tap twice." However, their basic verbal communications and understanding are usually intact.

The Motor/Expressive combination is seen in anterior left hemisphere injuries, usually arising from a relatively serious problem such as a stroke or a fast-growing tumor. Such clients have dysfluent speech.. They may slur their words, speak haltingly, repeat sounds, and substitute sounds which makes their speech unintelligible. In extreme cases they may be mute or unable to communicate verbally at any level, although nonverbal communication, reading and writing, may remain intact. Problems with naming are frequently present and may be consistent with expressive aphasia or Broach's aphasia.

The Motor/Writing two-point code is seen primarily in disorders where the dominant hand is dysfunctional. This result can be seen in lateralized subcortical disorders but can also be a peripheral disorder where the function of the arm is disrupted by spinal cord or nerve injuries or by fractures. When the disorder is in the brain, secondary attentional or arousal problems usually will be noted in the testing process. When the injuries are peripheral, the deficits are generally limited to items which tap motor speed, coordination and as tactile sensitivity. Thus, drawing and writing are often disrupted, along with the speeded items. Secondary elevations may be seen on the Tactile, Right Hemisphere, or Left Hemisphere scales. The Motor-Reading combination is rarely present in a normal person who has had a brain injury, but does occur in people who had a learning disorder (dyslexia) prior to a brain injury. This situation is most often seen in teenagers and young adults who have had a head injury and have a history of school problems. The occasional exception to this tendency is seen in individuals with multiple strokes, who may develop an acquired dyslexia, along with more general motor problems, from a small stroke. This condition is usually a precursor to a more fully developed multi-infarct dementia.

The Motor/Arithmetic two-point code is seen in individuals with primarily subcortical lesions who have motor and attentional problems. It is also seen in many individuals with pre-existing arithmetic disorders, which occur in up to 30% of normal controls on the LNNB. In cases where an arithmetic difficulty is premorbid, it is best to ignore this scale and look for the two-point code with Arithmetic not included. This discrimination usually provides a more accurate picture of the impact of a current lesion, although the premorbid Arithmetic elevation may reflect a learning disability and early brain injury in some cases.

The Motor/Memory combination is nearly always seen in subcortical injuries. This deficit is common after mild to moderate head injuries. These clients have generally mild but pervasive motor problems as well as difficulty retaining information, especially with interference. They perform better with simple memorization tasks. They generally have little insight into their condition or the impact of their memory problems. Emotional lability and irritability are also common. The Motor/Intermediate Memory two-point code has a similar interpretation, but the condition tends to be somewhat milder than when Motor/Memory is the two-point code, although both may have serious consequences for day-to-day functioning.

The Motor/Intelligence two-point code is also rarely seen. As in the case of Motor/Reading, it may represent pre-existing problems or may reflect a multi-infarct or similar process (such as multiple tumors). It is very important with this and similar codes to discriminate what was pre-existing, particularly if the testing is administered to assess the effects of an injury, although this concern is less important when the test is used simply to determine the degree of a client's deficit. If this finding represents a new disorder such as a multi-infarct process, it generally represents a more advanced dementing process than does the Motor/ Reading code. However, these codes are very rare and will likely not be seen by most clinicians.

The Motor scale combinations provide a wide range of possible interpretations. A full consideration of the power of this technique would involve all possible two-point codes, as well as the common three- and four-point codes. A similar process may be used with the major factor scales. The reader is referred to the test manual for a more detailed consideration of these codes.

Item Analysis

The next level of interpretation involves the pattern of errors. Each scale can be divided into groups of items which explore a specific aspect of the overall scale area. Item analysis involves focusing on these specific item groupings to evaluate contributions to the overall scale elevations. Consequently, more specific hypotheses of the underlying deficits are generated. This information can be used to modify the more statistically based interpretations generated from the high point codes and to provide more precise detail of the specific problem.

The item analysis is conducted scale by scale, and begins with the highest (most impaired) T-score. In general, as the scale elevations decrease, the contribution of these scales to the item analysis also decreases. In many cases, the deficits seen on the more normal scales reflect the impact of the client's major deficits. For example, some items on the Intelligence scale may be missed not for a lack of intelligence but for visual or visual-spatial problems. Thus, if the Visual scale is poorly performed and Intelligence is relatively better except in this one area, such deficits are better explained on the basis of the deficits on the Visual scale.

By analyzing the more impaired scale first, we are able to avoid over-diagnosing such secondary problems which may appear to be additional problems. In making an analysis, the attempt is always to identify the fewest number of problems which can account for the full range of the client's errors. Such distillation yields a more parsimonious description of the client and leads to more accurate diagnoses and better-targeted treatment suggestions.

The analysis of any case will differ considerably depending on the exact items missed, but the general analysis follows the item subtypes listed earlier. For example, if the Receptive Language scale is the most impaired, the client's ability to discriminate phonemes is examined in the first section of the test. Half of the items require writing the phoneme, while the other half requires repeating the sound. If the client can do either half, then phonemic hearing is likely intact and the problem is attributed to pronunciation, writing, or sound-letter conversions. If the client is unable to do both types of problems, there may be confusion as to the task or an inability to discriminate phonemes. A finer analysis can be made to see if phonemes can be understood when presented singly, or whether problems show up only when they are presented in groups such as two or three sounds at a time. The ability to understand phonemes only individually or not at all may reflect a very basic phonemic discrimination deficit, whereas an inability to hear groups of phonemes may suggest a milder discrimination problem.

Performance on these items can be compared with the next set of items which require the client to follow simple commands. If the client can complete these items but not the phoneme items, they may be unable to discriminate sounds in isolation but be able to do so in context or with well-learned words. In such cases, there are likely to be problems both with single phonemes as well as unfamiliar words. Such clients may appear to understand more than they in reality do because they follow the simple or common elements of a communication.

However, if the client can manage phonemes but not simple commands, this deficit would suggest an inability to comprehend the meaning of sentences and words. The items may be analyzed to evaluate the complexity level at which the client fails: single concrete words, abstract words, similar-sounding words, simple sentences, or complex sentences. The level the person can achieve is indicative of the degree of impairment, as well as location of the injury. If the client cannot perform any of these items, there may be confusion, dementia, or a severe receptive language deficit (seen most often in infarcts, bleeding, aneurysms, or some forms of open head injury).

The last group are the more complex verbal-visual items. If the client has shown no problems up until this point, errors here often reflect injuries external to the language areas in the right hemisphere or anterior areas of the brain. Such deficits may reflect an inability to understand the relationship or spatial nature of some words or to follow the sequential learning required by such items. Such individuals appear to have intact receptive speech, but they develop misunderstandings when sentences are complex and require retention and analysis.

This limitation may be due to memory or to a direct verbal-spatial problem. Errors in these items that occur after failure to process simple commands, however, are likely due to an inability to follow speech. In cases where phonemes are impaired and simple items are intact but these verbal-spatial items are impaired, a language problem may exist which is not well-practiced or automatic which occurs in some left hemisphere injuries.

By combining this analysis with a similar analysis on each of the other scales along with the scale patterns, a reasonably detailed description of the client's problem areas can be developed and etiologic hypotheses may be formed. The accuracy of the analysis depends heavily on attentiveness to precise item patterns and recognition of differential emphasis of each item.

Qualitative Data

At this point, addition of the qualitative data enables the examiner to focus on the etiology of the client's deficits. These is more descriptive and rely heavily on the observations of the examiner. Familiarity with the range of client behavior permits more insights relevant to the neuropsychological diagnosis. The development of observational skills requires experience and appropriate supervisory instruction to avoid missing subtle aspects of behavior. The LNNB, through its qualitative scales, expedites this process by alerting the user to the general categories and specific types of qualitative information which have been useful in understanding neuropsychological deficits. However, observations should not be limited to these categories because more information may explain the client's behavior and enlighten the examiner.

Interpretation of the qualitative information can occur at two levels. The first is purely descriptive. Statements such as, "The client needed frequent redirection to attend to each item," or "Motor behavior was marked by severe tremors which occurred only when the client's hands were at rest," help clarify a client's performance. The rule of thumb should be that any deviant or unusual behavior or activity which necessitated a change in the testing procedures is not accounted for by the scoring system should be recorded and presented.

The second level is more complex and requires a working knowledge of how different brain injuries affect behavior. The goal at this level requires recognition of the neurological and neuropsychological implications of the observed behavior. To reach this level successfully, the user needs a wide range of knowledge in the areas of neurophysiology, neuroanatomy, neuropathology, and recognized neuropsychological "syndromes." This experience cannot be gained simply through administration of the test, but rather through study within these distinct areas. Such preparation is the essence of Luria's original evaluation approach. The second level is arguably the most difficult to master.

History

Although neuropsychology at one time emphasized "blind analysis," which transpired in the absence of any client information except age, education, gender, handedness and test scores, client history is now well recognized as an integral part of any neuropsychological evaluation or testing. Thus, in addition to generating the data, we must also become familiar with the client and the client's past. Background information that helps characterize the symptoms includes rate of onset, age of onset, duration, complicating factors, impact of deficits, and potential etiologies. In addition, issues such as nonneurological psychiatric problems which could alter the test results must also be examined. However, the patient history is not to be accepted without scrutiny. For example, prior head injury does not necessarily explain the patient's current complaint or neuropsychological status. There must be integration with test data to demonstrate that the history itself is reliable and related to the test results. In cases where forensic issues are involved, multiple methods of ascertaining the accuracy of history are advocated when possible.

Integration of Psychometric, Qualitative, Historical, and Medical Findings

The final and most complex step is the integration of these different sources of data. In some cases, this may be relatively simple if the lesion is localized, the data consistent, the history simple, and the quantitative and qualitative data concur. In many other cases, however, clients profiles will be inconsistent due to varying levels of motivation and arousal, the impact of their injuries, secondary emotional issues, pre-existing problems, ethnic and cultural variations, variable learning and educational experiences, and different premorbid strengths and weaknesses. Although in research reports the differences among lesions may appear to be straightforward, such reports often eliminate subjects with many of the complicating problems that are faced in real practice.

As a result, this final process is highly dependent upon knowledge, experience, and a rigorous examination of all of the data for patterns and inconsistencies which focuses on the client as an individual rather than as a diagnosis (such as "left hemisphere injury"). This is primarily a clinical process for which there are no consistent or unambiguous rules, but which represents the apex of neuropsychological training. Ultimately this analysis/assessment reflects the capability of the clinician.

CASE EXAMPLE

This diagnostic process is best illustrated by a detailed case example. The client, Mr. E.F., who was injured in an automobile accident three years ago, is a 42 year-old-man with 12 years of formal education. Hit while walking by a drunk driver who went through a red light, the client was initially unconscious and was taken to a local hospital. An MRI revealed hemorrhage in the right parietal area of the brain and clinical evidence of severe concussion. A small hematoma was detected over the left frontal-parietal area. This was initially treated conservatively but the hematoma continued to expand. Several hours later burr holes were drilled to drain the hematoma.

The client was unresponsive for approximately 48 hours. Subsequently, he reacted only to loud sounds and to his name. He did not respond with any language until four days after the accident when he requested water. One week after the injury, he was able to reliably recognize his family and staff members, but he tended to confuse people with similar features and was unsure of names. This was followed by brief periods of agitation but eventually progressed to self care tasks.

The client showed bilateral weaknesses, which were worse on the left side. As time progressed, his hand strength improved bilaterally but was clumsy and awkward with his left hand. He had some difficulty dressing initially, but this dissipated within a week. He was discharged from the hospital and rehabilitation five weeks after his injury. The current testing occurred approximately seven months post-injury as part of an evaluation related to settlement of an insurance claim. The client is a salesman and has reported more problems achieving his sales goals since his return to work four months before the evaluation.

Presence of Brain Damage

The client's scores on the basic scales of the LNNB are listed in Table 4.1. The client's critical level is 60, so nearly all the scales of the test are elevated and the profile can be considered abnormal. In addition, the range of scores from high to low is 37 points, also well into the brain-damaged range.

Scale Pattern

The highest scores are Visual (87) and Tactile (80), although this is not a clear-cut code. There is a clear-cut three-point high code of Visual, Tactile, and Rhythm (78). This three-point code is almost exclusively associated with right hemisphere injuries, usually in the posterior areas of the hemisphere. Such clients typically have substantial difficulty with spatial relationships, nonverbal communication, complex pictures, overlapping pictures, left-sided tactile sensation, left-sided motor awkwardness and slowness, bilateral coordination problems, and visual memory. In more severe cases, there may be neglect of the left side of objects and written material, along with difficulty drawing complex figures and many simple figures. Drawing ability, even when intact, may be slow. In some cases, there is difficulty with some everyday tasks like dressing. Tasks which require sequences of behaviors may be confused, as may verbal tasks which involve spatial or logical relationships. Some mathematical processes which involve sequencing doing mental arithmetic and processes such as "borrowing" may also be impaired. Emotional lability is common, as are problems understanding one's own emotions and those of others.

Item Pattern

The items within the highest scales are evaluated first. On the Visual scale, the client was able to identify real objects and simple representations of real objects (line drawings). However, when an object was obscured (as in a blurry photograph) or part of it missing, he was unable

Table 3.1. Scores on the Basic Scales of the LNNB for EF

Scale	T-Score
Motor	65
Rhythm	78
Tactile	80
Visual	87
Receptive Language	64
Expressive Language	58
Writing	61
Reading	64
Arithmetic	72
Memory	66
Intelligence	54
Delayed Memory	69
Pathognomonic	61
Left Hemisphere	50
Right Hemisphere	66

to recognize the object. When item drawings overlapped one another, he was unable to separate most of the objects out of the picture. Items requiring the completion of spatial patterns were poorly performed although he was able to complete one item where logical verbal analysis could be substituted for spatial analysis. He was unable to tell time on analog clocks or to draw the hands of the clock at a specific time. He was unable to visualize objects in three dimensions or to rotate objects in two dimensions in his head.

On the Tactile scale, he could perceive basic touch on both sides of the body. On the left side, however, he had difficulty identifying where he was touched, how hard he was touched, sharpness, or direction. On these items, he performed well above chance but poorly compared to normal controls. He had bilateral difficulty with identifying objects drawn on his wrist, but could recognize letters and numbers drawn in the same manner on his right side but not his left side. He was very slow to recognize objects by touch alone with the left hand compared to normal performance with the right hand.

On the Rhythm scale, he could discriminate basic sounds but had difficulty distinguishing patterns. Thus, if he were presented with two rhythmic patterns, he would have difficulty identifying and comparing them. This was evident both when he had to judge patterns similarity or whether he needed to reproduce the patterns. He was able to sing and recognize whether tones were high or low pitched. He was also able to count the number of beats or tones in a pattern without difficulty.

On the Arithmetic scale, he was able to recognize Arabic and Roman numerals. He could write and read numbers without failure. He was able to complete simple computations, but could not do computations in his head which required borrowing or carrying. He was unable to do serial sevens and serial thirteens. He was able to compare numbers without difficulty and understood how numerals in different places within the number had different values.

On Delayed Memory, he showed much stronger performance on the verbal as compared to the visual items. While he could remember words memorized during the test and describe procedures, he had difficulty remembering what pictures he had seen throughout the test and had difficulty remembering how words and pictures had been associated on the Memory scale. Verbal memory, with and without interference, was intact. The pattern of errors on the Memory scale was very similar, with visual items performed more poorly than verbal items.

On the Motor scale, his speeded movements with his left hand were somewhat slow, although right-hand items were performed at a normal speed. Bilateral coordination was clearly impaired and slow. He had several errors imitating hand positions by sight alone. He would make spatial distortions and mirror image the examiner by using his left hand instead of his right and vice versa. His drawings of simple figures (such as a square or circle) were intact but they were drawn slowly. However, his Greek cross was drawn very poorly and he was very slow drawing alternating m's and n's. He was able to perform motor movements on command, show how to carry out actions, and follow conflicting verbal commands without error. Oral-motor items were intact as well.

On Receptive Language, he was able to understand phonemes and simple statements and commands without error. However, he had difficulty with items involving spatial relationships ("Draw a circle to the right of a cross.") and verbal relationships ("Mary is taller than Beth, and Amy is shorter than Beth, who is the tallest?"). There were no problems of routine communication for the client.

On Reading scale, the client had difficulty reading complex words, but basic reading was intact as were letter-sound combinations. Writing was also generally intact except for a slightly higher than normal level of spelling errors. Expressive Language was performed well, except he had difficulty with the days of the week backwards, picture interpretation, and sequencing correctly mixed-up words.

Qualitative Observations

While the statements above could be generated from simply looking at the client's scores, the qualitative observations permit analysis of individual and comprehensive scale performance. Throughout administration, the client maintained adequate arousal and concentration and was not fatigued by the process. He did not become frustrated by failure. He appeared unaware of poor performance. There was no evidence of the neglect of the left side of words, sentences, or visual stimuli..

Any items which required visual-spatial transformations or analysis without external aids were performed very poorly. His basic drawings were adequate, but complex drawings were severely spatially distorted. Use of the left side of his body showed rigidity and awkwardness. He could perform speeded tasks while watching his hands and fingers, but "testing the limits" found that he slowed considerably when he was asked to do such tasks with his closed eyes. He showed great confusion when he needed to use any kinesthetic or proprioceptive feedback from the left side. While bilateral coordination was slowed, this was due entirely to interference from the left hand.

His difficulties with language occurred when visual interpretation, visual-spatial concepts, or relationship concepts were required. When describing pictures which were not overlapping or obscured, he could focus on concrete details but failed to observe the interrelationships of the pieces. This was evident across several scales including Receptive Language, Expressive Language, and Intelligence. Verbal processes were preserved. Arithmetic problems involved carrying and borrowing, especially when he had to do them in his head. Problems on Writing were greater than expected given his age and education, and consisted of difficulty with more complex words. His reading and spelling levels appeared to be below sixth grade but he did understand basic phonemic relationships to letters. He was able to integrate sounds to produce approximations of words and was able to spell phonetically, although not necessarily correctly. His expressive speech was fluent.

While he did not show any difficulty accepting failure (primarily because he seemed not to notice it), he did show some emotional reactivity when he desired a rest or the testing was accidentally interrupted. He regained composure easily, but his initial reactions were greater than expected.

History

The client's referring history has already been detailed, but in the course of the evaluation several salient additional points were uncovered. While the client graduated from high school, he did poorly in school, barely graduating with a low "C" average. He was never interested in school and made little effort. He worked from an early age, even while attending school, and he stated that work was always his focus. He was not in special education at any level. He had not taken any standard IQ tests as a child or adult. He remembered his scores on standardized school tests as "low" but could offer no more specific information.

There was no history of head injuries or any other neurological disorder. To the client's knowledge, he achieved normal developmental milestones and had no illnesses beyond the normal childhood maladies. He was never hospitalized, but was once seen in an emergency room for an uncomplicated fractured upper arm resulting from a "jungle gym" fall as a child. He did not hit his head in that accident and had not been unconscious. He consumed beer occasionally but denied heavy drinking or ever having passed out from drinking, although there were episodes when he got sick, especially as a teenager. He denied current use of drugs, but admitted to experimenting on a small scale as an adolescent. He denied drug abuse and stated he had never been treated for any alcohol or drug problems.

Integration

This is a reasonably consistent case which appears to follow a rational pattern. The worst of his injuries, per his medical records, was in the right posterior area. This is consistent with his visual-spatial problems and left-side tactile/kinesthetic/proprioceptive problems. The absence of any left sided motor problems that cannot be attributed to his sensory problems tell us that the lesion is relatively posterior and spares the more anterior motor areas of the brain. The absence of any visual field loss and the absence of left-sided neglect suggest that the lesion is circumscribed and so does not extend over wide areas of the brain. The occipital areas appear intact.

His poor verbal performance on some of the scales raises the question of the role of his left hemisphere hematoma. Most of his verbal problems, however, can easily be attributed to the spatial problems in the right hemisphere. Dysfluency was not evident. Verbal intellectual processes are intact. Several lines of evidence suggest that his reading and writing problems may have pre-existed. First, we have his own reports of performing poorly in school. Second, the data itself suggests that the brain-based basic processes required for achievement, such as phonemic discrimination, letter-sound matching, decoding, phonemic integration, and the like are all intact. His inability to do higher level words appears to be related more to a lack of schooling and practice than to a deficit in any underlying neuropsychological skill. Finally, there are no qualitative findings which we would expect with a left hemisphere injury.

All of these lines of evidence suggest that the impact of the hematoma was minimal and is currently so minor as to not be identifiable. This is consistent with the type of hematoma he had sustained, since it was treated properly and there was no bleeding or significant bruising in the same area.

His memory problems are restricted to nonverbal material, another indicator of a relatively focal right hemisphere injury. He clearly had difficulty with both immediate and delayed memory. Typically, victims of head injury on the LNNB show much worse delayed as opposed to immediate memory problems. The exception occurs in cases similar to this where there is actual destruction of brain tissue in a focal area, which may produce the current pattern rather than the more diffuse pattern seen in many head injuries.

There was no qualitative or quantitative evidence from the test of frontal problems. His logical processes and problem solving abilities were intact, as were his attention, concentration, and behavioral control. Perseveration and inflexibility were not present. Although there was some unawareness of his deficits, such unawareness is often seen in right parietal injuries. Some believe that such deficits imply a frontal disorder, but the author has seen this in cases with clear focal injuries of this type. There were no right-sided motor problems or evidence of any dysfluency or other Expressive Language problem.

Overall, the client clearly suffered a substantial brain injury whose residual impact is seen in the posterior right hemisphere. He has retained many intact skills, especially in verbal areas, but shows deficits in visual memory, visual-spatial skills, left side somatosensory (tactile) functions, and nonverbal problem solving. The client shows mild emotional lability which he generally controlled. These deficits are serious enough to affect many major functions, including driving. While driving itself may be overlearned and his dominant motor skills are normal, his ability to judge relative speeds and traffic patterns may be impaired. In heavy traffic or complex driving situations, he is likely to have a much higher chance of making errors.

His salesmanship skills would also be affected. While his verbal skills are well preserved, his memory for faces and other nonverbal stimuli is impaired. As a result, he may not be able to relate to customers as well which may interfere with his performance. He also may have difficulty understanding nonverbal communications from customers, a skill integral to salesmanship. These deficits would be consistent with the drop-off in his performance since the accident. While he can continue to work, his job requirements need to be reviewed or the expectations for his achievement lowered.

The evaluation does not reveal anything that should interfere with basic living skills, but such clients will have other social difficulties. For example, they also can be very irritating to others because of their lack of awareness of their impact on others. It is important for those close to this client to receive some feedback and perhaps some therapy so they can understand why this happens and the appropriate responses for them to make. Without such intervention, the likelihood of social disruption or marital problems increases significantly.

SUMMARY

This chapter has presented the basic clinical approach to the LNNB. The LNNB was designed to be used at several levels of expertise ranging from beginner to advanced user. The extent of the various interpretive approaches and the ultimate value of the information produced by the test is dependent on the skills and knowledge of the examiner and on the quantitative and qualitative indices from the test. It is extremely important to integrate the various types of information generated by the test to derive the most useful and specific information, but the novice user can start at more elementary levels of interpretation and develop skills to progress to advanced levels.

SUGGESTED READINGS

Code, C. (Ed.) (1996). *Classic cases in neuropsychology*. Mahwah, NJ: Lawrence Erlbaum.

Goldberg, E. (1990). *Contemporary neuropsychology and the legacy of Luria*. Hillsdale, NJ: L. Erlbaum Associates.

Golden, C. J., Hammeke, T. A., Purisch, A. D., Berg, R. A., Moses, J. A., Jr., Newlin, D. B., Wilkening, G. N., & Puente, A. E. (1982). *Item interpretation of the Luria-Nebraska Neuropsychological Battery*. Lincoln, Nebraska: University of Nebraska Press.

Golden, C. J., Purishch, A. D., & Hammeke, T. (1985). *Manual for the Luria-Nebraska Neuropsychological Battery*. Los Angeles: Western Psychological Services.

Golden, C. J., Zillmer, E., & Spiers, M. (1992). *Neuropsychological assessment and intervention*. Springfield, Illinois: Charles C. Thomas.

Incagnoli, T., Goldstein, G., & Golden, C. J. (Eds.) (1986). *Clinical application of neuropsychological test batteries*. New York: Plenum Press.

Luria, A. R. (1973). *The working brain*. New York: Basic Books.

Luria, A. R. (1980). *Higher cognitive functions in man*. New York: Plenum.

5

Rorschach Inkblot Technique

Barry A. Schneider

[handwritten: NOT UP TO DATE (Old Exner)]

[handwritten: missing scores]

INTRODUCTION

"What might this be?" With these few words a person is introduced to one of the most fascinating techniques in all of psychological assessment, the Rorschach. Developed by a Swiss psychiatrist, Hermann Rorschach (1884–1922), the test consists of ten abstract inkblots that are shown one at a time to the subject, who reports what is seen. The task may seem rather innocuous, but in the hands of a trained clinician, it can yield a veritable gold mine of information about personality style and structure, quality of thinking and affect, diagnostic issues, and can also facilitate in treatment planning and evaluation. In brief, what at first blush may seem to be a parlor game that hinges on imagination is actually a very sophisticated and complex way to examine the psychological world of patients and others deemed appropriate for evaluation.

TEST CONSTRUCTION AND DEVELOPMENT

Hermann Rorschach was not the first to explore the mind by resorting to associations to ambiguous stimuli. In 1857, well before Rorschach's work was published, Justinus Kerner authored a book titled *Kleksographien*. Written in German, Kerner's book presented a series of inkblots and a collection of poems inspired by associations to them. Kerner's work showed that inkblots were able to make rather unique impressions upon viewers. It should be noted, however, that Kerner did not appreciate that differing perceptions of people had implications for personality assessment. The critical relationship between perception and personality style was to be Rorschach's contribution. Nevertheless, because Kerner's book was popular, it is thought that it was known to Rorschach and was probably influential in his own work with inkblots.

Barry A. Schneider • Center for Psychological Studies, Nova Southeastern University, Fort Lauderdale, Florida 33314

Understanding Psychological Assessment, edited by Dorfman and Hersen. Kluwer Academic/Plenum Publishers, New York, 2001.

Also predating Rorschach's publication, Alfred Binet (1857–1911), perhaps the most noted French psychologist, used inkblots to facilitate diagnosis. Although, he was best known for the development of intelligence testing, Binet's work with blots influenced others in their exploration of the use of these ambiguous stimuli to aid in personality description and diagnosis. Most of the focus of these early investigators was directed to the content of the blots. That is, the inkblots were used to collect the subject's associations. One can readily discern the influence of psychoanalytic thinking on these endeavors. Additionally, some effort was made to examine some of the more cognitive aspects of personality style, such as those reflected in the perceiver's approach to the task. While there is relevance of these works to Rorschach's ultimate contribution, it is not at all clear whether any of these early explorations were known to him. Indeed, it has been suggested by some historians that Rorschach probably was not familiar with these studies.

Rorschach's own work may have been influenced by his father. It is known that the elder Rorschach was an artist and that young Hermann was also very interested in art. It has been reported that he enjoyed making ink sketches. Indeed, according to some historians, his interest in art was so strong that he struggled to decide whether to pursue art as a career or to study the natural sciences. Moreover, it is rather interesting to note that, when young Hermann was in high school, he was nicknamed "Kleck," which means inkblot. While perhaps only coincidental, this rather fortuitous experience may have in some way influenced his later research. Rorschach eventually chose science over art as a career. He received his medical education in Swiss and German medical schools. He finished his studies in Zurich where he did a dissertation under the supervision of Eugen Bleuler. It was while he was training in psychiatry that he first attempted to understand how people respond to inkblots. In collaboration with Konrad Gehring, a friend who was also an art teacher, he tried to determine whether gifted students engaged in more fantasy associations than did average students. Although this study was never published, its relevance to his later work seems apparent.

One might also speculate that Rorschach's time with Bleuler and later with Carl Jung, who was at that time Bleuler's assistant, helped young Hermann develop some appreciation for the Freudian concept of the unconscious. Indeed, Bleuler's descriptions of the psychotic, unlike the earlier French matter-of-fact protocols (not too unlike today's symptom-description checklists), operated in the sphere of the unconscious and the motivational. Also, it is known that Bleuler encouraged Jung in his word association investigations, and steered his associate in the direction of Freud. Thus, these important relationships involving both Bleuler and Jung appear to have influenced Rorschach by having introduced him to psychoanalysis. Even though he did not receive formal psychoanalytic training, his deep interest in this model of the mind is clearly reflected by his having been elected vice president of the Swiss Psychoanalytic Society.

Rorschach was intrigued by the idea that reactions to inkblots could reveal a great deal about personality structure. This fascination led to some fourteen years of intensive research developing an inkblot test. Ultimately, he presented inkblots to 405 subjects, 288 patients and 117 nonpatients. Their responses, as well as his efforts to distinguish among various patient and nonpatient groups through a scoring system, culminated in the now famous 1921 publication *Psychodiagnostik*. Interestingly, although he experimented with thousands of different blots, he settled on 15 for the monograph. However, since the cost of reproduction was high, the publisher suggested he select only 10. Those 10 blots are the same designs that are used today, more than 75 years after their initial printing. Unfortunately, Rorschach did not live to see the fruits of his labors. In February, 1922, eight months after the publication of his work, he died from complications following appendicitis. He was 37 years old.

The value of a psychological test ultimately rests upon three critical features: (a) standardization of administration, (b) reliability of measures, and (c) validity of interpretations. If a test is going to provide meaningful data, it should have clear instructions that ensure subjects will be tested in the same manner. Obviously, differences in how a test is administered can seriously alter the responses. Likewise, scoring must be designed so that trained raters will score responses in a similar way. Otherwise, one would not expect to get similar findings. A test is considered to be "good" if it yields consistent results from one administration to the next. For example, one would expect a 12-inch ruler to accurately measure 12 inches every time it was used. If, however, the ruler was somehow damaged so that it no longer was 12 inches in length, then it would no longer be a reliable tool to measure 12 inches. A "good" test is also one that measures what it purports to measure. If students enroll in a course in statistics, they would not expect to be confronted by exam questions about the American Civil War. Such an exam would not be valid for statistics.

A test that is standardized, reliable, and valid allows the examiner to feel rather confident that the resulting data are good indices of the variable(s) being measured (provided the examinee responded honestly to the test). Moreover, such a test can be re-administered at other times for comparisons. For example, will Mr. Jones, whose current responses yield scores consistent with persons who are both depressed and potentially suicidal, show any changes in his responses after treatment? Such a test can also allow for comparisons both among and within groups where appropriate data have been accumulated (e.g., comparison with others of similar diagnosis; comparisons with nonpatient groups). Despite much criticism regarding its value as a "real" test, the Rorschach does in fact meet criteria common to other popular assessment techniques, particularly with regard to standardization of administration, operational definitions for scoring, and norms for interpretation. For example, reliability research with the Exner Comprehensive System has shown high inter-rater reliability for scoring and correlation coefficients of at least .80 for so-called trait variables and of between .70 and .79 for state variables. Additionally, extensive norms have been collected for different diagnostic groups including outpatients with character disorders, inpatient depressives, inpatient schizophrenics, and nonpatient adults. Exner has also collected normative data for nonpatient children and adolescents, grouped by age from 5 to 16 years. Thus, depending on the characteristics of the particular person to be evaluated, one can compare and interpret scores in line with nonpatient norms with norms from patients with specific psychiatric disorders, or with both. These data clearly reflect that the Rorschach, administered, scored and interpreted via the Exner system meets criteria that psychologists deem necessary and appropriate for a psychological test. Even though the Rorschach inkblot technique does not call for typical objective responses (e.g., true-false; multiple choice), it is very much a real test.

ADMINISTRATION AND SCORING

The Rorschach inkblot technique involves the presentation of the same 10 symmetrical blots originally designed and researched by Hermann Rorschach. Five of the blots are in achromatic shades of grey and black, two blots include the color red in addition to grey and black, and the remaining three blots are composed of various chromatic colors. The blots are shown one at a time in the order of their number (i.e., I–X). In the Exner system, the examiner sits at the side of the subject. The rationale for this arrangement is to minimize possible body language cues by the examiner and also to facilitate seeing the blots as the subject perceives them. (This writer must confess that, at times, he has chosen to sit across from the examinee with a desk between himself and the subject, particularly when testing incarcerated, violent, forensic cases, and with some floridly psychotic inpatients. Years of experience in clinical and forensic settings has underscored the need to exercise caution in these situations or in any others where the examiner is at risk.) The basic task for the examinee is to respond to the question, "What might this be?" The examiner writes down the verbatim responses to each blot. Typically, a record will consist of about 23 responses. This part of the testing is referred to as the "Free Association" phase. (Note the minimal use of instructions or guidance.) After responses to all 10 blots have been collected, the examiner informs the subject that there is another part of the test (the "Inquiry"). The task now is to elicit information as to "where" (location), and "how" (determinants) the various contents expressed in the Free Association phase were perceived. The stated purpose is, "To help me (the examiner) see what you saw." Each response is read back to the subject, who then is asked to articulate where the percept was seen and what about the blot made it look that way. This information enables the examiner to code or score the responses. Then the data can be computer analyzed and/or manually transformed into various frequencies, ratios and indexes (Structural Summary) for interpretation via comparisons with data from patient or nonpatient groups, as well as for more idiographic interpretation based upon other clinical information and theoretical proclivities of the examiner.

Scoring and Interpretive Guidelines

It is interesting to note that a subject asked to recite what is perceived from the blots is really being asked to violate "reality." That is, in order to adhere to the task, the subject must actually misidentify the stimulus. Indeed, the perceptual-conceptual activities demand that subjects try to fit the blot (stimulus) to their internal store of percepts. These cognitive processes are quite sophisticated. At the very least, each response requires the subject to first scan the blot, then encode it, then consider the possible responses that are consistent with the stimulus as processed by that particular person given his or her age, range of experiences, culture, intelligence, etc., then choose to offer each response or not offer it (censorship). Moreover, all of these operations are influenced by the personality traits of the subject, as well as by the environmental situation. Responses may be simple or complex, common or unique. They might include movement, color, shading, and contour, singly or in combination. If a response includes more than one determinant, it is referred to as a blend. Production of multidetermined responses suggests a person who is psychologically complex. A person who constructs many blends, and/or includes many determinants in the responses is probably demonstrating an overactive ideational and emotional style. Some blends appear to reflect presence of conflict or pain (e.g., combining chromatic color and shading).

Description of the Blots and Common (Popular) Responses

While there are many possible responses to the blots, some occur with a high frequency and are therefore referred to as Popular(s). Exner has established the criterion of one occurrence every three protocols (from the records of nonpatient adults, nonschizophrenic outpatients, and inpatients who were neither schizophrenic nor psychotic) to warrant a Popular designation in his system. What follows is a brief description of each of the blots and the popular responses that are associated with them.

Card I is a fairly large black and grey mass with four conspicuous white areas. This structure can be perceptually divided into three parts: a center portion and two sides. Additionally, careful observation reveals small black spots outside the basic large structure. The whole blot is often seen as a winged creature, bat or butterfly.

Card II introduces color (red). Its structure is less massive than Card I. It consists of two large grey-black areas and three red areas (two above and one below). There is also a white area in the center. This blot often calls for percepts of animal forms such as the heads of dogs or bears. Whole animals are also very commonly seen.

Card III is made up of two distinct black-grey areas that are connected to a light grey area. In between the main areas is a distinctly shaped red area. On both sides above the main areas are two more red areas. The black portion of the blot often calls for percepts of human forms. The center red part is often seen as a butterfly or bowtie.

Card IV is rather massive looking in its design. It is black-grey with much shading. It is often seen as a human or humanlike figure, such as a monster, giant, or alien.

Card V is basically black and presents a shape and outline that is easy for subjects to address. Percepts of a bat or butterfly are quite typical.

Card VI is basically grey with much shading variations throughout. The upper part is differentiated from a large shaded portion. Either the whole blot or the main portion without the upper area is often seen as a rug, a hide, or an animal skin.

Card VII is largely light grey with a small darker area in the bottom center. The upper area is often seen as a face or human head. The figure is typically identified as a female, child, or Indian.

Card VIII is the first of three blots that are totally colored. For this blot, the colors are pastel. There are several distinct areas including the top which is blue-grey and green-grey, a blue center area, a pink and orange area at the bottom, and two pink portions on the sides. The latter areas are often perceived as whole animal figures such as bears, dogs, rodents or wolves.

Card IX is comprised of colors that appear to run into one another. The design of this blot is quite different than the others in that it does not present distinct differences in color or shape. The colors and their shading variants make this a rather difficult blot for many subjects, be they patients or nonpatients. There is a bottom pink area. The blot has upper orange areas on each side. These portions are often seen as human or humanlike, with typical designations such as witches, giants, monsters or aliens.

Card X is full of colors with very distinct shapes and areas. Looked at quickly, the array of colors might resemble an artist's palette with its daubs of different colored paints. Two distinct blue areas on the sides are often seen as crabs.

In brief, there are a variety of variables than can contribute to a response. These variables are distinguished by specific codes or scores. Scoring the responses by breaking them down into defined categories allows the examiner to understand what, where and how a response was developed, and thus, how the subject handled the task.

What follows is a brief introduction to some of the basic scoring categories and their interpretive place in the Exner system. The interested reader should consider examining the Exner texts and the workbook for the comprehensive system. Those with a penchant for computer-assisted assessment should also look into the Rorschach interpretation assistance program.

Location (W, D, Dd and S)

Where was the response seen? What part(s) of the blot was included? These questions are answered by carefully noting the exact portions of the blot that constitute the response. There are three main location scores: W for the whole or entire blot; D for a common detail or area; and Dd for an unusual or infrequently cited portion. (The D and Dd locations are based on normative studies.) Sometimes white space (S) is used either by itself, or more typically, in conjunction with the other locations. In any case, S is always scored with one of the three main scores (i.e., WS, DS, DdS). The examiner uses diagrams of the blots to carefully note the area(s) articulated by the subject. The part of the blot attended to can yield clues about cognitive style. For example, does the subject attempt to use the whole blot by integrating disparate parts? Does the subject opt instead for usual locations along with rather typical percepts? Or is this perhaps the kind of person who gets caught up in unusual areas tied to idiosyncratic material? Obviously, there are other possibilities as well. The point to be made is that where a person sees the percepts does reflect aspects of his or her perceptual style, which can also lead to hypotheses about the person's personality. Indeed, complex well-perceived whole responses suggest an integrative capacity and an ability to use abstract thinking. It's sort of like looking at a piece of modern art and being able to pull the various images, colors, and shapes together to yield an appreciation of the artist's message. Contrast this style with one where the subject is only able to note specific images without the ability to integrate them by some superordinate concept or theme. In brief, the capacity to combine areas to develop a complex whole response reflects an investment of energy and a quality of thinking that is distinct from a style that is essentially geared to seeing the obvious and simple (reliance on D and noncomplex W responses). The use of Dd locations suggests an investment in the less obvious, and might also involve an atypical or obsessive style. If a few white space responses are offered, this can suggest independence on the part of the subject. If, however, the frequency of S increases (e.g., 3 or more in a record of about 23 responses), then the subject is likely to be somewhat negativistic or appositional. In some sense it's like the examiner asking what the figure is and being given the ground as the reply. Indeed, as the number of such responses increases beyond 3 in an average protocol, the oppositional style is more likely to be characterological and can signal a tendency for hostility. In a typical record of a nonpatient adult, one should expect to find a balance among the location scores with about 9 W responses (some will be simple, some might be complex), 13 D or usual detail responses, and around 1 or 2 Dd or unusual detail responses. Additionally, one can expect about 1 or 2 white space or S responses. Also, it can be valuable to examine the parts of the blot used, as well as if the subject tends to use the same general parts to each of the cards. For example, does the subject tend to approach each blot in more or less the same systematic way (e.g., W, then D, then Dd), or is the style erratic? This type of assessment is referred to as sequence analysis.

Developmental Quality (DQ)

The interpretive value of location scores is enhanced by a code used to distinguish the quality of the processing involved in developing the responses. As indicated above, not all responses are the same. Some are complex, others are simple. Some are distinct, others are vague. Some responses indicate an effort by the subject to integrate portions of the blot, while others show a lack of such activity. Developmental quality (DQ) provides an operationally defined mechanism to facilitate scoring and interpretation of how responses were formulated. There are four possible scores. The symbol "+" is coded for synthesized responses. These are defined as responses wherein discrete parts of the blot were combined into a single response. That is, two or more objects, etc., are separately described, but are viewed as related to each other. At least one of the percepts must have a specific shape or form associated with it (e.g., bat versus dust). The symbol "v/+" is coded for a somewhat less distinguished synthesized response. This case is similar to the previous one regarding the separate percepts in relation to each other, but here none of the percepts have a specific form demand or shape. The third category is scored "o" for ordinary response. It is defined for cases where a discrete part of the blot is selected as the object. The object has a specific form associated with it, but it is seen alone. Finally, the score "v" is coded for a vague response, or one that is diffuse or reflects only a general impression of an object. In such a case, the object or percept has no specific form or shape.

Determinants

Perhaps the most difficult aspect of scoring involves coding the various determinants. These scores reflect both "how" and "why" a particular response was offered. In essence, these perceptual elements address the question, "What made it look like that?" In the Exner system, there are seven categories of determinants, each addressing some aspect of how the blot was perceived and processed. The categories and their respective codes are as follows:

1. **Form (F):** This determinant is scored for all responses, either as the sole determinant, or in conjunction with others. It reflects the use of shape or contour to delineate the responses. When used alone, it suggests the removal of affect from the situation. Not that no feelings or problems exist, but the subject has more or less been able to suspend the affect or its influence at this time. One would typically expect persons embroiled in emotional problems to produce fewer pure F responses. Such persons are unlikely to be able to compartmentalize their problems. Persons who produce F-only responses tend to be defensive and possibly constricted. However, as noted previously, many pure F responses might very well indicate a person with a capacity to control emotions. In a typical nonpatient adult record, one should expect around 8 pure F responses.

2. **Movement (M. FM, & m):** This category is divided into three subcategories: (a) human movement (M); (b) animal movement (FM); and (c) inanimate movement (m). In addition, all movement scores are further distinguished by a code noting the quality of the movement, either active (a) or passive (p). It is believed that human movement responses reflect a bridge between the inner world of fantasy and the outer world of reality. M responses have been associated with creativity and capacity for reflection. They can also reflect an ability to delay action and emotional response by substituting thinking and fantasy production. That is, people who produce M responses are often able to pause and use thought and their intellect when confronted by stressful situations. Movement is the only determinant not actually present in the stimuli. Whereas form, color, shading, etc., are elements of the various blots, the perception of movement is solely a function of the subject, something he or she adds to the interpretation of the blot. Thus, as part of the rather elaborate cognitive-perceptual processes involved in the perception of the blot leading to the offering of a response, there is, in the case of movement, the imposition of this determinant. The process of viewing humans in some kind of kinesthetic activity is believed to be intellectual in nature. In contrast, seeing animal movement is viewed as more developmentally primitive, involving internal need states, and is associated with impulsive behavior. Inanimate movement responses indicate feelings of situational stress or environmental pressures. These responses are viewed as being beyond the subject's control. In a typical nonpatient adult protocol, one can expect about 4 Ms, 4 FMs, and 1 m.

3. **Chromatic Color (FC, CF, C, & Cn):** This category includes four symbols. The appropriate designation reflects the extent to which form plays a part in the percept. FC (form-

FC

color) indicates form is primary in the percept and color is secondary (e.g., "a red rose...it has sort of the shape of a flower and it's also red"). CF (color-form) is coded when the opposite obtains; color is primary and shape or form is secondary (e.g., "it's red like a rose, and I guess that could sort of be a stem or leaf"). C (pure color) is scored when only color is used to form the response (e.g., "blood!"). Additionally, there is a special color code, Cn (color naming), that is used in the very rare instances where the response is the name of a color. In brief, color responses are believed to reflect aspects of the affective or emotional life of the subject. Furthermore, depending on how form is used (i.e., primarily, secondarily, or not at all), color responses can suggest how the person modulates his or her intellectual or mental controls in relation to emotional experiences. Not surprisingly, developmental studies show more CF and C compared to FC for young children compared to older children or adults. One should expect a typical adult record to have 4 FC responses, 2 CFs and no pure C or Cn responses.

4. Achromatic Color (FC', C'F, & C'): There are three possible scores for responses in which black, grey, or white are involved (e.g., "a black cat"). The specific score depends upon the use of form. The scheme is the same as noted above for chromatic color responses. Interestingly, this category is related to the notion of internalization or constraint of painful feelings. The idea is that use of achromatic color reflects the holding in of affect instead of overtly dealing with the environmental stimuli (the case with chromatic color responses). The capacity to handle these uncomfortable affects is related to the use of form (intellectual control); the less the control (C'F, C'), the more the person is experiencing the painful emotions and is not dealing with them very well. In a typical adult record one can anticipate few such responses. The average for all three achromatic scores is less than 2 with a mode of only 1 such response.

5. Shading (FT, TF, T; FV, VF, V; FY, YF, and Y): This category has three subcategories, each with three possible scores depending the use of form. The subcategories relate to different aspects of shading: (a) texture (T); (b) depth, vista, or dimensionality (V); or (c) diffusion (Y). Interpretatively, T scores reflect a need for emotional contact with others (e.g., "a bearskin rug"). Such scores also appear to reflect a need for acceptance and nurturance. V or vista scores reflect a very painful experience (e.g., "an aerial view of an island"). Such scores suggest looking inside oneself and feeling badly about what is discovered. V reflects a negative introspective self-evaluation. One takes a look inside and finds that he or she is bad or worthless. Feelings of guilt are also associated with vista responses. Diffuse shading or Y scores reflect a sense of helplessness (e.g., "an X-ray of a stomach"). Pure Y may reflect *Y* pressure from anxiety in relation to stressful circumstances. Again, in interpreting any of these shading responses, the role of form must be carefully considered. Thus, when form is primary, it suggests better control of these painful experiences. Shading responses are not readily found in the records of nonpatients. The expected frequencies are 1 texture score and no vista or diffuse shading scores.

6. Form Dimension (FD): This is a single symbol category used for responses where dimensionality or depth is perceived based on the size or contour of objects (e.g., "a tree up on a hill...it looks much smaller, so I guess it's very far in the distance"). (Note that dimensionality based on shading is scored for vista.) FD suggests a self-focus that is not as negative as V. While it also suggests an introspective looking inside oneself, the difference is that here there is less pain and negative assessment. This code appears to reflect a tendency to be self-evaluative, or philosophical about self-exploration. A nonpatient adult record might contain 1 FD response.

7. Pairs (2) and Reflection (Fr and rF): These categories are scored when the symmetry of the blot is noted as part of the response. The pair code is used for responses of two objects that are perceived as identical (e.g., "two bears fighting; there's one on each side"). Reflection scores are reserved for responses where the objects are reported as actual reflections or mirror images (e.g., "a girl looking at herself in a mirror"). The particular reflection code (Fr or rF) depends on the use of form (primary or secondary). In general, pair responses represent a reality-based self-focus. In comparison, reflection responses indicate an intense, egocentric self-focus. In a sense, use of reflection characterizes a person who sees the world revolving around himself or herself. Such a person might not be inclined to modify or correct his or her views based on facts or reality. Such people already have their minds made up and don't wait to confuse the situation with the facts. Whereas a typical adult nonpatient record might contain about 9 pair responses, one should not expect to find any reflection scores.

Form Quality

A most important code is scored for all responses in which form or shape is a determinant (primary or secondary). This score reflects how well the response conforms to the designated area of the blot. Some flexibility in performance is expected. After all, the subject is attempting to locate percepts in an inkblot and is not actually identifying pictures of real objects. Even so people with good reality-ties produce good form quality responses. Indeed, they see things pretty accurately. In contrast, people with serious psychological problems (e.g., schizophrenia) or who are laboring under extreme stress do not maintain the same hold on reality and do not perceive as well.

Form quality scores are intended to address the subject's reality-ties or perceptual accuracy. The Exner system provides a four-point scale to distinguish levels of quality. A score for superior form quality (+) is used when there is an unusually enriching use of form to articulate the response. A score of ordinary (o) is coded for common uses of form that define objects readily seen by others. A score of unusual (u) is used for low frequency responses that do not violate the essential contours of the blot. Finally, a minus (−) code is applied when there is an unrealistic or distorted use of form. In the latter case, it is as if the response or percept had been imposed on the blot without regard to the actual shape of the blot. Adult nonpatients use good form (i.e., scores of + or o) for about 80% of their responses. In sharp contrast, inpatient schizophrenics produce good form response for only 40% of their responses. Likewise, inpatient depressives also show diminished perceptual accuracy compared to nonpatients; they produce only 50% good form quality responses. These data suggest that protocols with many poor form quality responses should alert the clinician to expect poor or weakened reality-ties, possible eccentric behavior, and in extreme cases, psychotic dysfunctioning.

Contents

Coding for contents is one of the least difficult of the various scoring elements. It involves classifying what the subject reports having seen into its most appropriate category, or categories if more than one content is reported (i.e., primary or secondary). The categories include: whole human (H); human detail (Hd); whole human fictional or mythological [(H)]; human detail fictional or mythological [(Hd)]; human experience (Hx); whole animal (A); animal detail (Ad); whole animal fictional or mythological [(A)]; animal detail fictional or mythological [(Ad)]; anatomy (An); art (art); anthropology (Ay); blood (Bl); botany (Bt); clothing (Cg); clouds (Cl); explosion (Ex); fire (Fi); food (Fd); geography (Ge); household (Hh); landscape (Ls); nature (Na); science (Sc); sex (Sx) and X-ray (Xy). There is also a category for idiographic contents (ID); it allows classification of unusual responses that do not fit into any of the standard categories. Normative data indicate that animals and humans are most frequently reported. About 48% or 11 responses of a typical protocol of a nonpatient adult will involve animals. Around 24% or 5 responses will involve humans. As noted above in the section describing the blots and their common or popular responses, almost all of these readily seen and reported percepts are either animal or human.

Research shows schizophrenics produce fewer popular responses than nonpatients; depressed patients produce fewer human responses than either nonpatients or schizophrenics. Not surprisingly, an absence of human content suggests a significant lack of interest in people, or a sense of detachment from others. Failure to produce human content responses has also been associated with problems with identity, self image, or both. Botany, clouds, nature, and landscapes as content are also associated with a distant or isolated style in interpersonal relations.

In addition to the quantitative analysis of contents (e.g., percentages) evident in the Exner system, contents can be interpreted through their thematic characteristics. Here, the Rorschach is viewed somewhat like a TAT. From this perspective, the blots are seen as stimuli to fantasy material, rather than as stimuli for a problem-solving perceptual task. Some thematic elaborations can be formally scored using codes from the Exner system [e.g., morbid (MOR), aggressive (AG), or cooperative [COP]]. (These codes will be discussed in the section on special scores.) Other thematically-based scores have been developed by researchers outside the Exner system, particularly from the domain of object-relations theory. Approaching the Rorschach via themes can provide the clinician with valuable idiographic material regarding underlying personality dynamics. Thematic inferences used in conjunction with nomothetic hypotheses derived from the quantitative data of the Structural Summary can yield a rich and comprehensive picture of the individual.

Organizational Activity

Another possible code to be considered is the Z score. These scores relate to the extent to which the blot has been organized in the development of the response. For example, a whole (W) response that involves synthesizing the parts of the blot to include the entire stimulus field is a more complex production than is a response of a readily perceived common detail. The former response would receive a Z score, the latter would not. Specific numerical weights are assigned to each blot based on the degree to which organization of the stimuli has taken place. Z scores are coded for responses where integration has been a part of the construction of the percept. Such productions include integrated whole responses, integrated adjacent detail responses, integrated use of distant details, and integrated use of white space. The frequency of the Z scores (Zf) is then transformed to a weighted score that is based on normative data. One can compare the actual frequency sum to the normed estimate to address the amount of organizational activity in the protocol. Such comparisons can answer whether the subject organizes the blots within normal limits or perhaps tends to miss a lot of the stimulus field, or uses too much data. If there is too little organization (underincorporator), the person might tend to miss important elements of his or her world and might be inclined to behave inappropriately based on less than adequate information. Too much organizational activity (overincorporator) suggests a person who attends to lots of unnecessary environmental details. Such a person might become immobilized by a style of overscanning. Indeed, the task of decision-making might lead to considerable discomfort, since overincorporators might feel pressure to act on (what is to their minds) insufficient information. Such a person might be inclined to "miss the forest for the trees."

Special Scores

The last element to be considered when scoring a response concerns whether or not it meets criteria for a "special score." These codes reflect some unusual quality in the manner in which a response was offered, embellished, or both. For example, the subject may have used strange or peculiar language, employed nonsequitors, described morbid content, or imposed aggressiveness onto the percept. These codes allow for both quantitative and qualitative analysis of response features that earlier systems addressed only qualitatively. The codes with a brief description follow. (For a detailed explanation, the reader is referred to Exner texts).

1. **Deviant Verbalization (DV):** This code is scored for neologisms (i.e., use of new or self-coined words)

2. **Deviant Response (DR):** This code is applied where the subject uses an inappropriate phrase and describes a response in a circumstantial, overly elaborate, or rambling manner.

3. **Incongruous Combination (INCOM):** In this case, the response involves the inappropriate use of details that are condensed into one object (e.g., "looks like a bear with four testicles").

4. **Fabulized Combination (FABCOM):** This code denotes an implausible relationship between two or more objects in the blot (e.g., "two ants flying a rocket ship").

5. **Contamination (CONTAM):** This code reflects a very serious distortion that is the most pathological of the combination scores. Here, two or more percepts are imposed or fused together to create a single response. The process and product violate reality. It is as if two photographic negatives had been superimposed onto one another creating a new, albeit strange image. For example, the subject first reports seeing a "butterfly," then sees a "human." But the response to the blot is "a butterfly man."

6. **Inappropriate Logic (ALOG):** This code is applied when the subject has resorted to strained or unusual logic to explain a response (e.g., "it must be snow because it's all white").

7. **Perservation (PSV):** There are three different types of this code, although all receive the same designation. The first type involves within-card perseveration. It is coded when the subject offers consecutive responses comprised of the same location, DQ, determinants, FQ, content category, Z score and special score(s). The specific content may vary, but not the category (e.g., "bat followed by butterfly"). The second type, content perseveration, refers to reporting the same percept as seen before, but not as a consecutive response (e.g., "that's the same butterfly I saw a few cards ago"). The third variety, mechanical perseveration, is most associated with organically impaired or intellectually low functioning persons. Here, the subject mechanistically responds with the same percept to several of the blots.

8. **Confabulation (CONFAB):** This code is applied to responses where the subject focuses on a detail of the blot, but elaborates the percept to include a larger area or the entire blot (e.g., "there's a paw; it's a bear").

There are also several special content codes; they are as follows:

1. **Content (AB):** There are two instances when this code is applied. The first case involves responses with the content code for human experience (Hx). The other case is when the response is a symbolic representation (e.g., "a statue representing democracy").

2. **Aggressive Movement (AG):** This code is scored for all movement responses where the activity reflects aggressive action.

3. **Cooperative Movement (COP):** This code is applied to all movement responses wherein two or more objects are seen as interacting in a positive or cooperative manner.

4. **Morbid Content (MOR):** This code is scored for a response if either of two charac-

teristics are present: (a) the object is reported as dead, damaged, broken, ruined, etc. (e.g., "a decayed tooth"); or (b) an object is described in a dysphoric manner (e.g., " a very sad face").

   5. Personal (PER): This code is used for responses that include some self-reference or personal familiarity with the content. It is coded whenever a response is offered via the subject's own knowledge or experience. Such a response often includes the use of personal pronouns (i.e., I, me, my, or we).

   6. Color Projection (CP): This code is used for those rare instances when an achromatic blot or area is identified as chromatic. This type of response has been associated with an abuse of the defense of denial. It is as if the subject rejects "what is," and instead, imposes what he or she believes to be "true." In a phrase, this is the kind of person who reflects the notion, "Don't confuse me with the facts; my mind is already made up."

The Structural Summary

   After all the responses have been scored and coded, the examiner prepares the Structural Summary. The summary is an array of the data in various frequencies, ratios, and indexes. It is well beyond the scope of this chapter to present many of the important details regarding the Structural Summary, its components, and the arithmetical and tabular procedures. (The interested reader should refer to Exner.) However, in simple terms, the summary can be thought of as composed of two main sections, an upper part and a lower part. The upper section includes the following: location features (i.e., location codes, organizational activity, developmental quality); the determinants, form quality, contents, approach summary, and special scores. The lower section is divided into seven blocks of data and a bottom portion that notes special indexes that are scored from the Constellation Worksheet (a set of empirically-based criteria that are statistically associated with the indexes). What follows is a brief description of the scores, ratios, etc., that constitute the lower section of the summary.

   The first section to be considered is the Core section. It includes R, or the total number of responses in the protocol, and the total number of each of the determinants. Some of the other elements are:

   1. Lambda (L): This is an important ratio that compares the number of pure form responses to all the other responses. The ratio relates to how open the subject is to his or her emotions. The mean score for adult nonpatients is .58 with a standard deviation of .26. A high score suggests a person who is over controlled and emotionally constricted. In contrast, a low score suggests a person who is too emotional, perhaps even volatile, with poor control of feelings.

   2. Erlebnistypus (EB): This ratio compares human movement responses to the weighted sum of the chromatic color responses. The EB is very important since it reflects the problem-solving style. People who produce a lot of human movement responses tend to be what is called introversive; they think about solutions to problems, mulling over the various possible choices and potential consequences before taking action. People who load up on the chromatic color side tend to be extratensive; they solve problems by talking with others and are inclined to act quickly using a trial and error approach. There needs to be a clear preference (determined numerically) to designate one style versus the other (EB Per or EB Pervasive is a ratio that notes the dominant style). Interestingly, persons who approach problems from either of these styles use about the same amount of time and are similarly effective. Some persons, however, do not show a preference. Such persons are referred to as ambitants (M = Sum of C). They tend to show difficulty in coping with situations, and they show less efficiency in their ability to solve problems.

3. Experience Actual (EA): This is the sum of the EB components (M and Sum of C). It relates to the available resources a person has to solve problems in stressful situations. It involves organized ideation.

4. Experience Base (eb): This is a ratio of nonhuman movement scores to responses involving shading and achromatic color. The nonhuman movement data relate to internal and external stress; these data also reflect unorganized ideation. The shading variables relate to unorganized, negative feelings (e.g., guilt, neediness). Thus, eb can be thought of as a rather crude index of subjectively felt distress.

5. Experienced Stimulation (es): This score is the sum of both sides of the eb. It is an index of all the unorganized materials a person is confronting; es gets in the way of handling problems in a task-oriented manner.

6. D Score (D): This is an important score that provides information about the relationship between available resources and demands being made upon the subject. It reflects such concepts as tolerance of stress and control. Numerically, it is the difference between EA and es. The raw difference score is converted to a scaled difference score that is reported in standard deviation units. If the raw score falls within the standard deviation, D is valued at 0 and is deemed adequate. This suggests that available resources are potentially sufficient to meet demands. However, if the D Score is too much above or below plus or minus one standard deviation, then the person might have greater or lesser amounts of resources to deal with demands. A score that is too high (i.e., +2 units or more), could mean the person is less likely to profit from treatment. He or she might use resources to prevent confronting issues. Too little resources (i.e., –1 or lower) suggests a person who has only limited resources to meet demands, one who is overloaded without sufficient material to cope.

7. Adjusted es (ADj es): This score is a mathematical correction of the es to see what effect situational factors have on the resulting D Score. By literally subtracting the numerical analog of situational variables (i.e., all but one m and one y are subtracted from the es) the resulting score is thought to reflect the subject's usual fund of resources.

8. Adjusted D Score (Adj D): The raw difference score between EA and Adj es is calculated and transformed using the same conversion table as is used to determine the D Score. This score can then be compared to the D Score for indications of a usual versus an atypical fund of resources and the ability to deal with stress.

The Ideational section consists of human movement responses which are scored minus for form quality, or those special cases where there is no form quality score (i.e., human experience), the raw sum of the special scores, the number of Level-2 special scores (i.e., some special scores that are especially deviant receive weighted values to indicate the greater degree of pathology). Additionally, this section includes the following:

1. Active:Passive Ratio (a:p): This ratio reflects all movement scores and their active or passive codes. Typically, a ratio of 2:1 active to passive is expected. If the ratio is higher than expected on the active side, the person might not tend to profit from input from others. High on the passive side can indicate a person who is expecting others, perhaps the therapist, to take over and do the work. In brief, such a person tends to be dependant, or passive, or both in relations with others.

2. M Active:Passive Ratio (Ma:Mp): This ratio involves only human movement. It is typically about 3:1 active to passive. Interpretatively, it concerns aspects of thinking. If too skewed on the active side, it suggests a person who does not gather enough data. If too passively skewed, it suggests a tendency to fail to take action, perhaps lacking in assertiveness.

3. Intellectualization Index [2AB+(Art+Ay)]: As the name implies, this index, comprised of abstract, art, and anthropology scores, indicates use of an intellectualized defensive style.

The Affect Section includes data regarding pure C, space, and color projection. It also involves three affect-related ratios.

1. Form-Color Ratio (FC:CF+C): This ratio involves modulation of feelings. One expects a ratio of 2:1, reflecting the dominance of form or intellectual control over emotionality.

2. Affective Ratio (Afr): This ratio reflects the number of responses to the last three blots versus the number of responses to the first seven blots. In general, this ratio provides information regarding interest in emotional stimuli. Thus, a high ratio (mean = .69; standard deviation = .16) suggests overresponsiveness to emotional stimulation. Conversely, a low Afr suggests the subject is likely to back away from environmental stimulation.

3. Complexity Ratio (Blends:R): This ratio notes the number of multiple determinant responses, or blends, in the record. In brief, this ratio gives some information about the subject's ability to attack problems in different ways or the ability to entertain alternate ideas or hypotheses. Too few or no blends in a record suggest a person who cannot examine several possible avenues when addressing a problem. Too many blends or many determinants in a few responses may suggest an overly ideational style. Also, form quality and use of color and shading are of particular importance in interpreting these scores. For example, the use of chromatic color and shading in a single response has been associated with experiencing a painful conflict.

The Mediation section is next. It consists of the frequency of popular responses and five percentages. The latter are as follows:

1. Conventional Form (X+%): This percentage reflects the appropriate use of form. It is calculated as the sum of all responses in which form is both used and is scored + or o for form quality, divided by the total number of responses in the record. Basically, this percentage is a measure of how well or accurately things are seen. In this vein it offers some index of conventionality.

2. Conventional Pure Form (F+%): In this case, only responses based solely on form or contour are included. The percentage is calculated by adding all form-only responses that also have form quality scores of + or o and dividing the sum by the sum of all pure-form responses in the record. In essence, this score is a measure of psychological operations without the influence of affect (no determinants other than form are involved). This score can be compared with X+% to yield information regarding the influence of affect on functioning. For example, if X+% = .50 and F+% = .80 for a schizophrenic patient, one might infer that the patient functions better in structured situations that are devoid of much emotion. If, however, there is a lot of environmental stimulation, the patient's reality testing ability appears to suffer. If these scores were reversed and the patient in question was diagnosed schizoid or borderline, then one might expect that in a more or less affect-free environment that functioning would not be optimal. In contrast, if this person was in an environment where there was a lot of affect or many things going on, then this person would tend to function better, relatively speaking.

3. Distorted Form (X−%): This is a measure of reality testing. It reflects the proportion of perceptual distortion in the record. It is calculated by dividing the sum of responses with form quality scores of minus (−) by the total number of responses. One should expect a low percentage (mean = .07; standard deviation = .05). If the percentage is high (15–20%), the clinician should be concerned; the subject is seeing things others don't see.

4. White Space Distortion (S–%): This percentage that include white space. It is calculated by dividing the sum of the responses scored minus (–) for form quality that also include white space divided by the total number of responses scored minus. Only .08% of a typical record is scored S–. High scores suggest strong negativism or anger leading to perceptual distortions.

5. Unusual Form (Xu%): This percentage notes the proportion of responses wherein the contours of the blots are used appropriately, although they are not statistically conventional. It is calculated by dividing the sum of scores coded unusual (u) for form quality divided by the total number of responses in the record. One can expect an Xu% of .14 for a typical nonpatient.

The next grouping to be presented is the Processing section. This portion of the Structural Summary consists of frequency data (i.e., Zf, DQ+, and Dqv), two ratios, and a difference score. The latter three entries are as follows:

1. Economy Index (W:D:Dd): This ratio notes the relationship among the various location scores. In an adult nonpatient record a typical ratio is 9:13:1.

2. Aspirational Ratio (W:M): This ratio compares the total number of whole responses to the total number of human movement scores. Nonpatient adult records typically yield a ratio of 2:1. If the ratio is higher than expected on the W side, this might suggest an individual who is overly involved with trying to organize his or her world or perhaps very high in need for achievement. High loading on the M side reflects a person more prone to thought-oriented activity. Whereas the high W person might be viewed as inclined to reach out to the world, the high M person is disinclined to make this kind of contact. Indeed, such a person might actually be defensively limiting such activity.

3. Processing Efficiency (Zd): As indicated above, this score reflects the difference between the sum of the Z scores, or ZSUM, minus the estimate of Z based on the frequency of Z in the record (Zest). (See discussion of Organizational Activity.)

The next grouping is the Interpersonal section. In this portion of the summary, there are several frequency data entries (i.e., total number of COP responses, total number of AG responses, and the number of primary or secondary Food contents). There are also four ratios which are as follows:

1. Isolation Index (Isolate/R): This score relates to social isolation. The numerator is composed of the number of primary and secondary content scores from the categories of Botany, Clouds, Geography, Landscape, and Nature. (Both Clouds and Nature have their raw scores doubled.) The notion of isolation is suggested by all of the contents being nonhuman, inanimate, and typically static. The mean score is .20 with a standard deviation of .09.

2. Interpersonal Interest [H:(H)+Hd+(Hd)]: This score reflects interest in humans. Both primary and secondary contents are used. If the loading is on the right side, it might indicate a distorted view of others.

3. (H)+(Hd):(A)+(Ad): This ratio suggests the extent to which views of others are fantasy based rather than reality oriented. Both primary and secondary contents are used in the construction.

4. H+A:Hd+Ad: This ratio can yield information regarding how the person views the social environment. If it is high on the right side, the subject might tend to view the environment in an unusual or guarded manner.

The next portion of the summary is the Self-Perception section. There are four frequency scores (i.e., sum Fr+rF, total Form Dimension scores, total number of Morbid content responses, and the sum of responses that involve Anatomy or Xray contents, either primary or secondary). The other entry is a ratio.

Egocentricity Index (3r+(2)/R)

This index relates to self focus or self concern. It is a measure of how one thinks about oneself. If the score is low, the person is probably not particularly self-focused. The person might not feel he or she measures up well. This situation is usually referred to as low self-esteem. In contrast, a high ratio indicates an investment in self-focus, but likely not involving others. Really high scores necessitate reflection responses as well as pair responses. The former are not readily found in Rorschach protocols. Such responses usually note a narcissistic tendency.

Finally, the bottom of the summary contains reference to six special indices. Each is composed of several variables that are scored "present" or "not." A specific number of positive scores is required for an index to be deemed operative. The indices are particularly important for the variables they reflect, and several of them are so-called Key Variables for determining the search sequence among the sections of the Structural Summary (the interested reader is referred to Exner for details regarding this interpretation scheme). The special indices are: the Schizophrenia Index (**SCZI**), the Depression Index (**DEPI**), the Coping Deficit Index (**CDI**), the Suicide Constellation (**S-CON**), the Hypervigilance Index (**HVI**), and the Obsessive Style Index (**OBS**). Each index relates to its title. Moreover, the more the scores that comprise each variable exceed the statistical cut-off, the greater is the probability the index is a good reflection of that problem.

Interpreting a Rorschach Protocol

Rorschach interpretation cannot be fully addressed within the limits of this chapter. (As noted above, the reader interested in interpretation according to the Exner system should consult volumes written by Exner and by Exner and Weiner.) Nevertheless, for the purposes of this presentation, there are some basic points to bear in mind. This author believes that to best appreciate the potential richness of Rorschach data, one should examine the Structural Summary, engage in thematic analysis, and evaluate the test-taking behavior of the subject. In interpreting structural data, one can follow Exner's current suggestions to search for key variables (e.g., positive SCZI or DEPI) that set a perspective on the subsequent data analysis. Moreover, presence of these key variables dictates the order of examination of the various sections of the Structural Summary. Another interpretive strategy involves beginning with the Core section and proceeding through the other sections based upon significant findings within each specific domain. In any case, careful exploration of Structural Summary data allows the clinician to make interpretations relative to the subject's ability to cope with a cognitive-perceptual task, and to compare these findings with empirical data from both patient and nonpatient groups. For example, interpretations/hypotheses can be made regarding how this person is likely to think, feel and behave in other problem-solving situations.

As noted in the body of this chapter, the various scores, as well as relationships among scores, can yield a variety of information about the subject's cognitive-emotional status. It has also been noted that full appreciation of a Rorschach record should include interpretation of the thematic and symbolic characteristics. In this case, rather than being viewed as stimuli to cognitive-perceptual activity, the Rorschach blots are considered to be stimuli to fantasy material. This approach seems particularly valuable in exploring responses where the subject has elaborated the percepts beyond identification and description. In brief, these instances indicate projection has played an integral part in the process. Such responses include those involving movement, those where form quality has been grossly distorted, and those instances of elaboration attributed to the percept by the subject versus descriptions of elements that are actually part of the blot. The interesting and potentially valuable hypotheses regarding underlying attitudes, preoccupations, self-concept, and interpersonal issues are but a few of the areas tapped by such a thematic approach. Another thematic strategy involves reading each response and its inquiry and proceeding through the entire record to explore response style, projections, sequential issues, symbolic representations, etc. Again, this approach can yield some very interesting and useful information, particularly when such card by card analysis also includes hypotheses derived from careful examination of structural data.

Finally, how the subject interacts with the examiner can furnish valuable clinical information about interpersonal style. For example, does the subject press for help, structure or both? Does the client display confidence, or is he or she tentative or anxious? Does the client become irritated or angry? Behavioral displays and interpersonal style can be especially meaningful and helpful to the examiner who is attempting to understand and appreciate the world of the client.

This writer has long maintained the belief that virtually all assessment techniques are special forms of the clinical interview. In the case of the Rorschach, the examiner asks specific questions (e.g., "What might this be?"; "What makes it look like that?"), follows a semi-structured format for eliciting data, and attempts to measure and evaluate the findings against norms and in light of the characteristic style of the subject. These processes are much in line with many of the tasks carried out by a therapist in the course of conducting diagnostic and therapeutic interviews.

CASE EXAMPLE

The case to be presented was chosen for several reasons. First, although there has been considerable modification of identifying data to ensure confidentiality, the protocol is real, having been obtained from a former graduate student. Second, the record is replete with rich structural, thematic and symbolic material. In light of the information presented above, it is believed that the reader will be able to appreciate a good deal of the discussion that follows.

Background and the Presenting Problem

The client, a twenty-one-year old, Caucasian male, was, at the time of testing, an undergraduate at a small, private, out-of-state college. He presented himself to the college counseling service with complaints of "overwhelming feelings of stress." He reported experiencing both suicidal and homicidal thoughts and fantasies, although he stated he would never act upon them unless he felt "desperate enough." Interestingly, he recalled that as a young child he told other children in his class to "go home or I will slit your throat with a knife." Additionally, he reported being both intrigued and impressed with the "genius" of a serial killer seen in a popular movie. He attributed his current difficulties to a chaotic home environment and academic pressure. He lived with five immediate and extended family members, including his blind mother, a sister and a half-sister. Both sisters he described as "hot-tempered." The other two residents were described as elderly extended family members. He reported that when he was four years old his father was asked to leave the house after he was caught engaging in an extramarital affair that had produced a female child. The current household was depicted as "tempestuous, with constant arguments that generally ended in screamfests." The academic pressures related to his having a triple major (premedicine, music, and philosophy). He was currently taking 18 credits, and had been doing fairly well, especially in light of the course load. (He was administered only the first two subtests of the WAIS-R, Information and Comprehension, and achieved perfect scores on both! These scores indicate an estimated I.Q. of 150, well above the 130 mark used to denote the Very Superior category.) His grades have dropped somewhat due to some short-term illnesses. He reported studying well into the night, getting only about five hours of sleep. The client was referred to the counseling service by his academic advisor. The student's complaints, along with the historical information, prompted the assessment. The testing was directed to his current level of functioning, with particular emphasis on his tolerance for handling stress and his ability to modulate and control aggressive impulses. He was also given an appointment for the following week to see a therapist and was informed about local crisis hot lines and facilities he could contact if his status changed and he needed immediate attention.

Card I

1. Did you see the movie Silence of the Lambs? This is a bee. Like on the poster—where it is a female with a bee on her (indicated mouth)—it is all based on this psychopath's fascination with the bees. I'm not sure if it is more of a bee or a moth—some flying creature that is very rare.

E: (repeats S's response)
S: This is the poster that—it has a female's face and this moth or bee is placed on her lips, her lips are gone. The whole movie is focused around this killer that leaves this moth behind and Hannibal Lecter knows who it is.
E: What makes this look like that moth?
S: The markings, in the movie it is yellow and black with triangular markings like this and it has its wings extended. This part up here looks like the head with the little claws here that it has.

2. The head of a cat with an evil grin. The cat's eyes are very uh slanted. Kind of with a grin—like right now I am reading a book called Killer Clown—The murders of John Gacy on the cover there is a picture of a mug shot where he was arrested and he just had this smile on his face as if he didn't really care and that's the kind of smile.

E: (repeats S's response)
S: Here are its ears, a little deformed. The cat might have gotten his ears cut or something. Here are his eyes, evil looking eyes.
E: Evil?
S: Slant of the eyes?
E: Eyes?
S: Symmetrical, shape.
E: Evil grin?
S: Looks like a smile, like he is laughing—like a laughter you always hear in the movies—like a Vincent Price laughter, like he is making fun of you because he knows something that you don't—that kind of grin—he knows something you don't. Like he is going to get you or something like that.

E: Anything else?
S: Am I allowed to turn it around?
E: Anything you like.
S: (turns the card several times) Nope. (hands card back)

Card II

3. (client's jaw tightened—long delay before responding) Back when I was about twelve we had a pretty large bird cage and there were usually mice that would hang around and would eat the seeds and occassionally eat a bird. So when we caught a mouse it was more of a—we would try to get rid of them. And I saw this mouse and with a simple rubber band and a sharp metal object I shot at it like a bow and arrow and I killed it. And when I pulled it out I was interested in it so I split it open and so this I guess would be a rat in half, laid open.

E: (repeats S's response)
S: When I killed the rat it was with a little metal rod and when I shot it it went right through the side and out the other. When it was dead I got a real sharp knife and I just cut it in half to open it up to explore but I found that I couldn't cut the head so I—whoosh (gestured cutting the throat) slit the head off.
E: (points) So this is where the head?
S: Would be. The blood has just leaked out. This would be his legs. Once again from being cut open this is the blood.
E: Laid flat?
S: Cut the head off, sliced it open and flat so that the back is up. Kind of like when I skinned a cat in 11th grade where you had to lay the cat flat down and cut around and eventually take the skin off.
E: Part of a biology course?
S: Yes. The teacher actually let me keep the skin too.

Card III

4. Two females, some kind of African ritual um, making a sacrifice. The red part being the blood of an animal.

E: Repeats S's response)
S: See the heads here, females because of the breasts. The arms. This would be like a sacrificial alter or something. They are standing and arching their butts back. Whatever they are sacrificing, this would be considered as the blood marks, that they might make usually when they kill something they like smear it on their faces.
E: Blood?
S: Because it is red. Were it black I might say it was motor oil.
E: You are using this part here?
S: Yes and this could be part of the ritual where on the outside around them someone else might be holding up a dead animal or if this is a wall they have to make some kind of drawings on the wall.

5. Beetle—just the head of a beetle or like a black widow spider.

E: Which one?

S: Black widow spider—because the red in the middle resembles the pattern that is the symbol of the black widow, the red triangular shape on the back. Very sharp jaws.

E: (repeats S's response)

S: Sharp jaws, you can only see its front two legs. I see this as the remainders of a–no not exactly because spiders don't exactly kill—they inject their digestive fluids which decompose the animal. Then they ingest it back in. So I m not sure what that could be. This would be the spider's eyes.

E: Eyes?

S: They look in any direction you look at it; it is still looking at you. Spiders have eight eyes. The only direction they cannot see you is if you come at them from the bottom.

E: This part of it?

S: No just this area here.

E: Black widow spider?

S: The blackness and the design, that is the marking that they have.

E: Design?

S: Shape of the design and the red.

Card IV

6. (turns card several times)

   A creature that you would probably read about in a J. R. Tolkein story line. An evil creature. Not exactly with arms—like what you would see on a Tyrannosaurus Rex, useless forearms, very strong tail and hind legs.

E: (repeats S's response)

S: You can see the very useless forearms, rather small head, large body, large feet.

7. Turned around it still looks like a creature from one of his stories—more like a dragon with wings opened up ready to take off in flight.

E: (repeats S's response)

S: You can see the dragon's neck curving.

E: Head is here, the mouth is open wide.

E: Neck curving?

S: Like how a snake is ready to strike, It kind of curves back and all of the sudden it whoosh (uses hand to demonstrate) like that. So his neck is actually in like this.

E: Mouth?

S: A little lighter—looks like an opening.

E: Ready to fly?

S: Wings are spread open but not completely open. Kind of curved to catch the wind.

Card V

8. Bat

E: (repeats S's response)

S: Ears, body, wings extended.

E: Extended?

S: Extended like in flight. Could be a vampire bat that Dracula turns into in all of these stories.

E: Vampire bat?

S: Could be any kind of bat, just a bat. I have a fascination with vampires though, so I could say vampire bat.

Card VI

9. Some kind of a like a—
   Excaliber in a stone

E: (repeats S's response)

S: Sword, this is the handle wedged into this rock and yet the handle has the sharp edges so whoever is the one to take it out has to be careful.

E: Rock?

S: Solidness and the color.

10. Or a magic wand, an Indian wand.

E: (repeats S's response)

S: I wasn't taking this into consideration. Indian chiefs and medicine men ornate their wands with feathers of a bird—eagle or falcon, some bird of some importance or power and this is their um their sign of authority.

E: Feathers?

S: Not fixed, random lines shape.

11. There are a lot of sharp edges it just um—somewhat like a crucifix type thing. Jesus Chris on a cross.

E: (repeats S's response)

S: This is like the mountain side with the cross, the head, body, with the arms sticking out. Kind of like has an aura around the head like the aura that you see, that angel type of aura goes around there.

E: Aura?

S: The lightness, it looks like glowing.

Card VII

12. (leans forward, puts head on hand) Do you know who Betty Boop is? - 2 Betty Boops (said after response # 13: "Although Betty has a chunk of her butt missing.")

E: (repeats S's response)

S: Betty. Betty is the sexual figure of the 40's and 50's. Small waist. Very innocent. "I love my man, my man is my life" type of thing an uh there are two of them. Their hair is touching here. She is in a very innocent type of pose (demonstrates hands together curved away from body).

13. Like a a Indian relic of two um females looking at each other. Only from a, only the bust. (Rubbing card with thumbs) More of a family type of relic because the arms are pointed out and not toward each other like at war. Something that a mother would pass on to her daughter.

E: (repeats S's response)
S: Two females figures and maybe a feather up here. Only the busts—this the joining part of the two, not actually a part of the body. The hands are pointed away from each other. If they were pointed toward each other it would be more a sign of aggression.
E: Mother to daughter?
S: This doesn't seem to be something a male would have, considering the Indian culture where males are encouraged to hunt and do this and that.

Card VIII

14. Inside a dissected human being. An open heart, lungs spread out, gall bladder cut in half. (rubbing card with thumbs) Could be a female (points) the uterus. Small inclination of a spinal cord but more like an autopsy type thing and apparently something was inserted in her—to u—to kill her.

E: (repeats S's response)
S: Open heart here.
E: A heart?
S: Were this closed up. It is not as it is often pictured like a valentine but rather has an apricot shape. If you were to slice it down the middle you would get more of a valentine interpretation of a heart. This would be the different chambers.
E: What about it made it look like chambers?
S: The different tone colorations, since it would be a chamber. Light wouldn't be coming into that chamber as you look at it; it gets darker inside. The lungs just look like they were parted.
E: Lungs?
S: The shape.
E: Gall bladder?
S: The gall bladder is bluish green in color and sits right about here. It looks like it is cut open and spread open.
E: Uterus?
S: The shape.
E: Small inclination of the spinal cord?
S: Right here. This could be part of the back bone. It stops right here. It might have been that the spinal cord was torn off. It ends here.
E: Something inserted into her that killed her?
S: Did you see the movie *Seven*? Do you remember, I think it was lust that he had a leather maker make a certain phallic symbol. It was a leather strap-on but at the very

edge it had a knife and at gunpoint this guy had to make love to this prostitute with this thing on and it eventually killed her because of the knife stabbing her and that um reminded me of the woman.

E: What part of this looks like the wounded part?

S: The knife—here. (points)

E: What about it made it look like a knife?

S: The sharp edges.

15. Two tigerlike creatures trying to climb a tree, a very thin tree, from a rock of some kind.

E: (repeats S's response)

S: Looks like a Chinese bonsai tree.

E: What about it made it look like a bonsai tree?

S: Usually bonsai trees grow in very unusual places, like out of rocks. This is a rock and it has a very tiny root and it just sort of sprouted out. They make their own very distinct patterns like this one.

Card IX

16. (turns card several times, rubbing card with thumbs) Something like a blooming flower with leaves possibly coming from a fruit or a reddish type of plant like what a carrot looks like while it is still under the ground.

E: (repeats S's response)

S: This, looks like the flower here with the pistil, the leaves like a rose type of leaves coming out of a fruit, an apple or some sort of red fruit. Also makes me think radishes and carrots look like that before you pick them out. This is what is under the ground.

17. It also looks like a swatted mosquito put under a microscope slide with the only real part of the mosquito being left is the—what would you call it. I know it is not the nose—what they use to sting you and suck out your blood.

E: (repeats S's response)

S: Well, the mosquito that I swatted was kind of crushed and the only part that I was able to see was the blood that had been pushed out of the animal like this and, it was kind of a greenish, grayish type color. You couldn't tell very much except for a needle that they use. This is like the mosquito's own blood along with that of human blood, just scattered.

E: What makes it look like blood?

S: Where it is.

18. Atomic bomb destroying—like a Hiroshima type mushroom, but that is going underneath the ground and destroying that also. (rubbing card with thumbs)

E: (repeats S's response)

S: I look at the green stuff as the earth. The pink is the mushroom cloud. The atomic cloud is forming, kind of coming out.

E: Coming out?

S: Um, atomic bombs when they blow up and come up, they extend outwards creating the cloud.

E: What makes it look like it's coming out?

S: That direction and that direction and in this direction. See the lighter outside area and the darker' inside. (points) That is where the bomb actually hit and it looks like it went through the earth and is destroying the inner part of the earth.

E: Destroying?

S: I would imagine that this was once unified and this is a barrier that is moving away.

19. It also looks like what you would get if you take an apple, beets, and a carrot and put it in a—one of those—um—a blender.

E: (repeats S's response)

S: An apple here. You can see the heart of the apple here and the—um—center—core and the seed, the mashed up beets and carrots. See the colors; green apple of course.

E: What makes it look like seeds?

S: Um, ever eaten an apple down to the core? The seeds are long and thin. So am I normal?

Card X

20. Like a union of all different types of insects and arachnids and a crab.

E: (repeats S's response)

S: Crab, snail, worm, beetles, caterpillar getting ready for metamorphosis. You know how they create that silk that they wrap themselves in? They create it in the mouth and they are creating it to wrap themselves around in it and that gray is usually the color of it.

21. Also looks like a fishing lure. These are usually the colors that would attract certain fish. I don't like this one. (card) Too many colors.

E: (repeats S's response)

S: Um, usually fishing lures look like little feathers. Um, this would be the thing that holds it all together, but in the water it spreads out which would make it look like insects to a fish. This is what the fish might see as it is coming toward it.

E: Spreadout?

S: See. Opening up, spreading out in all directions.

22. I see a—like a western movie they have, um, cow's skull.

E: (repeats S's response)
S: Just that right there.
E: Help me to see it the way you do.
S: Usually what is left is the, a nose, the hole of the eyes—the two dark holes. The roundness of the skull, and these are overly exaggerated horns of a bull.

23. I see a face. Glaring yellow eyes. Green raised eyebrows, kind of like in an angry manner. Mouth closed but ready to explode. Face all red. He is biting down so hard on his lips that he is bleeding a little. Veins popping out of his neck.

E: (repeats S's response)
S: Two eyes glaring at you; they have red pupils like they are ready to explode. Eyebrows here. I'm not using this part. Mouth is like this. (demonstrates tight) Like something is being held back. Like biting down to keep from saying something. This part here looks like the blood.
E: Blood?
S: Because it is red. The redness of the face signifies anger also.
E: Veins popping out?
S: See, here and here, like when you get angry. See them to the side. They are like bigger coming out here.

Structural Summary Hypotheses

Even with an elementary background regarding the components of the Structural Summary and their interpretation, the reader should be impressed with a number of features in this client's record. First, the total number of responses (23) and the Lambda (.15) suggest a valid protocol. Despite the client's reported distress, he had been able to offer the average number of responses. The Lambda is very much in line with his interview presentation. That is, the very low Lambda suggests he is inclined to be overly emotional with poor control of his feelings, possibly even volatile. Positive indexes for both depression (DEPI = 5) and suicide potential (S-CON = 9) further indicated the seriousness of the situation and that it necessitated immediate attention and close monitoring. His basic problem-solving style is extratensive (EB = 4:10). Thus, he is the kind of person who is likely to act upon the environment by interacting with others and is prone to using trial-and-error tactics. He also might be rather quick to act. Despite his exceptional intellectual abilities, the quality of his problem-solving abilities appeared to be diminished due to an overload of internal and external factors (D = –1). When confronted by complex and stressful situations where the demands exceed his resources, he is vulnerable to disintegration and may react impulsively. His action-oriented, impulsive style is now rather unmodulated by his intellectual faculties (FC:CF+C = 3:8). Also, there is the added element that he can be rather negativistic or oppositional (S = 4; S-% = .20). Typically, he does appear to have adequate resources to handle or solve problems (Adj D = 0). Indeed, his apparent academic success would seem to reflect this. Now, however, there is just too much on his plate.

While the patient's current state does not preclude his ability to see common percepts (P = 5), the quality of his mediational functions is clearly poor. Indeed, this young man appears to be translating the stimulus field (the blots) in rather atypical ways (X+% = .57; X–% = .22; S–% = .20; Xu% = .22). In this case, it appears that he is unable to modulate either his affective responses or to adequately control his thoughts (MOR = 8). He is struggling to control both his feelings and cognitions. The former notion is lent support by his apparent ability to deal with these stimuli when their affective components are not incorporated into the process (F+% = 100). (Since there is a considerable literature showing a strong relationship between a low F+% and severely disturbed psychiatric patients, it should be noted that the client's score is based on only three out of 23 responses in the record. Therefore, greater interpretive value is placed on the conventional extended form quality score (X+%), which in this case is very low.) Moreover, the client often handles the task of perceiving the blots in such a way as to violate their contours. In brief, at times he violates reality by seeing what others don't see. The configuration of a low X+% and elevated X–% indicates considerable impediments to his ability to respond appropriately. In further support of this notion, there is one very rare movement response where the form quality is poor (M– = 1). This particular score suggests inefficient social skills and poor interpersonal relations. Additionally, the client comes across as laden with anger and negativism (S–%=.20). Thus, his thinking appears peculiar, and his interpersonal style can be rather offensive and inappropriate.

In addition to deviant perceptual functioning there are signs that this patient engages in complex mental activity (Blends:R = 13:23), including the previously-noted preoccupation with both morbid imagery and negative affects. Some of his complex responses are especially indicative of conflict (color-shading), which is most consistent with his current very painful interactions with the environment. There is also concern that he inefficiently overincorporates in his efforts to process environmental stimuli (Zd = +14.5). It appears that he is a inundated by both internal and external forces and is not able to adequately organize this information. In this vein, he might very well believe that he does not have enough data to make a decision before acting. In line with his intelligence, he appears inclined to use intellectualization as a defensive strategy (2AB+Art+Ay = 7), although at this time he is unable to do so in a way that protects him from either his thoughts or his emotions. Not surprisingly, he also appears to feel socially isolated (Isolate/ R = .35) and seems to have a disturbed view of others [H+(H):Hd+(Hd)] = 2:4). In light of his preoccupations, emotional turmoil, etc., it follows that he would not be especially sociable. One would not expect this young man to have close friends or to be capable of engaging in deep intimate relations.

Although the patient has very high academic aspirations, he is perhaps too involved with a need for achievement. This need probably plays a part in his stylistic efforts to organize his world (W:M = 19:4). Indeed, the very high number of whole responses (19) reflects an intense use of psychological energy to organize information. As the findings show, however, he is not doing well in these endeavors. This notion is further reinforced by Rorschach responses replete with strange or peculiar qualities (Dr = 5; Lv2 = 4). The latter are particularly evident in the special scores (Wgtd Sum6 = 29; MOR = 8; AG = 3).

In brief, although some of his responses are "colorful" and he might even have some inclination to shock the examiner, this patient does not appear to be feigning his condition. His situation is extremely serious. His perceptual-conceptual abilities are severely compromised. His thoughts are morbid. His emotions are unchecked by intellectual control. He is depressed and potentially suicidal. He is also at risk for acting out against others. The little background information provided clearly highlights a chaotic home environment and considerable academic demands. These circumstances appear to enhance the psychological and emotional turmoil. Prognosis is guarded. While his record does not currently meet the criterion for a diagnosis of schizophrenia (SCZI=3), such a notion should not be ruled out.

Additional Thematic Features

The limited scope of this chapter necessitates keeping comments about thematic analysis rather brief. Nevertheless, one cannot help being both intrigued and struck by the vivid images and accompanying commentary that comprise this record. Indeed, the very first response of "a bee or a moth" is tied into the patient's bizarre fascination and preoccupation with serial killers. He then sees a cat with "an evil grin." Here too, his projections and associations lead to an infamous serial killer, one who is described as having a smile that is like an evil grin. His next response is a gruesome depiction of a killed and mutilated mouse; Furthermore, the percept lead to his recalling how he killed and dissected a mouse when he was twelve years old. The details of this response are chilling. The patient's investment in death and dismemberment, along with his admiration for the intelligence of high profile serial killers (real and fictional), is frightening. After all, the patient is himself exceptionally bright and at least some of his deviant thoughts appear to have a long history (reported incident of threatening school boys). Now that he is falling apart, there is ample cause to be concerned. The death theme is also evident in his 4th response of an "African ritual." In this response he also includes references to sacrificial rites, including the smearing of blood. The same blot (III) also elicits the response of "a black widow spider." As if the percept were insufficient, the inquiry highlights the deadly process the spider uses, " . . . the(y) inject their digestive fluids which decompose the animal. . . . " There are other interesting themes that emerge, including references to magic ("Excalibur," "Indian magic wand") and religion ("Jesus Christ on a cross"). The former might reflect a wish for power beyond that which mere mortals can obtain. The latter might very well reflect his feeling that he is like Christ, a misunderstood victim, and that he too is being "crucified" by the world. One might wonder if his condition worsens if he will adopt the belief that he *is* Christ. It is interesting to note that religious thinking, particularly when it is of delusional quality, is often found among schizophrenics. Skipping ahead, it is also quite noteworthy to examine his very last response. In this case, he reported seeing " . . . a face . . . angry . . . mouth closed but ready to explode . . . biting down so hard on his lips that he is bleeding . . . " This image is very likely a self description. He is telling us how he feels. He knows he's in trouble; his emotions are welling up and he fears they will burst out. This young man very much needs help. At least some of his responses seem to show that he is desperate for assistance. It may very well be that on some level he knows he has to reach out before it is too late.

SUMMARY

This introduction to the world of Rorschach has touched upon a number of elements. Some historical background has been discussed, with a focus on the young psychiatrist, Hermann Rorschach, who developed the inkblots, engaged in the initial research with them, and for whom the test is named. There has been discussion of the psychometric qualities of the test. The reader has also been presented with some of the basics regarding test administration, scoring, and interpretation. Finally, an actual case was presented to illustrate how responses to the ten inkblots can yield findings that are both interesting and revealing about the psychology of a person.

ACKNOWLEDGMENT: The author wishes to thank Amber Myers, Psy.D. for the clinical case and initial scoring of it, and Michael Marshall, Psy.D. for his efforts at scoring the protocol to ensure reliability, and assistance in interpretation of the data.

APPENDIX

Sequences of Scores

Card No.	Loc #			Determinant(s)	(2) Content(s)	POP	Z	Special Scores
I	1	WSo	1	FMpo	A		3.5	DR,MOR
	2	WSo	1	FMao	Ad		3.5	DR2,PER,MOR
II	3	W+	1	FC.mp-	Ad,Bl		5.5	DR2,PER,MOR
III	4	W+	1	Mp.Co	2	H,B1,Ay,Ad	P	5.5	AG,MOR
	5	DSo		FC:FC	Ad		4.5	DR2
IV	6	Wo	1	Fo	(A)		2.0	
	7	Wo	1	FMa.FD.YF+	(A)		2.0	
V	8	Wo	1	FMao	A	P	1.0	PER
VI	9	W+	1	FC:FTu	Ay,Ls		2.5	
	10	D+1		Fo	Ay,Ad,Art		2.5	
	11	W+	1	Mpo Fy+	H,LS,Ay		2.5	
VII	12	Wo	1	Mpo	2	(H)		2.5	MOR
	13	Wo	1	Fo	2	Art,Hd,Ay,Ad	P	2.5	
VIII	14	W+	1	CF,FV-	Hd,SX,SC		4.5	DR2,MOR
	15	W+	1	FMau	2	A,Bt	P	4.5	
IX	16	W+	1	ma.CFu	Bt,Fd		5.5	
	17	W^v/+	1	CF-	Ad,B1		5.5	MOR
	18	W+	1	FV.ma.CFo	Ex,C1,Na		5.5	AG,MOR
	19	W^v/+	1	CFu	Fd		5.5	
X	20	W+	1	FMa.FCu	A	P	5.5	
	21	Wo	1	ma.CF-	Id		5.5	
	22	Do		FY.CFo	An			
	23	DdS+		Ma.FD-	Hd,B1		6.0	AG,INC

Summary of Approach

I	:	WS.WS	VI	:	W.D.W	
II	:	W	VII	:	W.W	
III	:	W.DS	VIII	:	W.W	
IV	:	W.W	IX	:	W.W.W.W.	
V	:	W	X	:	W.W.D.DdS	

Structural Summary

Location Features	Determinants Blends	Single	Contents	S-Constellation
			H = 2,0	YES..FV+VF+V+FD>2
Zf = 22	FC.m	M = 1	(H) = 1,0	YES..Col-Shd Bl>0
zsum = 88:0	M.C	FM = 4	Hd = 2,1	YES..Ego<.31,>.44
ZEst = 73.5	FC'.FC	m = 0	(Hd) = 0,0	YES..MOR>3
	FM,FD,YF	FC = 0	Hx = 0,0	YES..Zd.+-3.5
W = 19	FC'.FT	CF = 2	A = 4,0	YES..es>EA
(WV = 0)	M.FY	C = 0	(A) = 2,0	YES..CF+C>FC
D = 3	CF.FV	Cn = 0	Ad = 4,3	YES..X+%<.70
Dd = 1	m.CF	FC' = 0	(Ad) = 0,0	YES..S>3
S = 4	FV.m.CF	C'F' = 0	An = 1,0	NO..P<3 or>8
	FM.FC	C' = 0	Art = 1,1	NO..Pure H<2
DQ	m.CF	FT = 0	Ay = 2,3	NO..R<17
........(FQ-)	FY.CF	TF = 0	B1 = 0,4	9.....Total
+ = 11 (3)	M.FD	T = 0	Bt = 1,1	
o = 10 (1)		FV = 0	Cg = 0,0	Special Scorings

				Lvl	Lv2
v/+ = 2 (1)		VF = 0	CL = 0,1		
V = 0 (0)		V = 0	Ex = 1,0	DV = 0x1	0x2
		FY = 0	Fd = 1,1	INC = 1x2	0x4
		YF = 0	Fi = 0,0	DR = 1x3	4x6
		Y = 0	Ge =0,0	FAB = 0x4	0x7
		FR = 0	Hh = 0,0	ALOG = 0x5	
Form Quality		rF = 0	Ls = 0,2	CON = 0x7	

Fqx	FQf	MQual	SQx	FD = 0	Na = 0,1	Raw Sum6=	6
				F = 3	SC = 0,1	Wgtd Sum6=	29
+ = 2	0	1	0		Sx = 0,1		
o = 11	3	2	3		Xy = 0,0	AB = 0	CP = 0
u = 5	0	0	0		Id = 1,0	AG = 3	MOR = 8
- = 5	0	1	1			CFB = 0	PER = 3
none = 0 –	0	0	(2) = 4			COP = 0	PSV = 0

Ratios, Percentages, and Derivations

R = 23	L = 0.15				
			FC:CF+c = 3: 8	COP = 0	AG = 3
			Pure C = 1	F ood = 2	
EB = 4:10.0	EA = 14.0	EBPer = 2.5	SumC:WSumC = 2:10.0	Isolate/R = 0.35	
eb = 10.8	es = 18	D = -1	Afr = 0.77	H:(H)Hd(Hd) = 2: 4	
	Adj es = 13	Adj D = 0	S = 4	(HHd):(AAd) = 1: 2	
			Blends:R =13.23	H+A:Hd+Ad = 9:10	
FM = 6	: C = 2 T = 1		CP = 13:23		
m = 4	: V = 2 Y = 3				
		P = 5	Zf =22	3r+(2)/R =0.17	
a:p = 9:5	Sum6 = 6	X+% =0.57	Zd =+14.5	Fr+rF = 0	
Ma:Mp=1:3	Lv2 = 4	F+% = 1.00	W:D:Dd =19: 3: 1	FD = 2	
2AB+Art+Ay=7	Wsum = 29	X-% = 0.22	W:M =19:4	An=Xy = 1	
M- = 1	Mnone = 0	S-% =0.20	DQ+ = 11	MOR = 8	
		Xu% =0.22	DQv = 0		

SCZI = 3	DEPI = 5*	CDI =1	S-CON = 9*	HVI = No	OBS = No

SUGGESTED READINGS

Exner, J. E. (1993). *The Rorschach: A comprehensive system. Volume 1: Basic foundations* (3rd ed.). New York: Wiley.

Exner, J. E. (1991). *The Rorschach: A comprehensive system. Volume 2: Interpretation* (3nd ed.). NewYork: Wiley.

Exner, J. E., & Weiner, I. B. (1982). The Rorschach: *A comprehensive system. Volume 3: Assessment of children and adolescents.* New York: Wiley.

Ganellen, R. J. (1996). *Integrating the Rorschach and the MMPI-2 in Personality Assessment.* Mahwah, NJ: Erlbaum Associates.

Rorschach, H. (1921). *Psychodiagnostik.* Bern Bircher (Trans. Hans Huber Verlag, 1942).

Schafer, R, (1954). *Psyhoanalytic Interpretation in Rorschach Testing.* New York: Grune & Stratton.

Weiner, I. B. (1966). *Psychodiagnosis in Schizophrenia.* New York: Wiley,

6

Thematic Apperception Test

Adam Conklin and Drew Westen

INTRODUCTION

Since first being introduced over 60 years ago, the Thematic Apperception Test (TAT) has remained an important instrument in clinical training, testing, and personality research. Among projective tests, it is often cited as the second-most-widely used in clinical practice, behind only the Rorschach Inkblot Test. Time has tempered its developer's original claim that the test provides an "X-ray" of the "inner self." Instead, contemporary proponents of the TAT tend to make more circumscribed claims, asserting its utility and validity in assessing specific aspects of a person's personality and inner experience. These include core psychological conflicts, defenses, self-concept, and the expectations that guide behavior in interpersonal relationships.

As with other projective instruments, the utility of the test lies in its potential to reveal things about people of which they may not be conscious or which they would be reluctant to disclose directly: that is, to reveal implicit, or unconscious, processes. Also as with other projective tests, however, critics have raised questions about the reliability and validity of inferences made from TAT responses. They have noted that approaches to both administration and interpretation of the TAT have, in practice, lacked standardization, and they have pointed to the absence of comprehensive norms for scoring the TAT.

This chapter focuses on the uses of the TAT in psychological assessment. Its goal is to provide a sense of the strengths and limitations of the instrument as well as practical guidelines for its application in clinical settings. After reviewing the development of the TAT and debates about its utility, the chapter shifts to approaches to administration and interpretation of test data. As an illustration, we include a detailed presentation of a system for assessing social cognition and object relations (that is, the cognitive, affective, and motivational processes that underlie interpersonal functioning in intimate relationships) from TAT stories, applying it to the protocol of a patient hospitalized for anorexia. The conclusion provides a

Adam Conklin • Austen Riggs Center, Stockbridge, Massachusetts 01262   Drew Westen • Department of Psychology, Boston University, Boston, Massachusetts 02215

Understanding Psychological Assessment, edited by Dorfman and Hersen. Kluwer Academic/Plenum Publishers, New York, 2001.

summary of the main points of the chapter and suggests future directions for the clinical applications of the TAT.[1]

TEST CONSTRUCTION AND DEVELOPMENT

Origins and Early Development

Christiana Morgan and Henry A. Murray first introduced the TAT in an article that appeared in 1935. Murray and the staff of the Harvard Psychological Clinic published the current version of the test and the manual for its use in 1943. The test itself is composed of a series of ambiguous pictures, depicting a range of different human situations and settings. The task for the test subject is to create a story about what could be happening in each picture. In the manual, Murray notes that the purpose of the test is to reveal "some of the dominant drives, emotions, sentiments, complexes and conflicts of a personality," particularly those of which the person may be unaware.

Murray believed that given the relatively ambiguous nature of the TAT cards, subjects would have to draw on their own experience, wishes, and feelings in creating a story. This is what makes the TAT a *projective* test. The central premise behind the TAT is that in creating stories from ambiguous pictures that *constrain* but do not *determine* their responses, people will "fill in the gaps" between perception and narrative with many of the enduring expectations, fears, and desires that are activated in interpersonal situations in their daily lives, but that may not be available to introspection. (Importantly, this approach is consistent with recent advances in cognitive science which demonstrate that people's enduring schemas, networks of association, and so forth, typically influence their responses outside of awareness). Given that most subjects will have some experience with storytelling and creative writing, the task is also thought to be more intuitive and less anxiety provoking than many other tests.

Although contemporary practice has varied widely, Murray's original instructions called for administration of a standard sequence of a total of 20 cards on two days, with each session lasting approximately an hour. Based on the notion that subjects would more readily project relevant information about themselves in responding to pictures composed predominantly of characters of their own gender and approximate age, Murray and his colleagues developed specific sets of cards for men, women, boys, and girls. In all, the TAT includes 31 cards (30 black and white images and one blank card). The cards themselves are primarily composed of redrawn and reproduced images from paintings and photographs, as well as some original artwork. In investigating the origins of the images for the TAT, Wesley Morgan notes that, in several cases, details from the original artwork were omitted or made more vague to maximize ambiguity and provide the person with freer rein to express his or her own idiosyncratic responses. Little is known about the exact method that was used for selecting the final series of images for the TAT. Murray provides a very general description of a process that resulted in three revisions, in which subjects' responses were examined to assess the contribution of each card to the diagnosis the patient was given thorough a more thorough battery of tests and interviews. In fact, one of the limitations of the TAT is that the pictures do not appear to have been selected to cover a comprehensive range of human relationships or situations (e.g., three

---

[1]We focus in this chapter primarily on thematic apperceptive methods using Murray's original set of TAT cards. As is discussed further below, a number of alternative thematic apperception tests have been developed based on their own sets of cards and guidelines for scoring and interpretation. It is suggested that interested readers consult the texts by Groth-Marnat and Dana in the recommended readings for further information about these approaches.

cards with mothers, three with fathers, three depicting loss or death, three depicting friend-ship, three depicting sexual romance, etc.).

Murray's Approach to Scoring and Interpretation

Murray's system for scoring and interpreting the TAT developed out of the theory of personality presented in his 1938 text, *Explorations in Personality*. His main interest was in studying the core psychological "needs" of a person and how these internal motivational fac-tors interact with forces in the environment ("press") to shape personality and behavior. His approach to scoring begins with what he refers to in the manual as an examination of the "motives, trends, and feelings" of the "hero" in each TAT response. The hero is the character in the story with whom the test subject seems most strongly identified, typically the character around whom the plot revolves. Murray's reason for focusing on this character stems from his assumption that the test subject will project onto the hero her or his own qualities and world view. (The conditions under which this assumption is accurate are, however, unknown.)

In looking at the hero, Murray focuses primarily on the needs that emanate from the hero and the "press" he or she encounters in the environment. His system includes 28 different needs; among the better known examples, which have influenced subsequent research, are needs for achievement, affiliation, aggression, autonomy, and nurturance. Murray defines a press as a force in the environment that either supports or challenges a person. As manifested in the TAT, press has to do with the situations with which the hero is confronted in a given story. Murray identified 30 different types of press, half of which pertain to the needs of characters other than the hero. Typical examples would be another character's need for achieve-ment or for nurturance. Other types of press are attributes of the situation itself, such as an atmosphere of danger or an interpersonal encounter in which the hero is rejected by others. In terms of scoring, each TAT story is assessed for the presence of each type of need and press. Each need and press is then rated as to its strength using a 5-point scale.

Once needs and press have been scored, the next step is to examine the outcome of each story. This primarily involves looking at the balance between needs and press; the crucial question for Murray is whether the hero is successful in pursuing her or his needs. At this stage in interpretation, the psychologist identifies the most salient combinations of needs and press that the subject exhibits. These interactions between needs and press are then examined in relation to their outcomes, forming a unit of analysis Murray refers to as a *thema*. A simple example of a thema would be the hero's need for achievement going against the press of rejection by others, with the hero ultimately overcoming that rejection and succeeding. (This system, in many respects, foreshadowed not only psychotherapy research pioneered by Lester Luborsky on "core conflictual relationship themes" in the interpersonal narratives that pa-tients tell to therapists during psychotherapy, but also the script theory of Silvan Tomkins.) The final step in interpretation is to examine the ways different themas are related to each other. Among the virtues of Murray's system are its (a) grounding in both theory and empiri-cal observation based on hundreds of TAT responses; (b) recognition of the importance of recurrent cognitive-affective units that repetitively emerge in people's narratives; and (c) its attention to person x situation interactions.

Criticisms of the TAT

Although the TAT itself has endured, Murray's guidelines for its administration, scoring, and interpretation have not faired as well, in large part for pragmatic reasons: Murray's approach is very time consuming. As Bellak has noted, Murray's guidelines for administration and scoring require approximately two hours divided over two sessions to administer the test and an additional four to five hours to score and interpret the resulting 20-story protocol. Virtually all psychologists who use the TAT today employ significantly fewer cards than Murray recommended (typically no more than 8 to 10), often based on the particular characteristics of the patient being assessed or the referral question. Murray's system has also been hampered by the lack of comprehensive norms. It is also likely that the reliability of the approach diminishes substantially as the level of inference required increases in moving toward the final stages of interpretation.

Although many different systems for scoring and interpreting the TAT have been developed since Murray's, no comprehensive, empirically based scoring system has emerged. Further, a sharp divergence has traditionally existed between clinical and research approaches to scoring TAT responses. In the absence of a dominant system (similar to Exner's Comprehensive System for the Rorschach), many clinicians have eschewed formal methods of analysis for more qualitative and impressionistic approaches that focus on the interpretation of thematic content based on clinical experience and psychodynamic theories. Researchers, on the other hand, have tended to operationalize constructs, such as need for achievement and affiliation, more carefully, but these scoring systems have typically had little clinical utility. The resulting (and, unfortunately, enduring) lack of norms and standardization for the administration, scoring, and interpretation of the TAT has played a major role in the criticisms that have been leveled against it.

Critics of the TAT have questioned both the reliability and validity of TAT measures, such as measures of achievement motivation, which code the number of achievement themes that emerge in a protocol. Although interrater reliability has proven unproblematic with virtually all measures devised for TAT stories, estimates of internal consistency (such as coefficient alpha or split-half reliability) tend to be lower for measures of variables such as achievement motivation measured from TAT responses than from self-report questionnaires. The reasons for this, however, are a matter of contention. Whereas detractors have argued that this reflects instability of measurement, proponents challenge this interpretation on a number of grounds. For example, as Cramer and other proponents of the TAT have noted, measures of internal consistency are based on the assumption that the items of a test are relatively homogeneous—that is, that each item on a questionnaire, or correspondingly, each story a subject tells for any card, should optimally offer equivalent information. Cramer and others point out, however, that the cards for the TAT were designed to be *heterogeneous* and to test different areas of personality functioning. For this reason, themes and motives seen on one card—as well as the emotional tone of the associated story—would not be expected to emerge in the same way across cards. Further, as argued by Westen and colleagues, a major difference between self-reports and projective measures (such as the TAT) is that self-report measures capitalize on cognitive processes and self-consistency motives that bias estimates of internal consistency upwards. When a subject is asked to respond to a series of related items (e.g., "achievement is important to me," "I think it's important to succeed"), not only are answers processed using the same consciously activated self-representations, but the person is likely to notice and avoid obvious inconsistencies.

Critics have also questioned the validity of TAT-based measures, arguing that self-report instruments correlate more highly with outcomes and have greater predictive validity than TAT measures when applied to the same constructs. Along similar lines, they have argued that weak (or nil) correlations frequently reported between self-report measures and TAT measures of the same construct (such as need for power) provide evidence for the lack of convergent validity of TAT measures. However, in a watershed article published in 1989, McClelland, Koestner, and Weinberger addressed these criticisms in a theoretically and empirically straight-forward way. Based on a review of studies of motivation using both types of measures, they distinguished between *implicit motives* (assessed by the TAT) and *self-attributed motives* (assessed by self-report). A host of studies suggest that implicit motives tend to predict spontaneous behavior over the long term; whereas self-attributed motives are more predictive of choices made in specific situations in the short-term, when people's conscious attention is focused on their motivation. In other words, motives can be unconscious or conscious. Those that are unconscious tend to dominate behavior over the long run, whereas those that are conscious tend to control people's actions when their conscious motives are activated.

The distinction between implicit and self-attributed motives suggested by McClelland and his associates has received empirical support from two meta-analyses of research on achievement motivation conducted by Spangler. These analyses also provide support for the validity of TAT measures of achievement motivation—finding that they are actually more strongly correlated with outcomes than self-report measures. Additional evidence for the validity of TAT-based approaches to the study of motivation has also come from research on power and intimacy. Studies on motivation for intimacy by Dan McAdams and his colleagues have provided some particularly interesting and convincing examples. One study found that motivation for intimacy assessed by the TAT at age 30 predicted marital enjoyment 17 years later. Another study used beepers to page subjects at different points during the day to collect samples of spontaneous behavior. Subjects with high intimacy motivation assessed by the TAT were more likely to be thinking about others, to be engaged in conversations, and to be having positive feelings while with others than were subjects rated low in intimacy. As we will see, similar findings on validity have emerged from more clinically oriented TAT measures.

Assessing Clinical Constructs Using the TAT

In terms of research, one of the most productive applications of the TAT has been the work on motivation described above, particularly research on achievement motivation by David McClelland and John Atkinson and their colleagues. Hundreds of studies from this tradition have demonstrated that need for achievement assessed by the TAT predicts a broad range of outcomes cross-culturally, such as entrepreneurial success over many years in both the United States and India. Only recently, however, have researchers developed more clinically relevant measures with similarly solid evidence for reliability and validity. Here we briefly describe three approaches: Phebe Cramer's method for assessing defense mechanisms; Drew Westen and colleagues' system for evaluating social cognition and object relations; and Bellak's comprehensive system for scoring TAT responses.

Assessing Defenses

Defense mechanisms are unconscious affect regulation processes, which people employ to protect themselves from unpleasant feelings such as anxiety and guilt. From a cognitive perspective, they can be understood as aspects of procedural knowledge or as skills employed automatically and implicitly to regulate feeling states. Recent research by Phebe Cramer suggests that TAT stories can provide data for the reliable and valid assessment of at least a subset of defenses, including denial, projection, and identification. Denial, for example, involves a failure to acknowledge painful feelings or realities. According to Cramer, this defense can be exhibited in TAT responses in several ways, such as the omission of important objects depicted in a TAT card that most subjects find obvious or salient or the inclusion of statements of negation (such as "he is *not* feeling hurt").

Cramer's approach includes a detailed scoring manual for training raters. Acceptable internal consistency and split-half reliability, as well as good levels of interrater reliability, have been reported for the scoring system. Several studies support the validity of the measure. One large-scale study conducted by Cramer of children and adolescents ranging in age from 4 to 17 found predicted developmental differences in the use of defenses, providing support for her claim that defenses follow a developmental progression, with denial being least mature, identification being most mature, and projection occupying an intermediate position. Supporting the findings of numerous studies by Vaillant and colleagues that assess defenses from clinical interviews, other studies using Cramer's measure link defenses assessed from TAT stories to psychopathology. For example, a study by Hibbard and associates found that psychiatric inpatients were more likely to employ denial and projection, and were less likely to use identification, than were normal controls. Supporting the utility of the instrument in psychotherapy as a measure of personality change, Cramer and Blatt found that hospitalized patients who underwent approximately 15 months of intensive psychotherapy used defenses less often after treatment. This decrease in defense use was significantly correlated with reduction of symptoms and corresponding changes in object relations as assessed from Rorschach responses.

The Social Cognition and Object Relations Scale (SCORS)

Another approach to scoring TAT stories that has attempted to bring together research and clinical methods has been Westen and colleagues' system for assessing social cognition and object relations. Although object relations theorists have presented a number of different frameworks, their basic contention has been that mental representations of self and others that develop in childhood tend to endure and guide interpersonal behavior throughout the lifespan. According to Westen and others, the interpersonal nature of many of the TAT cards and the tendency of subjects to produce stories that include rich descriptions of characters and relationships make the TAT a particularly useful instrument for assessing representations of self and others and for assessing the cognitive, affective, and motivational processes subjects bring to bear on these representations in relationships. Westen and colleagues argue that TAT responses may be especially useful in capturing implicit "working representations"—representations activated under specific interpersonal circumstances that guide thought, feeling, and behavior in close relationships—rather than the conscious beliefs about the self and relationships that are more readily assessed by self-report.

Westen and colleagues' approach to scoring the TAT was derived from an integration of clinical observation, research, and theory pertaining to object relations and from studies of social-cognitive development. Although many clinicians and theorists have treated object relations as a unitary construct following a single line of development, Westen has pointed out that object relations actually subsumes a number of different processes and functions, each of which may have distinct developmental trajectories. To this end, the scoring system he and his colleagues developed assesses multiple dimensions. The earliest and most researched of these systems is SCORS.[2] The SCORS assesses four dimensions of object relations: (1) Complexity of Representations of People (the degree to which representations of people are rich, complex, and differentiated); (2) Affect-Tone of Relationship Paradigms (the degree to which relation-

---

[2]What follows is a brief description of the SCORS. In the section on scoring and interpretation below, we discuss the latest version of the scale (the SCORS-R) in greater detail.

ships are seen as benevolent or malevolent); (3) Emotional Investment in Relationships and Moral Standards (the degree to which a need-gratifying orientation toward others is maintained or transcended); and (4) Understanding of Social Causality (the degree to which attributions about social interactions are accurate and logical). Each dimension is rated using a 5-point scale. With the exception of Affect-Tone, each of these dimensions is thought to follow a developmental progression (with Level 1 being less mature than Level 2, and so forth).

The SCORS includes a detailed scoring manual and instructions for training raters. Research using the scale has consistently reported interrater reliability above .80 as assessed by both Pearson's r and the intraclass correlation coefficient. The internal consistency of the measure (as assessed by Cronbach's alpha) has also been strong, particularly for the more cognitive dimensions. Research by Westen and his colleagues, as well as by others, has demonstrated the validity of the SCORS in a number of different ways. SCORS variables correlate in predicted ways with well-validated research instruments (e.g., the Loevinger Sentence Completion Test and Weissman's Social Adjustment Scale) as well as with interviews assessing similar dimensions. Studies on reliably diagnosed adolescent and adult samples have successfully distinguished patients with borderline personality disorder from psychiatric and normal comparison subjects. A study by Porcerelli and his colleagues successfully used the Emotional Investment in Relationships and Morals dimension of the SCORS to differentiate among subjects classified as normal, sociopathic, or psychotic based on responses to the MMPI. Further research by Westen and colleagues on normal school-age children has found predicted developmental changes in object relations between second, fifth, ninth, and twelfth grades. Along similar lines, a study comparing adolescents and adults who have borderline personality disorder also showed predicted developmental differences. Other studies have found predicted associations between SCORS variables (particularly Affect-Tone of Relationship Paradigms) and childhood experiences, such as disrupted attachments, family instability (indexed by the number of times the family moved while the patient was a child), and sexual abuse.

Bellak's Approach

Whereas Cramer and Westen have developed systematic methods to assess specific clinically relevant constructs, others have attempted to produce more comprehensive approaches to clinical assessment with the TAT. A notable example is the work of Leopold Bellak. Bellak began working with the TAT in the early 1940s with Henry Murray. His text on thematic tests is now in its sixth edition (currently coauthored with David Abrams) and is one of the major references on the clinical use of the TAT. Bellak's approach builds on Murray and incorporates many of the insights of psychoanalytic ego psychology as well as findings from empirical research with the TAT. His goal has been to develop a system for the test that is as standardized and comprehensive as Exner's approach to the Rorschach. To this end, his method of interpretation includes assessment of ego functioning, dominant conflicts, defenses, object relations, and other clinically relevant variables. Although his approach is primarily qualitative and has not generated a large body of empirical research, it is also systematic, attempting to harness clinical inference in a reliable and valid way. Bellak's work will be considered further in the sections that follow.

Multicultural Assessment and the TAT

Before moving on to look at approaches to administering and scoring the TAT, it is important to note concerns that have been raised about the applicability of the test to non-Anglo-

American subjects. The ethnic and cultural homogeneity of the TAT as a stimulus is obvious, composed of cards exclusively depicting Anglo-American characters primarily placed in middle-class settings and situations. Efforts to adapt the test for subjects from other ethnic and cultural groups have typically involved the development of culture-specific cards. An early example was Thompson's modification of the skin color of Murray's original cards for use with African-Americans. More recently, researchers have attempted more thoroughgoing revision of the test stimuli, depicting characters of the testtaker's ethnicity and incorporating culturally relevant situations and settings. Although this is a daunting task, the best examples are the Themes Concerning Blacks (TCB) and the TEMAS (developed for assessment of Hispanic-American children and adolescents). As Dana has remarked, the TEMAS is also noteworthy in that limited norms exist for the test on different cultural groups.

Concerns about the applicability of the TAT in multicultural assessment go beyond the ethnic and cultural homogeneity of the test cards. Some psychologists, such as Dana, have noted that the majority of systems for scoring and interpreting the TAT are based on personality theory developed primarily through the study of Anglo-American and European subjects. This at least raises the possibility that these approaches have a Eurocentric bias that may fail to illuminate important aspects of personality valued by other cultural groups as well as potentially pathologizing what may be healthy and normative for other groups. In this respect, it is important for the examiner to be well acquainted with the full range of issues involved in multicultural testing.[3] In particular, authorities on cross-cultural testing have contended that any approach to interpretation should take into account the cultural belief system of the test taker. Bellak and Abrams also emphasize the importance of the tester having acquaintance with culturally normative responses for the TAT cards that are administered. Overall, these and other considerations suggest the need for caution in interpreting TAT responses from subjects or patients of varied cultural and ethnic backgrounds.

The development of culture-specific cards also raises the more general question of whether the over-50-year-old images from the TAT are fully adequate or appropriate for use on any population. Many of the images are undeniably anachronistic. Even Anglo-American subjects are likely to struggle to identify with them. Although the TAT depicts a range of different role relationships, these roles are not comprehensive and are not presented in a systematic way. Many authorities on the test have also noted the tendency of the cards to pull for negatively toned stories (and for some cards to be more negative than others). Thematic apperceptive methods would certainly be strengthened through development of a new set of cards that addresses these issues and includes empirically validated parallel forms for a range of different cultural and ethnic groups.[4]

ADMINISTRATION AND SCORING

Murray and others have emphasized that the setting in which the TAT is administered should be friendly and comfortable. The goal of the examiner is to develop a rapport with the subject that puts her or him at ease. Typically, cards are administered individually with the

---

[3]Dana's text on multicultural assessment in the recommended readings at the end of the chapter provides a detailed discussion of these issues. Bellak and Abrams (also referred to in the recommended readings) include a chapter on these issues as they pertain specifically to the TAT.

[4]There have been several attempts to create new sets of cards to address the general limitations of the existing images. Thus far, none of these has gained significant popularity. (For further information see Groth-Marnat in the recommended readings).

subject telling each story out loud.[5] (Murray's original guidelines call for the examiner to be seated behind the subject, as in a psychoanalytic session, although this is never done today.) In the 1943 manual, Murray provides the following general instructions to subjects:

> This is a test of imagination, one form of intelligence. I am going to show you some pictures, one at a time; and your task will be to make up as dramatic a story as you can for each. Tell what has led up to the event shown in the picture, describe what is happening at the moment, what the characters are feeling and thinking; and then give the outcome. Speak your thoughts as they come to your mind. Do you understand? Since you have 50 minutes for 10 pictures, you can devote about five minutes to each story. Here is the first picture.

Although testers vary in the way they present the task, as Groth-Marnat has emphasized, the most important instruction to subjects is to include the key elements of the story: *what is happening currently, what led up to the situation, what are the characters thinking and feeling, and how does it end?* Some (such as Bellak) have suggested as well that the TAT not be characterized to the subject as a "test of imagination." In many ways, the core elements of the simplified instructions that Murray provides for children, adults of lesser intelligence or education, and patients with psychotic disorders seem clearer and better-suited to the realities of contemporary administration of the test:

> This is a story-telling test. I have some pictures here that I am going to show you, and for each picture I want you to make up a story. Tell what has happened before and what is happening now. Say what the people are feeling and thinking and how it will come out. You can make up any kind of story you please.

Murray recommends that, after the subject has completed the first story, the test giver should provide some encouragement and remind the subject of the instructions if she or he deviated from them. Murray and others have advised intervening as little as possible as the subject responds to the remaining cards. Exceptions to this include prompting the subject if she or he omits one of the key elements of the story. In such cases, a brief prompt such as "*what led up to the situation?*" should be given. In clinical practice, most psychologists also probe any words or parts of the narrative they do not understand, to be certain they do not misinterpret the data. As with other psychological tests, testers also frequently obtain additional information by testing limits, as when a subject gives a "happily ever after" ending, and the tester encourages the subject to take another minute or two to finish the story with a more meaningful ending. Comments beyond this are to be avoided, though, because they may unduly affect the stories that the subject tells, inhibiting or overstructuring the process and curbing projection.

The examiner should write down, as close as possible, a verbatim record of the subject's response. Because stories often exceed 200 words, this can be challenging, frequently necessitating use of some form of shorthand notation, but with practice it is surprisingly easy. Some testers opt to tape-record responses (which is acceptable if done with the subject's consent), although this doubles the tester's processing time, since it requires listening to the subject's

---

[5]Some authorities on the TAT have allowed written administration of the test. Opinions on the differences between written and oral protocols have varied. Groth-Marnat has suggested that writing allows subjects to audit their responses which may result in stories that are more stereotypical (and therefore less informative). Others have contended that it makes little difference whether written or oral administration is used. The focus here is on oral administration because this is the way the test is routinely administered in clinical settings. It is also important to note that this more clinical and interpersonal approach to administration provides the examiner with valuable information about the subject's emotional and behavioral response to the task and reactions to the themes that emerge.

responses a second time. Testers should also note any significant pauses or emotional reactions the subject has to a card. Some have suggested further that timing the interval between the presentation of the card and the beginning of the response can provide valuable information about possible conflicts related to particular situations or themes.

As noted above, few clinicians use as many cards as Murray recommended, and most use either an idiosyncratic sequence or construct a card set for each individual patient. Bellak has been a strong proponent of the development of a standard sequence of TAT cards for use with both male and female subjects. He and David Abrams recommend using the following 10 cards: 1, 2, 3BM, 4, 6BM, 7GF, 8BM, 9GF, 10, and 13MF. These cards depict a range of characters and situations, including children and adults as well as relationships between peers, men and women, and what are often seen as family members. Bellak also leaves open the option of administering other cards to address specific issues after completing the standard sequence. As Bellak notes, a standard sequence is an important step toward making the development of norms and the meaningful quantification of scores possible. Use of a standard sequence also has the benefit of helping the new tester develop her or his own database of characteristic responses to a limited set of cards.

Authorities on the TAT have varied in their views about an inquiry phase for the test. Bellak and Abrams have recommended that any inquiry be done after all the cards have been administered (similar to contemporary practice with the Rorschach). Also, questions should not be leading or suggestive. Murray advised inquiring about sources of the subject's ideas and any free associations she or he may have about a response. Bellak and Abrams, as well as others, have suggested focusing on what is unusual or idiosyncratic about a response. It may also be useful to inquire into unexplained transitions or unlikely attributions the subject makes. Making such inquiries after the subject has told a story, or has completed the entire test, has the advantage of avoiding a tradeoff between standardization of administration and the need to obtain as much data as possible about the meaning of responses, which helps rein in testers' tendencies to make wild or highly speculative inferences.

As has already been noted, there is little consensus about which—if any—formal system for scoring the TAT should be used. We illustrate here how TAT responses can be used to assess social cognition and object relations, using Westen's system. Although this choice is somewhat arbitrary, we do so for several reasons (other than our own familiarity with it). Object relations theory is one of the dominant theoretical frameworks guiding contemporary psychodynamic clinical thinking, and a focus on interpersonal schemas and attributions is central to many cognitive-behavioral approaches as well. Just as the Rorschach can be used to assess many aspects of personality and psychopathology, but is arguably best suited to assessing perceptual and cognitive processes such as thought disorder (using measures such as Johnston and Holzman's Thought Disorder Index), the interpersonal nature of the TAT readily lends itself to an approach that focuses on the psychological processes activated in relationships.

The Social Cognition and Object Relations Scale–Revised (SCORS-R)

In the previous section we briefly described the Social Cognition and Object Relations Scale (SCORS) along with some of the evidence for its reliability and validity. Here we describe the latest version of the measure, the SCORS-R,[6] which assesses six dimensions:

---

[6]At this time information on the reliability and validity of the new version of the measure is not available. As noted below, however, the revised version of the SCORS is very similar to the original version, with most of the modifications made simply to render the instrument easier to use and to provide additional clinically relevant information, notably thematic content.

1. Complexity of Representations of People
2. Affect-Tone of Relationship Paradigms
3. Emotional Investment in Values and Moral Standards
4. Emotional Investment in Relationships
5. Understanding of Social Causality
6. Dominant Interpersonal Concerns

The Complexity, Affect-Tone, and Social Causality dimensions of the revised scale have been taken from the original SCORS with little modification. For the SCORS-R, the original "Investment in Relationships and Moral Standards" scale has been broken down into two dimensions, one focusing on relationships and the other on values and moral standards. Also, a dimension composed of 50 thematic items has been added to assess the dominant interpersonal fears, wishes, and concerns that recur in the individual's narratives. The first five dimensions of the SCORS-R are each assessed using a 7-point scale anchored at Levels 1, 3, 5, and 7 by specific scoring principles. Similarly to the original SCORS, each of these scales except Affect-Tone follows a developmental progression, with Level 1 being relatively immature and Level 7 being relatively mature. Dominant Interpersonal Concerns[7] are rated as to their frequency and intensity, also using a 7-point scale, and are ranked for their centrality in the protocol. An overview of the scales of the SCORS-R is provided in Table 6.1. In the next paragraph begins a brief description of each dimension.

Complexity of Representations of People

Object relations theorists have tended to agree about three aspects of the development of representations of the self and others. First, representations tend to become more *differentiated* from each other through development; that is, children become progressively better at distinguishing their own thoughts and feelings from those of others and can more readily understand different people's personalities and viewpoints. Second, representations become more *complex* as children develop more sophisticated views of others' subjectivity and personality and of the ways that personality dispositions interact with situations to lead to patterns of behavior, thought, or feeling. Finally, representations become more *integrated*. Whereas early in development children tend to have difficulty integrating representations that include seeming discrepancies or that combine elements with different affective valences (positive and negative), over time their representations become more integrated.

Thus, the Complexity of Representations dimension assesses the extent to which the person differentiates between the perspectives of self and others and appreciates the unique and complex dispositions and subjective experience of others. At the lowest level, people tend to be highly egocentric and unable to distinguish their own perspective from others. At somewhat higher levels, representations lack complexity, ranging from unidimensional to stereotypical. At the highest level, individuals are psychologically minded and able to recognize the subtleties of a person's personality and subjective experience.

Affect-Tone of Relationship Paradigms

Another important aspect of object relations, assessed by the Affect-Tone of Relationship Paradigms dimension of the SCORS-R, is the tendency to experience relationships as rela-

---

[7]The numbering system of the Dominant Interpersonal Concerns is, unlike the other 5 dimensions, completely arbitrary and not linked to any continuum of development or pathology.

Table 6.1. Dimensions of the SCORS-R

Score	Dimension
	Complexity of Representations of People
1	Representations of people are poorly differentiated from each other; person tends to be profoundly egocentric or embedded in own point of view.
3	Descriptions of people's personalities and internal states have little subtlety or complexity; descriptions may be simple, unidimensional, fluid, inconsistent, or poorly integrated; person may see people as all good or all bad.
5	Descriptions of people's personalities and internal states have some depth but are stereotypical.
7	Descriptions of people's personalities and mental states are rich and complex; the person is psychologically minded, attending to the subtleties of personality and subjective experience.
Score	**Affect-Tone of Relationship Paradigms**
1	Descriptions of people and relationships are grossly malevolent, with little hope of comfort or kindness between people.
3	Descriptions of people and relationships are unpleasant or hostile; people may feel painfully alone.
5	Descriptions of people and relationships have both positive and negative elements but overall have a slightly positive or hopeful tone.
7	On balance, people and relationships are experienced as positive and enriching.
	Note: where affective quality is bland or defensive (e.g., the person appends "happy endings" to stories), code 4; for ordinary malevolent responses to cards that draw malevolent responses (e.g., 13MF), code 3.
Score	**Emotional Investment in Relationships**
1	Expresses a need-gratifying orientation toward relationships; relationships appear interchangeable, unimportant in themselves, useful for self-soothing, highly tumultuous, or absent but not valued.
3	Descriptions of relationships are emotionally somewhat shallow; relationships may be continuous but lack depth or are based primarily on mutual participation in shared activity or mutual self-interest.
5	Descriptions of relationships demonstrate evidence of conventional concern, friendship, altruism, caretaking, or love.
7	Describes deep, committed relationships characterized by mutual sharing, interdependence, and respect.
	Note: where only one character is described and no relationship is depicted, code 2.
Score	**Emotional Investment in Values and Moral Standards**
1	Evidences a relative absence of moral values and concern for needs of others; may describe antisocial, manipulative, or aggressive acts without any sense of these actions as morally problematic.
3	Generally tries to avoid wrongdoing but has little genuine emotional investment in values, capacity for guilt, or heartfelt moral standards; moral concerns tend to focus on reward or punishment rather than fully internalized moral standards; may have childlike views of right and wrong or views of morality that appear unconventional but are largely self-serving; may view authority as arbitrary and illegitimate; may apply excessively harsh moral standards to the self or others.
5	Appears invested in moral values or social norms and to experience guilt for hurting other people or failing to meet moral standards; has conventional moral views and respect for authority figures.
7	Thinks about moral questions in a way that combines abstract thought, a willingness to challenge or question convention, *and* genuine compassion; appears committed both to abstract ideals and values *and* to concrete others.
	Note: where no moral concerns are raised by a particular story, code 4; where the person experiences the self as globally bad or evil for who s/he is rather than what s/he has done (i.e., for a specific deed), code 3.

Table 6.1. Continued

Score	Understanding of Social Causality
1	Explanations of people's behavior or narrative accounts of interpersonal events are highly unlikely, illogical, or distorted; the person does not appear to understand why people do what they do.
3	Explanations of people's behavior or narrative accounts are slightly confusing; descriptions of interpersonal events have minor logic errors, unexplained transitions, or idiosyncratic attributions; descriptions of people's thoughts and feelings may be slightly incongruent.
5	Narrative accounts are sensible and coherent; stories include a relatively complete plot and comprehensible explanations of the way people think, feel, and behave.
7	Narrative accounts of interpersonal events are particularly coherent and compelling.
	Note: where subject describes interpersonal events as if they just happen, with little sense of why people behave the way they do (i.e., alogical rather than illogical stories that seem to lack any causal understanding), or if the subject essentially provides a concrete description of the card with little or no story, code 2. For stories that are relatively straightforward and sensible but do not have complete narrative structure (e.g., a true ending), code 4.

Score	Dominant Interpersonal Concerns
1	Probably present, but not entirely clear.
3	Clearly present but neither particularly central to the story or subject nor idiosyncratic (e.g., authority conflicts on Card 1).
5	Clearly present and central to the action of the story.
7	Clearly central to understanding who the subject is or what s/he is struggling with; theme is unusual for the card, idiosyncratically elaborated, or obviously highly charged emotionally.
	Note: Rate each theme scored on each card using this 4-point scale; all other themes receive no score. A typical story will be rated for 1–3 themes.

tively benevolent or malevolent. Psychoanalytic writers such as Kernberg and Masterson have emphasized the importance of this dimension in patients with severe personality disorders, notably patients with borderline personality disorder, who often have highly malevolent expectations of relationships that can be activated under conditions such as separations or perceived rejection. The significance of this construct has been corroborated by social-cognitive research on the aggressive or malevolent attributions of aggressive boys, abusive parents, and many trauma survivors. This scale does not follow a developmental progression like most of the other dimensions of the SCORS-R; rather, it describes a continuum of ways a person can experience relationships. At lower levels, people's expectations and attributions range from grossly malevolent to hostile, empty, or absent. At higher levels, individuals expect relationships to be more positive and enriching.

Investment in Relationships

The ability to invest emotionally in relationships with others is another important dimension of object relations. Both object relations theorists and researchers studying developmental social cognition have noted that as children mature they tend to move beyond relationships based on the immediate gratification of needs to relationships that are reciprocal and involve genuine concern for others. The Investment in Relationships dimension of the SCORS-R charts signposts in this developmental progression. At the lowest level, others appear to be interchangeable and exist primarily for one's own self-soothing. At higher levels, relationships endure across time but are relatively conventional in degree of concern and intimacy. At the highest level, the individual is capable of deep commitment to others and can form relationships based on mutual sharing, interdependence, and respect.

Investment in Values and Moral Standards

Development of values and morals has been a central concern of both psychoanalysts and students of human development. The Emotional Investment in Values and Moral Standards dimension of the SCORS-R is based on an integration of these perspectives. Researchers and theorists working from each of these traditions have contended that development proceeds from behavior governed by external control (i.e., reward and punishment) to truly moral behavior governed by internalized controls. As assessed by the SCORS-R, individuals at the lowest levels display a relative lack of moral values and may commit antisocial or manipulative acts without moral concern. Somewhat further along this progression, individuals tend to avoid wrongdoing, but their focus is on avoiding punishment or obtaining rewards. At still higher levels, in which internalization of moral standards is more complete, individuals display an investment in moral standards and experience guilt if they violate internalized moral standards. Ultimately, at the highest levels, individuals can think abstractly and question convention in confronting complex moral situations. This highest level reflects research by Kohlberg on moral development; however, it is not scored for strictly intellectual, abstract, or philosophical musings that do not include a clear sense of compassion for others and an *emotional* wrestling with questions of how to balance the needs of the self and others.

Understanding of Social Causality

Another important dimension that affects people's ability to negotiate interpersonal relationships successfully is their understanding of social causality. Through development, the understanding of social causality tends to become more complex, logically coherent, and accurate. This dimension of the SCORS-R was derived in part from clinical observation of individuals with severe personality disorders, notably borderline personality disorder, who often make highly idiosyncratic, distorted, or illogical attributions regarding the intentions of others. At the lowest level, understanding of interpersonal behavior tends to be distorted or illogical, or to include highly unlikely causal attributions. At higher levels, people's understanding of their own and others' thoughts, feelings, and behavior becomes more accurate and logical, and their descriptions of people's actions show a greater congruence among thoughts, feelings, and actions. The major difference between this dimension of the SCORS-R and the original SCORS variable of the same name is that the current version does *not* code for complexity of attributions. The reason for the deletion of the complexity dimension from this variable was the unacceptably high correlation in virtually all studies between this variable and Complexity of Representations. Understanding of Social Causality now assesses exclusively the coherence, logic, and accuracy of attributions and of the overall narrative.

Dominant Interpersonal Concerns

The Dominant Interpersonal Concerns dimension of the SCORS-R is the newest dimension of the scale and is composed of 50 thematic items. Examples include themes of nurturance, friendship, dominance, rejection, victimization, and betrayal (see Appendix for complete list). These items were derived from a number of sources, including Murray's classification of motives, Erikson's theory of psychosocial development, Luborsky's work on core conflictual relationship themes, and contemporary research on interpersonal concerns. The themes have been tested for their comprehensiveness and nonredundancy through examining TAT protocols, Early Memories Test protocols, and clinical interviews.

Scoring

Scoring for the SCORS-R is relatively simple. Each story in a subject's protocol is scored for each of the first five dimensions using the guidelines summarized in Table 6.1. In addition, any theme present on any card is indicated and rated on the scoring sheet (see Appendix). For each of the first five dimensions, scores for each card are averaged to provide an overall level. For the Dominant Interpersonal Concerns, Westen and colleagues are currently experimenting with two scaling methods. The first is simply to sum the scores for each theme across all cards. The second is to rank-order the nine most prominent themes in the protocol, assigning a 7 to the three themes that appear most important, a 5 to the three that are next most important, and a 3 to the third most important set of three. The rest of the items are assigned a score of zero, unless the tester believes this misses significant information, in which case they can be assigned a value of 1 or 2. This second approach approximates a simplified Q-sort procedure, with a quasi-fixed distribution.

INTERPRETATIVE GUIDELINES

Before a clinical example is presented, several general guidelines for interpreting TAT responses should be outlined:

1. Interpretation is a process of hypothesis generation and hypothesis testing. Any hypothesis formed must be considered tentative and must be refined as it is supported or refuted by further information (from subsequent TAT responses as well as data from other tests administered). In general, it is not advisable to make claims based on one response to a test, unless that response is so salient and idiosyncratic (e.g., a suicide theme that is well elaborated and unusual) that the tester is relatively certain of its importance. Strong claims should be corroborated by multiple responses, similarly to the way scale scores on questionnaires are based on multiple items.

2. Interpreters since Murray have emphasized that what is unique or unusual about a subject's response generally yields more useful information than what is conventional or stereotypical. To know the difference, one often has to know the characteristic responses for different TAT cards. As many have noted, the cards are not as ambiguous as Murray had first contended. Different cards elicit different themes and particular emotional responses. For example, a story with prominent themes of anger and victimization in response to a card depicting a woman with her hands clenched around the neck of another woman (Card 18GF) is likely to mean something very different from a story that expresses similar themes in response to a card with a young boy looking at a violin (Card 1). In the absence of systematic norms for each of the cards, the description of typical responses in the texts by Groth-Marnat and by Bellak and Abrams provide helpful information (see recommended readings at the end of this chapter).

3. Interpretation involves careful scrutiny and scoring of each story, not just a cursory glance across a set of responses. Furthermore, as Bellak has noted, significant information is often gained by analyzing the sequence of responses. If a subject provides an emotionally

charged response to one card, is she able to regain her composure on the next? The answer can provide important information, not only about emotionally charged themes, but also about the person's ability to regulate her or his affects.

4. The TAT is not a diagnostic test, at least not in terms of the type of descriptive diagnosis presented in DSM-IV. It can provide important information that supports or strongly suggests a given diagnosis; however, to make a diagnosis, the tester usually needs to draw on information from clinical interviews, history, and other test data.

5. Predicting particular behaviors based on test data alone is a risky enterprise, whether the data are Rorschach responses or TAT stories. TAT stories filled with aggression are certainly meaningful; however, that alone cannot be used to predict how the person will behave in any given circumstance, because (a) most behavior reflects person x situation interactions, (b) most behaviors are multidetermined, and (c) the TAT represents a single stimulus situation, which does not typically allow prediction of the conditions under which the individual will behave aggressively, except insofar as particular themes or emotions are repetitively linked to aggressive responses.

CASE EXAMPLES

In this section, we present five stories from the TAT protocol of Ms. A, a 16-year-old hospitalized for anorexia. We focus on the SCORS-R for scoring and interpreting the protocol but will provide more general comments and hypotheses as well.

TAT Card 1

Ms. A's first response is to TAT Card 1, which depicts a boy sitting in front of a table that has a violin on it:

> The boy's parents made him take violin lessons, but he didn't want to. His parents just told him to go practice. He feels angry because he doesn't want to. So he just sits down and decides not to practice. Then his parents come in and they're angry because he's not practicing. So he starts practicing, but he doesn't like it. I guess that can be the end.

Scores for Card 1

Complexity: 3. The subject does not describe what the boy is like, other than in this specific situation, and only describes relatively superficial subjective experiences (feeling angry). Level 5 (stereotypical representations) is not scored here because the situation, not the people, is stereotypical; the characters themselves have no substance.

Affect-Tone: 3. This interaction is not extremely unpleasant (and hence does not score 1 for gross malevolence), but it is entirely negative. To receive a 4, the subject would have needed to include at least *some* mixture of positive and negative emotional tones, such as a sense that the child cared about what his parents felt or vice versa.

Investment in Relationships: 3. This story scores a 3 for a description of enduring relationships that are emotionally relatively shallow. The only relationship depicted is with the parents, which lacks depth.

Investment in Values and Morals: 3. The protagonist appears to have little investment in his parents' or any other particular moral standards and instead avoids disobedience primarily to escape punishment.

Social Causality: 4. This story is simple but sensible; the character at first resists his parents and then caves in under pressure. The plot is not well enough developed, however, to receive a 5, particularly because of its lack of a real ending; hence the default score of 4. There are no unexplained transitions or illogical features, which is why it does not receive a 3.

Dominant Interpersonal Concerns: d34, rated 3; d15, rated 1. The primary theme of the story is authority conflict (d34). This is, of course, a common theme for this card and would mean little if it did not recur within the protocol; hence a rating of 3. Item d15 (disappointed authorities) could also be given a rating of 1 (somewhat present), but it would not receive a rating beyond that because the parents are really more demanding of obedience than critical. The tester should be alert, however, to future instances in the protocol if they emerge. One would not score d25 (feeling misunderstood/lack of empathy) unless other indications suggest that this is the way the subject experiences the plight of the protagonist (as opposed to his simply being forced to meet parental demands, which is a normal intrusion on the life of a child).

Hypotheses

From a single card, all hypotheses are necessarily tentative, particularly given the strong pull of this particular card for stories of this sort. One would, however, wonder about oppositional trends, although this hypothesis could be easily discarded if the rest of the protocol did not bolster it.

TAT Card 3BM

The second response is for Card 3BM, which depicts a person lying on the floor leaning against a couch. Next to the person is what is often seen as a gun.

> The person was taken away to a concentration camp and one of his relatives was just killed, so he feels really sad that someone he loves is dead. Um...and he also feels sad because he thinks he's going to die . . . but he doesn't, because after a while, some troops come in to save him. (Why in a concentration camp?) Because it's World War II and he's a Jew in Germany. (What relative died?) I guess his wife maybe. (Any idea what this object is?) I thought it was a ring of keys. (How does that fit into the story?) I guess maybe that he had stolen them to get out of his cell, but they didn't work, so he's sad about that, too.

Scores for Card 3BM

Complexity: 4. The subject describes simple feeling states and provides, only with prompting, minimal identifying information about the character (a Jew in Nazi Germany). The response would receive a 3 for the very simple subjective life of the protagonist. It does not, however, reach a stereotypical level (5) because, even though the character is a Jew in Germany, he could be any Jew in Nazi Germany; nothing distinguishes his individuality, either in personality or internal states. Presence of descriptive material about a character typically brings a response to a rating of 4.

Affect-Tone: 3. The character is profoundly alone and threatened, but is saved by nonde-script troops. This is an ordinary malevolent response to Card 3BM and hence does not score for gross malevolence (1).

Investment in Relationships: 3. Once again, the subject describes enduring relationships that appear to be relatively shallow emotionally. The character is in part sad because someone he loves is dead; however, that someone does not appear to be specified in the subject's mind until the subject is specifically asked, and even then it remains hazy. The story is primarily about the character's being sad, imprisoned, and saved, with only secondary thought given to the interpersonal context. The subject appears to know that someone would feel sad if he lost a wife, but not to resonate with the feeling. This is now the second response that appears interpersonally shallow, and hence begins to build toward a hypothesis about the quality of this subject's emotional investments.

Investment in Values and Morals: 4. No items are applicable; hence a default score of 4. There is no real condemnation of the Nazis, which would bring it to a 5 for conventional morality, although the subject appears implicitly to believe what they did is wrong, or at least made people unhappy.

Social Causality: 4. Once again the story receives a 4 because it is relatively straightfor-ward but does not include much elaboration of the plot; the ending is again somewhat tacked on. It cannot be coded 5 or above because the subject was not operating from a well-articu-lated schema of the event of the story, as she required persistent prodding to produce it and showed little certainty about specifics.

Dominant Interpersonal Concerns: d12, rated 5; d44, rated 5; d20, rated 3. Themes of victimization (d12) and death of a significant other (d44) are clear in this story. A theme of rescue (d20) is also present, but not central to the story. One could score d24 (helplessness), but it would only receive a rating of 1 because this is not an angle with which the subject herself explicitly emphasizes.

Hypotheses

The subject has twice concluded negative stories with minimalist endings, suggesting, perhaps, an avoidant defensive style in which unpleasant feelings and experiences are simply wiped away. Both stories also have a depressive flavor, although again, given the nature of the stimuli, this should only be considered a weak hypothesis unless further evidence emerges in the rest of the protocol.

TAT Card 4

The next story is in response to Card 4 of the TAT, which depicts a woman holding the shoulder of a man who appears to be pulling away from her.

> Well, it's a married couple and...uh, a man comes in to take their home, but the man in the picture is angry, so he says, "Let me at him." But the woman doesn't want to see a fight so she tries to keep him back and says, "It won't do any good." So the man who came to their home leaves and says, "If you don't give me any money in a few days, I'll have to throw you out." (Why is the man taking their home?) Because they couldn't pay for it. (Who's

the man?) The man they borrowed money from to pay for the home, so I guess they're paying him back. (Why does the man leave and give them more time?) Maybe he feels sorry for them, or he'd rather have the money than throw them out and not have any money. (Why haven't they paid?) Because they don't have good enough jobs that they earn enough.

Scores for Card 4

Complexity: 3. The subject describes the interaction of the characters with plenty of dialog but offers little about their internal states or enduring dispositions, other than describing simple feeling states. If one tried to take these characters out of the story and imagine what they were like or imagine them in another situation, one would have a very difficult time forming a picture of them and their potential actions. This is a good indication that a rating of 3 is applicable. This has also been a pattern thus far in the subject's stories.

Affect-Tone: 3. The relationship with the landlord is clearly hostile. The subject does not say enough about the relationship between the spouses to score a 4 for mixed tone; that is, the only emotional tone in the story is negative. This is reinforced by the cynical alternative she offers as to why the man let them stay a little longer ("he'd rather have the money than throw them out and not have any money"). Clearly people do not seem very compassionate.

Investment in Relationships: 3. This story receives a 3 for the highest-level response the subject offers, namely a relatively shallow relationship between the spouses. Typically the highest level is scored unless the response is "spoiled" by an elaboration that makes clear something important about the subject's personality. The subject almost offered a higher-level response by having the landlord show some compassion (which would receive a rating of 5) but then spoiled it with "or he'd rather have the money than throw them out and not have any money." Once again the subject's story says little about the quality of the relationship between the characters, which is itself diagnostic. The couple appear primarily united by shared self-interest.

Investment in Values and Morals: 2. The subject describes, without moral commentary, a character who behaves aggressively without concern for others. In addition, the protagonists do not seem concerned about their failure to pay the rent. One could make a case for a rating of 5 (conventional moral concerns) in that the woman "doesn't want to see a fight," but the subject does not elaborate on why this is the case; she might simply be afraid that her husband will get hurt, rather than have any conventional moral qualms about fighting.

Social Causality: 4. Once again the subject provides a story with a relatively simple narrative structure and a half-ending.

Dominant Interpersonal Concerns: d12, rated 5; d39, rated 3. The main theme of the story is victimization (d12), although it is a relatively mild version because the exploitation is not life threatening or particularly harrowing; it is, however, threatening the protagonists' security in a serious way, which is why it would not simply be scored for aggression. An important point to note is that the subject added the element of victimization to a story that could have been told very differently (e.g., about a poor couple who could not pay the rent and a landlord who was trying to help out or who at least had compassion for their plight). The "let me at him" comment warrants a code of d39 (stereotyped sex roles), although it would only be rated a 3 because it is drawn by the stimulus and is very common with this card. The comment, on inquiry, about the couple not being able to pay the rent could lead to a score on d48 (frustrated by circumstance), although, like helplessness in the earlier response, it is only implicit and not central to the subject's understanding of the action of the story; this potential theme also only emerged in response to considerable (and perhaps excessive) inquiry on the part of the tester. Note that the subject could also easily have interjected issues around power and status (d09) but did not; a coder could *interpret* this story in terms of the efforts of the landlord to dominate the couple, but that would be projecting something into the story that the subject may not herself have intended.

Hypotheses

Once again, the lack of an ending to a negative story and the general sparseness of the response are striking given that the subject has an IQ in the 130s. This would suggest a fairly severe constriction of imagination, a more generalized cognitive and affective constriction, a lack of mental energy related to depression, or all of these.

TAT CARD 13MF

The fourth response is to TAT card 13MF, which depicts a man with his arm across his face covering his eyes. In the background there is a woman lying on her back on a bed.

> The man comes into the room and finds that the lady's dead. So he feels really sad. Then he leaves and goes to the police to find out who killed her. (What led up to it?) I guess the woman was sleeping, and someone came in and killed her. (Why?) Maybe it was rape. (Did the man in picture know the woman?) Probably her husband. (Did the killer know her?) No. (How does it end?) The police find the man who killed her and they put him in jail. The lady's husband is still sad. (What is he thinking?) "Oh, what happened? Who did this? And why?"

Scores for Card 13MF

Complexity: 3. Once again the character has minimal complexity. The subject only begins to elaborate on internal mental states (the "Oh, what happened" speech) after very extensive probing, and even then the internal states are simple and stereotypical. The language used to describe the man's subjectivity upon seeing his wife raped and murdered is remarkably child-like, especially given that the subject is a very bright 16-year-old.

Affect-Tone: 3. This is an ordinary malevolent response to this card and hence is rated 3. It could also arguably be rated 4 for defensive warding off of unpleasant material: The subject requires constant probing to produce a complete story, and this has not been the case in prior responses. This defensiveness is likely, however, to have as much to do with the sexual content as it does with the aggressive content, particularly as this has not been as much the case on prior cards, including 3BM.

Investment in Relationships: 4. The character "says the right things," and the subject offers stereotypic comments ("so he feels really sad") that indicate her knowledge about how people are supposed to feel in such circumstances, but the response shows a lack of depth of relationship. A man is sad about the death of an unspecified woman who only with inquiry becomes his wife. This is now a clear pattern in the protocol. If this character were less wooden and were clearly mourning for a specific other (rather than an initially unspecified "lady"), 5 would be an appropriate rating.

Investment in Values and Morals: 3. This response scores a 3 for "crime and punishment." The only moral theme in the story is that a man commits a rape and is punished. Not only was his punishment an afterthought, but the subject avoids any moral commentary, and the perpetrator experiences no moral emotions.

Social Causality: 4. Once again the subject provides a sensible but bare-bones outline of a story.

Dominant Interpersonal Concerns: d12, rated 5; d13, rated 4; d44, rated 5; d29, rated 3; d28, rated 2. This story is about victimization (wanton murder; d12), loss (d44), and sexual victimization (d13). All three themes are central to the story, although the rating on sexual victimization would be lowered slightly because it came out only on inquiry and may or may not have been central to the subject's underlying story schema. A secondary (but still clearly present) theme is that of punishment (d29), which is rated a 3 because it was clearly not central to the subject's "story schema" in creating the response and was only elicited after substantial inquiry. Sexual conflict (d28) is likely but not definite in the subject's uncharacteristically strong tendency to shut down on this card in comparison with previous responses; hence it would receive a rating of 2.

Hypotheses

The subject seems to distance herself from this card, both providing a very minimal story (even more so than her others), requiring a lot of probing, and then at the end describing the protagonist's subjectivity in a very emotionally distant, stilted way. This likely reflects her discomfort with the sexual content, which she only acknowledged in inquiry. It would be useful, however, to see her responses to other cards with sexual themes before drawing this conclusion. Unfortunately, the TAT cards themselves do not offer this kind of redundancy in content.

Card 7GF

The final response is to Card 7GF, which shows a girl sitting uncomfortably on the lap of a woman, who is usually seen as her mother, holding a doll:

> It's a little girl and her grandmother. Um, the girl is sad because one of her pets died, so she goes to her grandmother and the grandmother holds her and says not to cry and that it's okay to miss her pet, and she explains that she had pets that died, too, and it's really sad when it happens. The little girl's still sad and she wonders why it had to die. I guess the grandmother rocks her to sleep. (What led up to the pet dying?) I think old age. (What kind of pet?) A horse. (Why did the grandmother say not to cry?) Because she doesn't like seeing the little girl cry. (What is the grandmother feeling?) She feels sad because she had known the horse for a long time too, and she remembers how sad she was when she was little and pets died. (How does it end?) They have a funeral for the horse and the little girl still feels sad, but she learns to accept it.

Scores for Card 7GF

Complexity: 5. This response is substantially of a higher level on a number of dimensions. The image of the grandmother is fairly stereotypical, although it has a richness absent from the previous responses, including a richer sense of her subjectivity and her life history (thinking back to when she was a child). One could consider a rating of 6 for a complex subjective state because the granddaughter at the end experiences two contradictory emotions (sadness and acceptance); however, it is not entirely clear whether these are really simultaneous or are merely sequential, which is less developmentally advanced.

Affect-Tone: 5. The girl is consoled after a loss, leading to mixed affect tone. The grandmother is clearly comforting, and the little girl gradually mends her broken heart.

Investment in Relationships: 5. This response scores a 5 for the grandmother's conventional concern and considerable empathy for the little girl. The subject almost spoils the response, however, by turning the grandmother's empathy into egocentrism ("she had known the horse for a long time, too"), but having had a similar feeling in the past oneself can be a genuine source of empathy.

Investment in Values and Morals: 5. This response scores a 5 for the theme of the wise older figure and the girl's internalization of her grandmother's approach to loss. It could also receive a 5 for conventional moral concerns, as one could construe the grandmother as feeling that she is carrying out her conventional grandmotherly duties, although this is inferential and not necessarily immanent in the subject's response.

Social Causality: 5. Like the subject's other responses, this one lacks any gross causal problems. Unlike the others, however, it shows a much stronger ability to form a representation of a social situation and describe the action unfolding in a sensible and coherent way.

Dominant Interpersonal Concerns: d01, rated 5; d44, rated 5. The story is primarily about the loss of a loved one (a pet; d44) and the nurturance of the grandmother in response to this (d01). This is the first instance we have seen in the protocol of a positive interpersonal theme.

Hypotheses

The most striking aspect of this response is that the subject received much higher scores on every scale. Precisely why this is the case is unclear; it could be that something about mother-daughter or grandmother-daughter scenes activates higher-level functioning in this subject; alternatively, this card may not have appeared as gloomy to her as the other cards. In either case, it tells us something about the upper limits of her object-relational functioning. At the same time, one might wonder about a very idiosyncratic aspect of the subject's response, namely that she saw the woman as the girl's grandmother instead of mother. Although again, without further data one can only speculate, one hypothesis is that something about the subject's relationship with her own mother is conflictual and leads her to move away from either the closeness or the apparent tension depicted between the girl and the woman by skipping a generation.

Comment

This brief example of a protocol suggests some of the ways TAT responses can be coded for psychological dimensions such as social cognition and object relations. Two points about this example are worth noting. First, unlike most protocols, this one was unusual in that the scores across dimensions on each card tended to be highly correlated. In most studies to date, the more cognitive dimensions such as Complexity and Social Causality have been highly correlated with each other but not with more affective dimensions such as Affect-Tone. Correlations tend to be substantially lower between the cognitive and affective dimensions in developmental samples, where a child might, for example, provide a simplistic representation of the characters (e.g., 3 on Complexity) with shallow Emotional Investment (e.g., 2) but highly positive Affect-Tone (e.g., 6 or 7). Second, this is an abbreviated protocol, and it should be emphasized that five cards cannot provide a comprehensive portrait of an individual's personality, defensive style, object relations, and so forth. Nevertheless, if a report were written from these data alone, it would likely offer hypotheses such as the following (see also Table 6.2, which summarizes scoring of the protocol):

The patient tends to think about people in relatively simple ways. Her understanding of people's internal states, such as their emotions, is relatively underdeveloped for a young woman her age. The inferences she makes about people's actions are also relatively simple, but they tend to be accurate. Emotionally, her expectations of people and relationships tend to be negative but not malevolent; her world seems sad and empty interpersonally, but she does not expect gross abuse from relationships. Her capacity to invest in others tends to be relatively weak. She does not treat others simply as gratifiers of her needs, and she seems to understand what people feel in relationships, but she does not seem to have much depth in her capacity to invest in other people or in her ability to form intimate relationships. This likely relates in part to the constriction in her ability to get inside other people's heads and prob-

Table 6.2. Summary of SCORS-R scoring for Ms. A (including abbreviated listing of Dominant Interpersonal Concerns)

Scale	1	3BM	4	13MF	7GF	Mean
Complexity of Representations	3	4	3	3	5	**3.6**
Affect-Tone of Relationship Paradigms	3	3	3	3	5	**3.4**
Investment in Relationships	3	3	3	4	5	**3.6**
Investment in Values and Moral Standards	3	4	2	3	5	**3.4**
Social Causality	4	4	4	4	5	**4.2**

Dominant Interpersonal Concerns						Sum
d01. **Nurturance**					5	**5**
d12. **Victimization**		5	5	5		**15**
d13. **Sexual victimization**				4		**4**
d15. **Disappointed authorities**	1					**1**
d20. **Rescue**		3				**3**
d28. **Sexual conflict**				2		**2**
d29. **Punishment**				3		**3**
d34. **Authority conflicts**	3					**3**
d39. **Stereotyped sex roles**			3			**3**
d44. **Loss**		5		5	5	**15**

ably to think about her own mind as well. In terms of moral development, she appears to be someone who would not behave in aggressive or antisocial ways, although the extent to which she has well-developed internalized moral standards is unclear. To the extent that she does, her values appear relatively conventional. The major themes that recur in her narratives about interpersonal events focus on loss and on ways people hurt, aggress against, or victimize others.

More generally, the patient seems emotionally and cognitively constricted and somewhat depressed. To what extent her constriction reflects her currently depressed state or an enduring way of thinking and feeling is unclear. Given her high IQ, it is likely that the cognitive constriction seen in her responses is limited to the interpersonal realm, and that she will need considerable work in learning to look inward. She appears to be someone who shuts down in response to unpleasant feelings rather than dealing with them directly or lashing out.

SUMMARY

The goal of this chapter has been to provide a sense of the strengths and limitations of the TAT as well as guidelines for its application in clinical settings. Although criticisms have been raised about the psychometric properties of TAT scoring systems, a number of systematic approaches to scoring and interpreting the TAT have demonstrated adequate to high levels of both reliability and validity. Many of the problems raised by critics of the TAT have resulted from the lack of standardization in the way the instrument has been administered, scored, and interpreted in clinical settings. Future development of thematic apperceptive methods should address these issues. Nevertheless, the TAT is likely to remain—and, we believe, for solid reasons—important in personality assessment, particularly in the assessment of patterns of thought, feeling, and motivation in interpersonal functioning that may not always be readily accessible to introspection.

SUGGESTED READINGS

Bellak, L. & Abrams, D. (1997). *The TAT, the CAT, and the SAT in clinical use* (6th ed.). Boston: Allyn and Bacon.

Cramer, P. (1991). *The development of defense mechanisms.* New York: Springer-Verlag.

Cramer, P. (1996). *Storytelling, narrative, and the Thematic Apperception Test.* New York: Guilford Press.

Dana, R. H. (1993). *Multicultural assessment perspectives for professional psychology.* Boston: Allyn and Bacon.

Groth-Marnat, G. (1997). *Handbook of psychological assessment* (3rd ed.) . New York: Wiley.

McClelland, D. C., Koestner, R., & Weinberger, J. (1989). How do self-attributed and implicit motives differ? *Psychological Review, 96,* 690–702.

Murray, H. A. & The Staff of the Harvard Psychological Clinic. (1943). *Thematic Apperception Test manual.* Cambridge, MA: Harvard University Press.

Smith, C. P., Atkinson, J. W., McClelland, D. C., & Veroff, J. (Eds.). (1992). *Motivation and personality: Handbook of thematic content analysis.* New York: Cambridge University Press.

Westen, D. (1991a). Clinical assessment of object relations using the TAT. *Journal of Personality Assessment, 56,* 56–74.

Westen, D. (1991b). Social cognition and object relations. *Psychological Bulletin, 109,* 429–455.

Westen, D., Feit, A., & Zittel, C. (1999). Methodological issues in research using projective techniques. In P. C. Kendall, J. N. Butcher, & G. Holmbeck (Eds.), *Handbook of research methods in clinical psychology* (2nd ed.). New York: Wiley.

APPENDIX:
SCORING SHEET FOR THE SCORS-R (INCLUDING LISTING OF DOMINANT INTERPERSONAL CONCERNS)

Scale	Card									Mean
Complexity of Representations										
Affect-Tone of Relationship Paradigms										
Investment in Relationships										
Investment in Values and Moral Standards										
Social Causality										
Dominant Interpersonal Concerns										**Sum**
d01. **Nurturance**, dependence, trust, security, or mentorship, where the relationship is not between peers, and the experience is emotionally positive										
d02. **Emotional intimacy** or closeness between marital partners or lovers										
d03. **Sexual intimacy**, sexual desire, or romance										
d04. **Affiliation**, friendship, belongingness, or closeness with friends or family										
d05. **Mastery**, achievement, self-control, skill acquisition, or knowledge seeking (must be pleasurable to code)										
d06. **Autonomy**; self-assertion, independent thinking, or pleasure in behaving autonomously										
d07. **Admiration**, exhibition, recognition, sense of specialness, basking in acclaim, or having followers										
d08. **Identity**, self-definition, or reflecting upon or searching for one's place in the world										
d09. **Dominance**; striving for or struggling over power, control over others, status, or class										
d10. **Rejection**, abandonment, or being sent away										
d11. **Tumultuous relationships**										
d12. **Victimization**, gross exploitation, asymmetrical violence, severe verbal cruelty, deliberate infliction of harm, gross negligence, or physical abuse										

d13. **Sexual victimization**, rape, or sexual abuse										
d14. **Conflictual dependence** (such as overdependence, clinginess, or fear of commitment)										
d15. **Disappointed authorities**, critical parents, or characters who chronically worry about meeting high parental standards										
d16. **Loners**; depicts people who seem schizoid, unrelated, or unconcerned about their lack of connection to others										
d17. **Guilt** (moral guilt evoked by breaking a particular moral rule or standard; guilt must be explicit and tied to a particular deed)										
d18. **Self-loathing** or global badness of the self (sense of badness must be general, not tied to a particular action)										
d19. **Failure**, incompetence, inadequacy, or inferiority in comparison to others										
d20. **Rescue;** depicts characters who are rescued										
d21. **Fears** about safety, survival, or protection										
d22. **Competition**										
d23. **Sexual competition** (love triangles, competition for mates, etc.)										
d24. **Helplessness**										
d25. **Feeling misunderstood**; depicts people who feel that significant others misunderstand or do not respond empathically to them										
d26. **Loneliness**, isolation, or lack of meaningful relationships (must be distressing to the subject)										
d27. **Fear of losing self-control**, fear of one's own impulses, or disdain for others' acceptance of or submission to their own desires										
d28. **Sexual conflict** (e.g., preoccupation with, or avoidance of sexual themes; notable anxiety about sexual content)										
d29. **Punishment** or worry about being punished										
d30. **Harsh morality**; depicts characters who judge themselves or others very severely, who morally crusade, etc.										

d31. **Role reversal**											
d32. **Self-victimization** (not to be scored for suicide unless includes self-defeating or masochistic elements)											
d33. **Aggression**; depicts aggressive acts that fall short of victimization, or people struggling with aggressive impulses											
d34. **Authority conflicts**											
d35. **Conflicted identification** with a person or group											
d36. **Neglect**; depicts characters who are physically neglected, or whose basic needs for food, shelter, or clothing are unmet											
d37. **Low self-esteem**											
d38. **Shame**; depicts people who feel ashamed, humiliated, dishonored, or slighted											
d39. **Stereotyped sex roles**											
d40. **Concern about sexual orientation;** characters are concerned or confused about orientation											
d41. **Not belonging** , being an outcast, outsider, or scapegoat											
d42. **Sadism**, describes aggression with attitude of enjoyment or satisfaction											
d43. **Self-blaming**; attributes characters' misfortunes to their own enduring psychological traits or attributes											
d44. **Loss**; depicts characters who have lost, or fear losing, a significant other through death											
d45. **Suicide**											
d46. **Defectiveness**, handicap, or something being mentally or physically wrong											
d47. **Emptiness** or meaninglessness											
d48. **Frustrated by circumstance**; depicts characters who are frustrated or impeded by social circumstances that obstruct attainment of goals											
d49. **Betrayal**											
d50. **Resignation**; characters are resigned or fatalistic											

7

Sentence Completion Test

Michael I. Lah

INTRODUCTION

The term s*entence completion test* refers to a broad category of tests rather than to any one specific test. Use of sentence completion tests in psychology dates back to the very beginning of the discipline. Herman Ebbinghaus, who is primarily remembered for his pioneering work on human learning and memory, first used a sentence completion test as early as 1897 to assess the reasoning ability and intellectual capacity of school children in Germany. Alfred Binet and Theodore Simon later included a sentence completion test in their intelligence scale developed to assess intellectual deficits in children in France.

Another historical root of the sentence completion test is Carl Jung's use of the word association technique to study personality. Later researchers found use of a single stimulus word and subjects responding with a single word too limiting, however, and began to use phrases and parts of sentences to elicit responses. In the early part of this century, researchers used sentence completion instruments to study a variety of issues and groups of people. For example, sentence completion tests were developed to study normal college students, public works employees, emotional states of people, and the thought processes of senile and schizophrenic patients. From these early roots, a wide range of sentence completion tests has been developed over the years to assess various aspects of people's achievement, intelligence, and personality. In discussions of the clinical psychological assessment of an individual, however, mention of a sentence completion test most often refers to an instrument used to assess thoughts, feelings, and attitudes characteristic of a person's personality and relevant to his or her level of adjustment. In fact, sentence completion tests used for personality assessment are among the most frequently used psychological assessment instruments. (See Suggested Readings at the end of the chapter for several references.) It is this type of sentence completion test upon which this chapter will focus. Specifically, this chapter focuses on the *Rotter Incomplete Sentences Blank* (RISB), the most widely-used and researched standard sentence completion test currently available.

Michael I. Lah • Middletown, Connecticut 06457-6215

Understanding Psychological Assessment, edited by Dorfman and Hersen. Kluwer Academic/Plenum Publishers, New York, 2001.

TEST CONSTRUCTION AND DEVELOPMENT

The *Rotter Incomplete Sentences Blank* ("Rotter" is pronounced like the word "rotor") is a semistructured projective measure of adjustment. The instrument requires the subject to finish 40 sentences for which the first word or words are provided. It is assumed that an individual's statements about himself, his activities, and his relationships reflect his level of adjustment or maladjustment. The RISB was originally developed by Julian Rotter and colleagues with two goals in mind. First, it was developed in an attempt to standardize the sentence completion method for use with college populations. The thought was that a person's responses could be evaluated according to empirically derived scoring examples to obtain a total score that would provide an objective overall index of adjustment. This overall index of adjustment could be used as a screening method to identify students in need of therapy or counseling or to identify those students who should be observed for evidence of problems in their adjustment to campus and academic life.

The second goal of developing the RISB was to provide the clinician information of specific diagnostic value for treatment purposes. The RISB was designed so that it might save the clinician time by providing information useful for structuring initial interviews. Thus, the RISB elicits from the person statements about work and other activities, relationships with people, and other aspects of himself.

The RISB is a revision of an early experimental version of the instrument that was developed by Rotter and colleagues for use in Army Air Force convalescent hospitals. This early version was, in turn, adapted in part from several other versions of similar personality tests that had been used in army hospitals during and following World War II. Items were selected to elicit responses about a variety of content areas. Items were eliminated that tended to get stereotyped responses or that only got a narrow range of response. Further, the beginning sentence stems were kept generally short and unstructured based on early work that showed that these items provided the best responses. The sentence stems are either neutral or first-person.

After initial development of the RISB for college populations, Rotter and colleagues modified the RISB college form for use with nonstudent adults and high school students. The adult form of the RISB is identical to the college form except for two items where the wording is changed slightly. The high school form of the RISB has eight items that differ slightly from that of the college form. For example, the item "In high school" on the college form reads "In school" on the adult form and "In the lower grades" on the high school form.

The RISB was originally validated using groups of male and female college students at Ohio State University. Rotter and colleagues compared teacher ratings of adjustment to the overall adjustment scores obtained from the RISB. They found good support for using the RISB adjustment score to classify students as adjusted or maladjusted. They also evaluated RISB scores of a group of women rated as well adjusted and maladjusted by advanced graduate student clinicians and a group of male students who were self-referrals or had been referred to the campus psychological clinic for treatment. Again, they found good support for the RISB overall adjustment score as a means to correctly classify students.

In two more recent studies, validity of the RISB was again substantiated. In the first study, RISB scores for 120 university students (60 men and 60 women) were compared to those of 120 students (60 men and 60 women) who had sought help at the campus student mental health clinic. There was a highly significant difference between the RISB scores of the control and clinic samples in the predicted direction. In the second study, members of two fraternities and two sororities rated each other using a sociometric measure of adjustment. These ratings were then compared to RISB overall adjustment scores. The sociometric measure contained adjustment items that were designed to reflect different aspects of adjustment, aspects that would vary in the degree to which they correlated with overall adjustment. Some of the socio-metric items included assessed anxiety, self-acceptance, overall level of happiness, and sense of humor about oneself and life's problems. The results showed that students' sociometric scores were significantly related to the RISB overall adjustment scores. Readers are referred to the RISB Manual (see Suggested Readings), which provides an extensive review of a variety of studies that support the RISB's validity.

ADMINISTRATION AND SCORING

The RISB response sheet consists of 40 sentence stems that are presented on the front and back of a single sheet of white paper 8-1/2 by 11 inches. At the top of the front of the sheet is room for the person's name, age, and other identifying data. Below this are printed the in-structions, which tell the person to complete the items to express his or her feelings and to make a complete sentence. Subjects are instructed to try to complete each item. Space for fifteen of the items is on the front of the sheet, and the remaining twenty five items are on the back.

Administration of the RISB is relatively easy. The response sheet can merely be handed to the person. If desired, the administrator can briefly restate the instructions on the sheet. Some-times a person will ask if she must complete every item or do them in order. The person should be encouraged to try to do every item but, if she leaves a blank, she can proceed on to the other items and return later to any skipped items. If a person asks what she should say, one should state that there are no right or wrong answers and encourage her to do the best she can to complete every item with her true feelings. It is also helpful to remind people that there are more items on the back of the sheet. The average time to complete the RISB is about 20 min-utes; the range of times people take to complete it is about from 10 to 40 minutes.

Because administration of the RISB is easy, it can be administered by paraprofessional or nonprofessional staff. For example, the RISB is often given to new clients at campus or com-munity mental health clinics along with other initial paperwork. The RISB can also easily be administered to groups of individuals at one time.

Scoring

There are two main ways to use the data provided by the RISB. One way is to assign scores to each response using the objective scoring manuals to obtain a numerical Overall Adjustment Score. The second way to deal with the RISB data is to interpret or draw inferences from the content of the person's responses. Interpretation of subjects' responses will be dis-cussed in the next section of this chapter.

In using the objective scoring system, subjects' responses to the 40 sentence stems are scored for the presence or absence and the degree of conflict or maladjustment. Subjects' responses are scored by comparing them to the empirically derived scoring examples in the RISB Manual. Each response is scored on a scale from 0 (most positive) to 6 (most conflict), with a score of 3 being assigned to neutral responses that do not fall into one of the positive or conflict categories. *Positive* responses are those that express a healthy or hopeful frame of mind. Such responses include optimism, positive feelings about oneself or other people, statements of happy or enjoyable experiences, humorous responses, and so forth. *Conflict* responses are those that indicate an unhealthy or maladjusted frame of mind. Such responses include pessimism, hostility, hopelessness, mention of symptoms, personal fears or problems, statements of unhappy experiences, and so forth. *Neutral* responses are those that do not clearly fall into the positive or conflict categories. Such responses usually are simply descriptive, are common sayings or catch phrases, or are lacking in any personal reference. For example, in response to the item "People," completions such as "are great fun to be with," "are the cause of all that is evil on the earth," and "usually sleep eight hours at night" clearly reflect different frames of mind (positive, conflict, and neutral responses, respectively). Although exactly into which category a response falls is not always so easy to determine, the vast majority of responses are fairly easily scored. Items that are not completed or are only partially completed and do not provide a complete thought that can be evaluated are not scored. In addition to extensive lists of scoring examples, the RISB Manual provides general scoring principles for scoring subjects' responses and discusses scoring difficulties such as partial completions, unusually lengthy responses, and statements that are qualified or contain both positive and conflict elements. Although men's and women's responses often are similar, they cannot be scored using the same scoring examples. Therefore, separate sets of examples are provided for scoring men's and women's RISB protocols.

After all the items of an RISB protocol have been scored, the individual item scores are added together to obtain the total score for those items that were completed. If any items were left blank or not done with a scorable response, the total score for all completed items is prorated to obtain an Overall Adjustment Score that is comparable to those of other RISB protocols that have 40 completed items. For example, if a person left five items blank, the total score for the 35 completed items should be divided by 35 then multiplied by 40 to arrive at a prorated Overall Adjustment Score. With scores for 40 items ranging from 0 to 6, the Overall Adjustment Scores for the RISB can theoretically range from 0 to 240. In practice, however, the range of scores is usually from about 85 to 195. The RISB Manual provides normative data for college students. Currently no data are provided for adult or high school student norms.

For the objective scoring of items, the RISB Manual provides general scoring principles as well as numerous scoring examples for each item. Scoring of the completions does require some judgment on the part of the scorers, however. The reliability of scoring items has been found to be very good. The RISB Manual reviews the literature on interscorer reliability. Rotter and colleagues found 40 interscorer reliability coefficients reported in 31 different studies. A median reliability coefficient of .93 was found (range of .72 to .99). Usually it is relatively easy to obtain good interscorer reliability coefficients similar to those reported in the literature. More often, what may be problematic is preventing high or low scorer bias. High or low scorer bias is the tendency for someone to score items in one direction such as towards conflict (higher scores). For example, if one scorer of five protocols arrived at scores of 90, 110, 120, 140, and 150 and a second scorer arrived at scores of 96, 115, 128, 147, and 159, the correlation of their sets of scores would be very high (.99). There is a difference in their average scores of 7 points, however. When tested statistically, this difference would be significant and would indicate scorer bias. To prevent such an occurrence, scorers must try to closely follow the guidelines and scoring examples in the RISB Manual. Two other strategies help to improve scorer reliability. First, when one is having difficulty deciding into which scoring category a response falls (e.g., whether the response should be scored 4 or 5), one should not consistently chose the lower (or higher) score. Rather, when unsure of the scoring, alternate on difficult items, selecting the higher score one time, the lower the next time, and so forth. Second, it is helpful to score several RISB protocols in one sitting, which helps one keep the general scoring principles and specific scoring examples in mind. In addition, scoring the same item across several protocols can help improve scoring reliability. For example, scoring item one on several protocols, then scoring item two on all of them, and so forth can help scoring reliability.

INTERPRETIVE GUIDELINES

Although normative data are provided in the RISB Manual, Rotter and colleagues encourage users of the RISB to develop local norms for use of the objective scoring system with local populations of interest. For example, if one were using the RISB to screen students at a small private college, it would be more useful to know the average score and the range of scores for students at that college and perhaps at the college's student mental health service than to know the average score based on a variety of colleges and universities from across the nation. Similarly, someone in private practice who primarily sees educated, upper-middle-class clients would be interested in different normative data than a colleague working at a community mental health center in a large city or someone else working at a state psychiatric hospital.

In determining whether persons are adjusted or maladjusted, the RISB Manual reports that a cutoff score of 145 was found most efficient in correctly identifying a clinical and a control sample. The score of 145, however, does not guarantee that one will select the truly adjusted from the truly maladjusted, and this score should not be slavishly used. Again one's purpose and the specific population of interest should guide one in choosing a cutoff score. For example, if one were screening college students to select people to refer for guidance counseling, one might select a lower score, for example 135, to ensure that anyone who may be in need is identified and referred for further assessment or follow-up. For research purposes where one wanted to select relatively homogenous groups of adjusted or maladjusted subjects, one might use scores below 130 to select the "adjusted" group and scores above 155 to select the "maladjusted" group. The RISB Manual provides data on the percentage of clinical and control subjects correctly identified by RISB scores ranging from 125 to 160.

Whereas the numerical Overall Adjustment Score is useful for screening or some research purposes, in most clinical settings one is more interested in specific clinical and diagnostic information that can be obtained from a person's RISB responses. In fact, anecdotal evidence indicates that the RISB is most often used for this latter purpose. Whether the RISB is completed by itself, as part of intake paperwork before an initial interview, or as part of a battery of tests, the RISB can provide useful clinical information based on a *qualitative* analysis of the person's responses. The RISB Manual does not provide one specific method for clinical analysis or interpretation. One reason for this is that the RISB is used in such a wide variety of settings that it would be difficult to prescribe one method that would be useful in all settings. A second reason is that there is such a wide variety of theoretical orientations among clinicians that one method of interpretation would not be seen as appropriate for all. In addition, the clinician's training and experience play a role in determining how the material will be used.

Rotter and colleagues make a few general comments about interpreting the RISB. They note that a person's RISB completions can be interpreted at different levels of inference. They may be taken at face value on a literal level, at a common sense level, or at a much more symbolic, psychoanalytic level. Further, they note that the information provided by RISB completions primarily enables the clinician to analyze or interpret the *content* of the responses, what the person actually said in his or her completions. In addition, some *formal* aspects of the completions may contribute to one's interpretations. Formal aspects include such things as omissions, language use, spelling or grammar errors, the length of responses, handwriting, and erasures or crossed out words. The goal of interpretation is to arrive at an overall picture of the person and his thoughts and feelings about himself, his relationships with people, his life activities (e.g., work, school), his goals, and any problem areas. In addition, one may be interested in information about more enduring characteristics such as major needs, conflicts, defenses, attitudes, or patterns of behavior.

Following are some general guidelines to use in the interpretation of RISB protocols. First, one should read over the entire protocol to get an overall impression of the person. Does one come away with an overall sense that the person is being defensive, matter of fact, fairly candid? Does the person sound fairly well adjusted or is he or she expressing much conflict? Is there an overall mood or feeling tone of anxiety, depression, or something else?

The second step is to do a more detailed and careful review of each item. One should go item by item and note the specific content of each response, whether it is positive or reveals some conflict, and the specific nature of the conflict. Are specific emotions or problems mentioned? How common or unusual are the responses? During this careful analysis one should also note formal aspects of the completions that are noteworthy.

Third, one should review the items again and one's notes from step two and begin to look for certain themes or patterns between items and responses. For example, how frequently are certain topics or feelings mentioned, or is something conspicuously not mentioned? Is there a pattern of word or language use in association with certain RISB items? Are there patterns among items that have to do with similar content such as items that refer to people, one's family, achievement situations, worries, the past, or the future? Is there a pattern to items where the person tried to squeeze in very long responses in the space allowed? Conversely, is there a pattern to items that were completed with very brief responses or with flippant responses that suggest that the person was perhaps avoiding responding with his or her true feelings? Is there a pattern of items that were not completed?

Finally, one would try to integrate all one's thoughts and inferences into a coherent description of the individual. One would want to identify specific areas of adjustment or maladjustment as well as consistent themes that emerged. Of course, inferences and interpretations obtained from the RISB should be confirmed with other sources of data from other assessment instruments, interviews, background data, and so forth.

CASE EXAMPLE

The following case example illustrates clinical interpretation of a person's responses to the college form of the *Rotter Incomplete Sentences Blank*. The case concerns a female college student that completed the RISB as part of a series of group administrations to students at a small private college. A verbatim record of her responses is presented in Table 7.1. When her responses were scored using the objective scoring system, her total score was 157, which is more than a standard deviation above the norms for college students and which is similar to the scores of clinical samples reported in the literature. In addition, the content of her responses reveals considerable information that would be useful in a counseling or therapy situation. In the discussion that follows, the number of the item that is being discussed is noted in parentheses. Although all of the RISB item stems could not be reproduced, the reader should still be able to get a sense of how the person's responses are analyzed.

Table 7.1. Responses of a Female College Student to the *Rotter Incomplete Sentences Blank*[a]

Sentence Stem	Response
1. *I like . . .*	hairy chests.
2. *The happiest time . . .*	was when I won a pageant.
3. *I want to know . . .*	who I will marry.
4. *Back home . . .*	I don't get along with my sister.
5. *I regret . . .*	taking accounting.
6. *At bedtime . . .*	I go to sleep.
7. *Men . . .*	are snakes.
8. *The best . . .*	men are foreigners.
9. *What annoys me . . .*	men who screw around behind their girlfriends' backs.
10. *People . . .*	are generally moody.
11. *A mother . . .*	never gets along with her children.
12. *I feel . . .*	people aren't too honest.
13. *My greatest fear . . .*	is snakes.
14. *In high school . . .*	I was more innocent.
15. *I can't . . .*	stand business courses.
16. ———— *. . .*	aren't for me.
17. ———— *. . .*	I fell on a manhole.
18. ———— *. . .*	are frazzled.
19. ———— *. . .*	annoy me.
20. ———— *. . .*	from man-itis.
21. ———— *. . .*	my economics exam.
22. ———— *. . .*	stinks.
23. ———— *. . .*	is frizzled.
24. ———— *. . .*	excites me.
25. ———— *. . .*	money and a man who will spoil me.
26. ———— *. . .*	will be a full-time job.
27. ———— *. . .*	I am happy.
28. ———— *. . .*	I can't deal with my friends.
29. ———— *. . .*	when my dog was hit by a car and when I say [response left unfinished]
30. ———— *. . .*	economics.
31. ———— *. . .*	is bad in my major.
32. ———— *. . .*	obnoxious.
33. ———— *. . .*	I have is with accounting.
34. ———— *. . .*	I could travel every summer to foreign lands.
35. ———— *. . .*	thinks too much about my career.
36. ———— *. . .*	have a crush on my boss.
37. ———— *. . .*	want to enjoy life and not worry too much.
38. ———— *. . .*	is great fun.
39. ———— *. . .*	grades.
40. ———— *. . .*	gossip too much.

[a]The RISB sentence stems (in italics) are reproduced from the *Rotter Incomplete Sentences Blank* by Julian B. Rotter, copyright 1950, renewed 1978 by The Psychological Corporation. Reproduced by permission. All rights reserved. The sentence stems for items 16 through 40 are not reproduced here in order to protect the security and validity of the instrument. For the remaining item stems, readers are referred to the RISB form itself or the RISB Manual (Rotter, Lah, & Rafferty, 1992).

On initially reading over this person's responses, one gets the impression that this individual ("Kathy") is experiencing a lot of conflict in several areas of her life. Regarding some of the formal aspects of her completions, her responses are mostly short or moderate in length; on only two items (9; 29, referring to what pains her) did she have to squeeze in words to fit the space. Her responses are articulate, and there are no oddities in her language use. Her handwriting is legible, and only once did she cross out words (two) and then begin her response again. She appears quite candid in her comments, and she completed all forty items.

Regarding the content of Kathy's completions, she is experiencing conflict in several areas of her life. First, she appears unhappy with her academics. She regrets taking one of her courses (5) and mentions it a second time as being only trouble for her (33). She also hates her economics course (30) and failed an exam in that course (21). She goes on to state that she can't stand business courses (15) and feels that her school is bad in her chosen major (31). At the same time, her biggest worry is her grades (39). One wonders if some of the pressure she feels to get good grades comes from her father and his interest in her academics and future career (35). Another reflection on the degree of conflict she is experiencing in her academics is her general statement that reading stinks (22). With so much conflict surrounding her academics, one would want to explore with her how well she is doing academically as well as to discuss her chosen classes and major.

Another area of conflict is Kathy's relationships with men. Although she finds men attractive (1, 8), plans to marry (3, 26), and has a secret crush on her boss (36), she also has very strong negative feelings about men (7). One reason for this criticism of men may be that a current or recent boyfriend was unfaithful to her (9). Such a betrayal and being disappointed by other people (12) may point to why she is not as innocent as she once was (14). Based on her statement that she needs a man who will spoil her (25), one also would want to explore whether Kathy had some unrealistic hopes or expectations that contribute to her frustrations with men. Kathy is at least aware of some of her conflicts about men as indicated by her saying that she suffers from "man-itis" (20).

Besides men, other people do not appear to be much of a source of support or positive experiences for Kathy. She notes that people are moody (10), are not very honest (12), and that they annoy her (19). She also criticizes women as gossiping too much (40). She has some friends, but sometimes feels that she can't deal with them (28). In addition to other people, her family is a source of much conflict. Kathy notes that she does not get along with her sister (4), and we can infer that she also does not get along with her mother (11). Her father may be the person in her family with whom she best gets along, but she feels he is too concerned about her career (35), something she probably experiences as pressure to get good grades, a source of worry for her (39).

With so much conflict in her life, Kathy is experiencing considerable stress. She states that her nerves are frazzled (18) and that her mind is "frizzled" (23). She worries too much and is not enjoying life as much as she wants (37). She states that she is at her best when she is happy (27), but it seems that she probably is not happy very often. Rather, when given an opportunity to describe herself, she responds that she is very obnoxious (32). Although such a comment may have been made facetiously, Kathy made no other humorous comments in completing the RISB, so it seems likely that she was being serious. Such a comment also suggests that she may be fairly self-critical in general, something that would contribute to the stress and conflict that she experiences.

In light of so much conflict, what positive influences or coping strategies Kathy has is an important issue. Unfortunately, there appears to be little that is positive in her life. She does not like sports (16) or reading (22). She has friends but, as noted earlier, she sometimes cannot deal with them. In addition, her family of origin and other people appear mostly to be a source of conflict for her. Dancing appears to be one of the few positive outlets for her (38). In addition, her pet dog (if still alive) may be another positive thing for her (29). Despite so much conflict in her life, she appears to have some optimism and excitement about the future (24). Her coping strategies would be an important area for inquiry.

In summary, Kathy is a college student who is experiencing a considerable amount of conflict in her life. She appears to have much anger and she directs criticism at other people and at herself. Men, women, people in general, and her family all are sources of conflict and disappointment. The possibility that she expresses her anger and criticisms may explain why she perceives herself as "obnoxious." In addition to people, her academic life is problematic. Here too she is disappointed in her courses and her major and is unhappy and stressed. In a counseling or therapy setting one would have a wealth of information from Kathy's RISB completions to explore further with her. Although other interpretations are possible, the above discussion illustrates how one may gather considerable useful clinical information and hypotheses from a person's RISB responses.

SUMMARY

In this chapter, the sentence completion method of psychological assessment and, in particular, the *Rotter Incomplete Sentences Blank*, a semistructured projective measure of adjustment were introduced. The RISB is easily administered to individuals or groups, and the administration time is relatively short compared to most other psychological assessment instruments. One unique thing about the RISB is its objective scoring system that provides a numerical overall index of adjustment that can be used for screening or research purposes. In addition, the content of a respondent's sentence completions can be interpreted along with other thematic projective instruments to obtain useful clinical information about the individual. Finally, there is excellent research evidence in support of the validity of the RISB. The RISB and other sentence completion instruments have many advantages, and they fill a unique place in the continuum of psychological assessment instruments that are available to the clinician. The reader is encouraged to explore this useful and versatile assessment method.

SUGGESTED READINGS

Boyle, G. J. (1995). Review of the Rotter Incomplete Sentences Blank (2nd ed.). In J. C. Conoley & J. C. Impara (eds.), *The twelfth mental measurements yearbook* (pp. 880–882). Lincoln, NE: The Buros Institute of Mental Measurements.

Goldberg, P. A. (1965). A review of sentence completion methods in personality assessment. *Journal of Projective Techniques and Personality Assessment, 29,* 12–45.

Lah, M. I. (1989a). New validity, normative, and scoring data for the Rotter Incomplete Sentences Blank. *Journal of Personality Assessment, 53,* 607–620.

Lah, M. I. (1989b). Sentence completion tests. In C. S. Newmark (ed.), *Major psychological assessment instruments* (Vol. 2, pp. 133–163). Boston: Allyn & Bacon.

Lubin, R., Larsen, R. M., & Matarazzo, J. D. (1984). Patterns of psychological test usage in the United States: 1935–1982. *American Psychologist, 39,* 451–454.

McLellan, J. J. (1995). Review of the Rotter Incomplete Sentences Blank, 2nd ed. In J. C. Conoley & J. C. Impara (Eds.), *The twelfth mental measurements yearbook* (pp. 882–883). Lincoln, NE: The Buros Institute of Mental Measurements.

Piotrowski, C., & Keller, J. W. (1984). Psychodiagnostic testing in APA-approved clinical psychology programs. *Professional Psychology, 15,* 450–456.

Piotrowski, C., & Keller, J. W. (1989). Psychological testing in outpatient mental health facilities: A national study. *Professional Psychology, 20,* 423–425.

Rotter, J. B., Lah, M. I., & Rafferty, J. E. (1992). *Rotter Incomplete Sentences Blank Manual* (2nd ed.). San Antonio, TX: The Psychological Corporation.

Watkins, C. E., Jr. (1991). What have surveys taught us about the teaching and practice of psychological assessment? *Journal of Personality Assessment, 56,* 426–437.

Watson, R. I., Jr. (1978). The sentence completion method. In B. B. Wolman (Ed.), *Diagnosis of mental disorders: A handbook* (pp. 255–279). New York: Plenum Press.

8

The Minnesota Multiphasic Personality Inventory-2 (MMPI-2)

William I. Dorfman and Sean Leonard

INTRODUCTION

The Minnesota Multiphasic Personality Inventory (MMPI) is among the most widely used and best-researched assessment devices in clinical psychology, with over ten thousand studies addressing the test existing in the literature. Over the past 60 years it has been used in developing diagnostic, treatment, and occupational placement decisions, assessing personality structure, obtaining prognostic information, and detecting relative psychological strengths and weaknesses across a variety of clinical and normal populations. The purpose of this chapter is to provide the reader with an overview of the development, psychometric properties, and the clinical interpretation of the instrument, supplemented with a case study reflecting the application of the MMPI-2 in a psychiatric population.

TEST CONSTRUCTION AND DEVELOPMENT

MMPI

The original MMPI was developed in 1943 by Starke Hathaway and J. C. McKinley of the University of Minnesota Hospitals. Their goal was to design a reliable assessment device which would allow the clinician to assess progress and outcome in treatment and to diagnose and gauge the severity of pathology in their patients.

Their "empirical" method of test construction was unique at the time and was a significant departure from existing personality inventories. Historically, inventories were composed of lists of personality traits or symptoms which *theoretically* were thought to distinguish

William I. Dorfman and Sean Leonard • Center for Psychological Studies, Nova Southeastern University, Fort Lauderdale, Florida 33314.

Understanding Psychological Assessment, edited by Dorfman and Hersen. Kluwer Academic/Plenum Publishers, New York, 2001.

between pathological and normal individuals. Patients would endorse descriptors which they felt applied to them and based upon their self-report were diagnosed as having a particular disorder or personality style. While particular clusters of traits and test responses theoretically were predicted by the test author to differentiate between one diagnosis or personality type and another, they frequently did not. Also, these trait lists were obvious in terms of what they were measuring and their transparency allowed test takers to characterize themselves in any way they desired. It became quite clear that many individuals would not or could not describe themselves very objectively and that a different approach to personality test construction was needed which was less susceptible to defensiveness and distortion.

As an initial step in construction of the MMPI, based on empirical methods, Hathaway and McKinley collected a pool of over 1000 items from a variety of sources and reflecting a broad spectrum of symptoms, behaviors, medical problems, values, and attitudes. Once reduced to 504 items, the test was administered to several criterion groups of patients as well as to a large normal population consisting of relatives and visitors to the University of Minnesota Hospitals. Each clinical criterion group represented a distinct psychiatric subpopulation which had been assessed independently and was homogeneous and relatively pure in terms of diagnosis. Criterion groups included clinical subjects diagnosed and characterized with the labels "hypochondriasis," "depression," "psychopathic deviate," "paranoia," "psychasthenia," "schizophrenia," and "hypomania."

Those items which analysis reveal to actually differentiate statistically between specific reference groups, normals, and other clinical groups were included on the scales measuring that criterion group. In this way, MMPI scales of items were created which could be employed to differentially diagnose patients in the future. The authors later added two more scales, one labeled Masculinity-Femininity, the other labeled Social Introversion-Extroversion, bringing the total MMPI clinical scales to ten.

Four additional scales, referred to as the Validity Scales, were developed to address the problem of distortion and defensiveness in test-taking. A scale called "Cannot Say" simply measured the number of omitted items on the test; the "L scale" was designed to detect unsophisticated attempts by clients to present themselves in a favorable light; the "F scale" was constructed to identify deviant responses on the MMPI; and finally, the "K scale" was created to identify clinical defensiveness. The meanings of each of these scales will be described below.

Originally, Hathaway and McKinley expected that these scales could be considered as independent, with each scale measuring a different diagnosis. It was expected, for instance, that a client with hypochondria would receive an elevated score *only* on Hyponchondriasis (Hs), with other scales remaining within the normal range. It was soon discovered, however, that patients with a particular diagnosis obtained high scores not only on the relevant clinical scale, but on other scales as well.

While the developers set psychodiagnostic labeling as an important goal for the test, researchers over the years found that the MMPI performed poorly in this role. Rather than to yield a specific diagnosis (i.e., depression, hysteria, etc.), the test has been used to *describe* patients with characteristics, behaviors, symptoms, and traits that have been correlated with each scale in well over 10,000 studies over the past 50 years. For example, a client who received a high score on one or more scales would be best described *not* with the clinical label of the MMPI scale (i.e., psychopathic deviate), but with characteristics, symptoms, traits, and behaviors established in the literature as extra-test correlates that have become associated statistically with that scale. The meaning established over the years for individual scales as well as patterns of scale elevations are discussed later in the chapter.

MMPI-2

The normative group for the original MMPI is known as the "Minnesota Normals." These individuals were Caucasian with an average education of eight years and average age of 35; most of the women were housewives, and most of the men were blue-collar workers. This normative group certainly became less generalizable over the next several decades, and it was partially for this reason that researchers restandardized the normative sample in the late 1980s. Another consideration was that some of the items on the original MMPI were no longer in the popular lexicon, so that items had to be either omitted or rephrased. Finally, it is important to note that the domain of psychopathology has broadened significantly over the past fifty years, so that the MMPI had to consider issues such as substance abuse, eating disorders, post traumatic stress sequelae, and so on.

The MMPI-2 used a much more representative group of normals, which was obtained using 1980 national census data as a guide. The new normal comparison group, which was derived from the test results of 2,600 individuals in seven states, was therefore much more generalizable than the original MMPI on many demographic characteristics (e.g., ethnicity, educational and occupational background, marital status, etc.). The restandardization project also sought to retain as much of the core elements of the original MMPI as possible, which would allow for substantial research based on the original MMPI to be continued.

ADMINISTRATION AND SCORING

The MMPI-2 may be administered to patients who are eighteen years or older, and it has been estimated that the required reading level for the test is about the eighth grade level or higher. The test is available in several forms, including soft cover, hard cover, and audio-taped versions, each containing a total of 567 true-false items.

The MMPI-2 test booklet contains simple instructions explaining how to take the test, but the clinician should make certain that the client understands these instructions. Most clients will be able to complete the test without further assistance in about 60 to 90 minutes. It is recommended that the clinician provide no direct assistance to the client in interpreting meanings of specific items.

Currently there are no acceptable short-form substitutes for the MMPI-2, and attempts to find such measures for the MMPI were also largely unsuccessful. However, when time is short, it is possible to administer an abbreviated form of the MMPI-2 comprised of the first 370 items, which yields complete scores only for the basic clinical and validity scales.

The MMPI-2 can be hand-scored with templates provided by the test publisher or through computer scoring services available through NCS. Computerized scoring services are easy to use, save a great deal of time, minimize the potential for errors which are easily made during hand scoring, and yield printouts of test results which contain valuable but relatively uncommon scales. Special answer sheets published by NCS are available for this purpose and are sent and returned by mail. Online scoring and profile interpretation are also available through NCS.

After the raw scores are obtained, the first step in plotting the profile is to fill in the blanks on the bottom of the MMPI-2 profile forms with the corresponding scores for each scale. These blanks are located directly under each scale, along the row labeled "Raw Score." The second step involves adding K-corrections for scales 1, 4, 7, 8, and 9. Note that the K-corrections differ across these scales and that a conversion table exists for this purpose along the left-hand margin of the profile sheet. With this information, the clinician is able to complete the rows marked "K to be added" and "Raw Score with K." The third step is to plot the K-corrected raw score on the profile sheet. T-score equivalents are marked along the extreme left and right of the profile. For example, an examination of the profile sheet will reveal that a K-corrected raw score of 35 on Scale 8 corresponds to a T-score of 65.

The final step is to connect the dots. The plotting convention with the MMPI-2 is to connect the three validity scales (L, F, and K), and then connect the ten basic clinical scales. This produces separate validity and clinical profiles. Raw scores for each of the other MMPI-2 scales including the Harris-Lingoes, Content, and Supplementary scales, should be plotted on the relevant profile sheet in a similar fashion.

Description of the Scales

The Validity Scales

The validity scales are invaluable in gauging the test-taking attitude of the client as well as some demographic and personality characteristics. In the context of the MMPI, validity refers to the extent to which the client appears to have responded to test items openly and consistently. Therefore, validity is a primary concern in interpreting profiles; if the validity indices suggest that the client distorted information, exaggerated the self-report, or responded inconsistently to the test, then it is difficult or impossible to accurately interpret the test results. One of the strengths of the MMPI-2 is its inherent ability to provide the clinician with critical information about whether or not the client's profile allows for meaningful interpretation.

Cannot Say (?) Scale. The Cannot Say scale is simply the raw number of items that the client omitted or responded to with both true and false on the test. As the number of omissions becomes greater, so does the possibility that the profile is distorted and invalid. Omission of more than 30 items raises serious doubt about the value of the rest results. More than ten omissions should signal that the protocol be interpreted with caution. This problem may be remedied by asking the client to complete the omitted or ambiguous items.

L Scale. The L scale is designed to detect clients who are unwilling to admit to even minor faults; this is commonly referred to as the "Lie" scale, although this is an oversimplification of its role in MMPI-2 interpretation. The L scale was constructed because it was assumed that some clients may wish to represent themselves in an overly favorable light, either deliberately or unconsciously. Elevations on L suggest that the client is uninsightful, represents himself or herself as being above common human shortcomings, and is very moral and religious. Not surprisingly, these clients are viewed by others as overly conventional and unable to get along well with others.

Raw scores on L from zero to four (0-4) are indicative of a client who responded honestly to the test items and is sufficiently self-confident to freely admit to minor faults. Raw scores greater than four (4) are associated with increasing defensiveness or denial, lack of psychological sophistication, and limited insight into one's current situation. Extremely high scores on L may invalidate the profile and may even suggest that the test taker is simply lying about himself or herself and attempting to deceive the examiner.

F and Fb Scales. F (Infrequency Scale) and Fb (F Back) are essentially the same scale, except that F items are at the beginning of the test while Fb items begin at item 281 (there is some overlap, however). The Fb scale alerts the clinician to evaluate how deviantly the patient responds to the latter half of the test and helps in assessing test-taking attitudes on the Content and Supplementary scales. The F and Fb scales tap into peculiar experiences or beliefs which few normal people or even psychiatric patients endorse. F items were endorsed in the scorable direction by fewer than 10% of the standardization group.

Extremely high scores on F (T-score of 100 or greater) will in most cases indicate that the profile is invalid. Scores in this range may reflect a random, all-true, or all-false response set. However, such scores may also accurately reflect the presence of extreme, disabling psychopathology. More typically, a high F indicates an over-reported response set, where the client attempted to malinger or exaggerate or malinger psychopathology.

T-scores in the high range (between 80 and 99) may also be invalid, so other validity indicators should be checked. However, it is often the case that scores in this range reflect the true severity of the client's dysfunction; the clinician should be alerted to the possible presence of severe emotional problems or profound characterological disorders such as borderline or antisocial personality. In some cases, scores in this range indicate that the client was exaggerating his or her symptoms in an attempt to ensure that the clinician would take their condition seriously; this is known as a "plea for help."

T-Scores in the moderate range (between 65 and 79) suggest presence of bona fide psychopathology in the client. These clients may also be described as moody, dissatisfied, opinionated, restless, and somewhat unstable. The client may be unconventional in his or her attitudes and beliefs.

T-scores below 65 are associated with individuals who are functioning well and are not responding in a deviant manner. Very low scores may indicate that the client is overly conventional and conforming or that she or he attempted to appear in a very positive light.

K Scale. K is commonly referred to as the defensiveness scale, and it is similar to L in purpose except that it is more subtle. The original purpose of this scale was to correct for underreporting of psychopathology; early MMPI studies showed that in some cases the basic clinical scales alone would falsely identify a patient as "normal," so K, or a fraction of K, is added to scales 1, 4, 7, 8, and 9 to improve classification rates. These scales are now routinely plotted out as K-corrected. That is, defensiveness is corrected for, insuring a more accurate clinical profile. In addition to compensating for defensiveness, K also provides prognostic information and information on some relevant personality traits.

High scores on K (T-score of 65 and above) reflect sophisticated defensiveness, a tendency to respond in socially desirable ways, denial of problems, and inhibition of emotions. These clients are typically described as overly defensive and lacking in insight. Due to that lack of insight, clients who score high on K may be resistant to therapy or psychological interpretations of their problems.

Clients with moderate elevations on K (T-scores between 56 and 64) tend to minimize and overlook faults in themselves, their families, and their circumstances. These clients appear for treatment only because they are in acute distress. Clients who score low on K (T-scores between 41 to 55) are considered to be within normal limits and in possession of good ego-strength. These clients are usually considered to be good candidates for psychotherapy because of their capacity for insight and their ability to tolerate critical introspection. Low scores on K (T-scores between 35 and 40) suggest the client is openly conveying severe distress, pessimism, and the feeling that they are unable to handle their problems. Very low scores on K (T-score below 34) strongly indicate that the client is overreporting his or her distress, but it also may be that the client is suffering from great deterioration in his or her defenses.

Variable Response Inconsistency (VRIN) Scale. VRIN is a new scale added to the MMPI-2. VRIN helps detect whether the client responded consistently to items which are essentially the same in content. The VRIN scale is composed of 67 pairs of items scattered throughout the test, with similar or opposite content. It is expected that a client who attends to items and responds to them consistently will receive a low score on VRIN.

If VRIN is too high (T-score of 80 or higher), this indicates that the patient responded randomly to the test and that the clinician should consider the profile as invalid. VRIN can help clarify elevations on F. High scores on both of these scales would indicate profile invalidity, while high scores on F coupled with a moderate or low score on VRIN would point to either an accurate representation of disabling pathology or an organized attempt to exaggerate and over-report pathology.

True Response Inconsistency (TRIN) Scale. TRIN is composed of 23 paired items which are opposite in content; if a client is responding consistently, then he or she should respond "True" to one of the paired items and "False" to the other. In this way, TRIN clarifies a tendency to respond to items always in one direction (either true or false), regardless of the item content. Clients who tend answer in the true or false direction indiscriminately ("yea-sayers" or "nay-sayers," respectively) produce high T-scores on TRIN, typically above 80.

Validity Configurations

Now that the reader is familiar with the nature of the standard validity scales, it is appropriate to describe how the three scales work together. This task is relatively easy, because in practice there are three types of validity configurations which appear most commonly.

The most common configuration is referred to as the caret; it takes the shape of an "inverted V," and typically reflects an honest and valid profile. Here, L and K are in the moderate range (below a T-score of 50), while F is elevated (above a T-score of 65). This configuration suggests that the client is experiencing distress, which he or she admits, and indicates that the client would be amenable to psychological treatment. The client's defenses are somewhat compromised, and he or she may feel unprepared to handle the situation independently. Of course, as F becomes more elevated, so does the level of distress in the client.

With extreme elevations of F, especially when L and K are very low, the clinician should suspect overreporting or malingering. When F is greater than 100, while L and K are both below 50, the clinician should suspect that the client is exaggerating his or her distress, or "faking bad." However, note that extreme low scores on L and K are indicative of very compromised defenses and are commonly associated with correspondingly high elevations on F. Thus, such a validity configuration may in some cases accurately represent the critical breakdown of defenses and resulting psychopathology.

The validity configuration which is shaped like a "V", or an inverted caret, is often described as a defensive profile. Here, F is low (a T-score of about 50 or lower), but L and K are comparatively elevated (T-scores at about 65 or 70). These clients are invested in appearing normal. They may be seeking to appear normal for personal gain (such as in employee evaluations), or, they may be described as highly defensive individuals reluctant to acknowledge having any psychological problems or shortcomings. As L and K increase, while F remains low, it becomes more likely that the client is defensive and perhaps making a deliberate attempt to deny emotional problems and to appear in a very positive light.

The Basic Clinical Scales

Scale 1: Hypochondriasis. This scale is intended to differentiate hypochondriacs from normal individuals. All of the items are health-related, to include such areas as generalized aches and pains, gastrointestinal distress, and respiratory, vision, and sleep problems. Very high elevations on Scale 1 (T>80) suggest that the client is likely to have a long history of vague and nonspecific somatic complaints and has probably seen many medical doctors. Such clients may be resistant towards the idea that there is a psychological basis to their physical symptoms and tend to be frustrating to work with; they may be seen as a "help-rejecting complainers." These clients are described as immature, egocentric, and narcissistic, and they tend to rely on somatization and repression to cope with tension and conflicts. They lack insight into their tendency to use these complaints to control others, as well as to disguise hostility and resentment. In addition, the client may be sour, whiny, defeatist, cynical and struggling with frustrated dependency needs.

Scale 2: Depression. This scale taps into symptomatic depression, and it differs from most of the other basic clinical scales in that it tends to be more of a state than a trait measure. In other words, elevations on this scale are more sensitive to the client's immediate satisfaction and comfort in living and may fluctuate over time. Items on this scale tap into anhedonia, feelings of worthlessness, social withdrawal, despondency, psychomotor retardation, and concentration problems. Very high elevations on Scale 2 (T>80) indicate that the client may be severely depressed, withdrawn and introverted, overly self-critical, hopeless, and timid. These clients may also exhibit psychomotor retardation and may be indecisive. They tend to feel guilty, lack self-confidence, and feel pessimistic and hopeless. Very high scores on this scale have also been associated with suicidality. Moderate scores on Scale 2 (T between 60 and 80) reflect that the client may be mildly depressed, fretful, timid, cautious, and dissatisfied about themselves or their lives.

Scale 3: Hysteria. This scale taps into the classical definition of hysteria, which is the tendency to overly rely upon denial and repression and to experience stress through involuntary loss of sensory or motor functioning. Clients who score very high on scale 3 (T>80) tend to exhibit circumscribed somatic symptoms which develop and then remit suddenly. These clients deny emotional problems, lack insight into the cause of their symptoms, and tend to react to pressure and conflict by converting stress into physical complaints. Clients who score high on this scale (T between 60 and 80) tend to deny and repress impulses and may give the impression of being overly nice, naive, and Pollyanna-like. These clients prefer to deal with others on a superficial level and tend to feel extreme discomfort in situations which may elicit anger or require originality or self-assertion. These clients may be described by others as dramatic and manipulative.

Scale 4: Psychopathic Deviate. This scale surveys the client's tendency to be amoral and asocial, although it does not directly measure criminal tendencies. Rather, it is a gauge of the client's capacity to behave and think in accordance to conventionally upheld standards. Very high scores indicate radical rebelliousness which may reach destructive or criminal proportions, while low scores suggest strictly conventional behavior. Clients who score very high on scale 4 (T>80) tend to be described as rebellious, impulsive, irresponsible, demanding, careless, and emotionally unstable. They have poor adjustment to societal conventions, and it is not unusual for such clients to have extensive criminal histories, poor work histories, and unstable relationships. Thrill-seeking behavior is also common, as well as a tendency to become easily frustrated and consequently lash out towards others, at times violently. Sexual maladjustment, deviant sexual behavior, or both may also be present due to the client's lack of impulse control coupled with disregard for the rights of others. Unstable family relationships, marital strife, and perhaps domestic violence are correlates of very high scores on scale 4. High scores on scale 4 (T between 60 and 80) are indicative of a client who may operate according to unconventional standards. These individuals tend to be chronically dissatisfied with others, including their families, friends, and society in general. They tend to avoid intimacy or close interpersonal relationships and are prone to impulsive and thrill-seeking behavior, although these behaviors may not reach criminal proportions. Note, however, that well-educated individuals may score in this range, which is perhaps a function of intellectual skepticism or independent thinking.

Scale 5: Masculinity–Femininity. This scale was originally devised to identify homosexual clients, who were until relatively recently considered to be suffering from a psychological disorder. However, the current utility of scale 5 is that it detects gender-stereotyped interests and behaviors. In light of converging gender roles over the past several decades, it may be more useful to conceptualize scale 5 as measuring a client's tendency to either engage in active or passive behaviors. However, extreme scores on scale 5 may also indicate gender role or sexual orientation confusion which may warrant clinical attention. Females who score high on Scale 5 (T>80) are described as aggressive, vigorous, assertive, confident, and uninhibited. They may be described by others as unfriendly, unemotional, and rough. Corresponding high scores on this scale for men correlate with artistic and aesthetic interests, good judgment and common sense, and show effeminate interests and behaviors. In some cases, high scores for men may indicate sexual dysfunction, while high scores for female psychiatric inpatients may suggest psychotic disturbances. Low scores (T<40) for females suggest that the client is passive, submissive, highly constrictive, self-pitying, and fault-finding. Corresponding low scores for men have been correlated with a tendency to be "macho," with an overemphasis on physical strength and athletic prowess. Such men tend to avoid dealing with feelings and emotions and employ a stereotyped approach towards resolving problems; others may describe these men as being intellectually limited, crude, and unoriginal.

Scale 6: Paranoia. This scale measures paranoid ideation and behavior in the client, which may reach delusional proportions. Extreme scores (T>80) usually reflect a disabling level of pathology; these clients may have feelings of persecution and maltreatment, demonstrate delusions of reference, and may feel that they are being controlled by others. These clients may be psychotic, and the clinician should consider that the client may be suffering from a serious psychiatric illness. Clients who score high on this scale (T between 60 and 80) tend to project blame and hostility onto others and tend to be described as rigid, stubborn, touchy, and overly sensitive. They tend to brood a great deal and are resentful of others. High scores indicate that the client is probably suspicious, distrustful, rigid, and hypersensitive. These clients tend to express anger and resentment in an indirect manner.

Scale 7: Psychasthenia. Psychasthenia is a term which refers to what is currently known as obsessive-compulsive anxiety. It may be helpful to consider scale 7 as the psychological analogue to a fever: Most anyone with psychological discomfort will have at least a little Scale 7, because feeling compromised tends to induce anxiety. In this way, Scale 7 may best be considered as an overall indicator of psychological discomfort. In evaluating prognosis for psychotherapy, some elevation on Scale 7 may be desirable as this would indicate the client is in sufficient discomfort as to be motivated for positive change.

Extreme scores on scale 7 (T>80) usually indicate the presence of disabling anxiety; these clients tend to have an entrenched cycle of obsessing, which may reach disabling proportions. These clients may ruminate and obsess over their situation to the point where day-to-day tasks are overwhelming. Additionally, they are described as phobic, apprehensive, and dissatisfied. High scorers (T between 60 and 80) tend to worry excessively over minor problems, are overly self-critical, and may be indecisive, perfectionistic, and fearful of failure. These clients may rely heavily upon intellectualization and rationalization, which begins to fail them as 7 increases in elevation. They may become preoccupied with morality and religiosity and struggle in their interpersonal relationships. They are seen by others as being immature, shy, unassertive, dependent, and insecure.

Scale 8: Schizophrenia. This scale is comprised of items which reflect bizarre mentation, feelings of social alienation, unusual perceptual/sensorial experiences, and feelings of persecution. The reader will recognize that these themes are directly related to schizophrenic symptomatology, and very high elevations on this scale (T>80) tap into other common characteristics of individuals who suffer from this disorder, such as poor family relations, profound apathy, aberrant sexual behavior/ideation, concentration difficulties, impulse control problems, and an overall subjective feeling that life is stressful and overwhelming. Such clients may be disorganized or disoriented, and experiencing psychotic symptoms. High scores on scale 8 (T between 60 and 80) are indicative of schizoid mentation or at least social awkwardness. Such clients are perceived by others as socially introverted with poor social skills and tend to respond to internal and external stress by retreating into their very elaborate fantasy systems. They seem genuinely puzzled by what is expected of them in social situations and may often behave in eccentric or bizarre manners in social situations. These clients tend to have abstract interests, such as philosophy, religion, and science, and may be described as aloof and creative; this may be to the exclusion of more practical concerns, similar to the stereotype of the absent-minded intellectual.

Scale 9: Hypomania. This scale taps into the presence of manic or hypomanic symptoms in the client. However, scale 9 is sufficiently sensitive as to detect more diluted forms of manic symptoms, such as high energy levels, stimuli-seeking behaviors, impulsivity, and overreactivity. The secondary contribution of scale 9 to overall profile interpretation is that scale 9 may be considered the catalyst for other pathology detected on the profile; when scale 9 is elevated, the clinician may assume that other detected pathology is active and energized.

Very high scores on scale 9 (T>80) may indicate that the client is overactive, consistent with the diagnosis of mania: He or she may exhibit flight of ideas, pressured speech (including hostile joking), grandiosity, sleep disturbances, and accelerated psychomotor activity. These clients tend to be ambitious, zealous individuals who express an internal pressure to achieve, yet they tend to work in transient spurts. They may flare up belligerently when they feel obstructed or crossed, and their impulse control in this area is very limited. They may be overextended in their work and relationships, and in some cases they may be hypersexual. The clinician should expect that clients who score very high on scale 9 also have experienced depression; these clients are reluctant to slow down because they associate doing so with depression. High scorers on this scale (T between 60 and 80) are described as energetic and emotionally labile. They may respond to poorly to structured environments and may be described by others as narcissistic and grandiose.

Scale 0: Social Introversion. This scale is a rather gross but useful index of how comfortable a client feels in social situations. Clients who score very high on this scale (T>80) tend to be withdrawn, aloof, or anxious in social situations. These clients also tend to deny many impulses, temptations, and mental aberrations, but will report low self-esteem and feelings of interpersonal inadequacy. Clients who score high on this scale (T between 60 and 80) tend to be described as cold and distant and appear to prefer being alone over being with others. Such clients are likely to report that they have concern about their social introversion and are likely to be unassertive and overly compliant in their social interactions.

INTERPRETIVE GUIDELINES

Codetypes

A codetype is a way of describing the shape of the profile and summarizing the entire configuration by listing to the two or three highest clinical scales above a T-score of 65. The previous discussion of the basic clinical scales considered the case where only one clinical scale was elevated; this is known as a spiked profile (e.g., if Scale 4 has a T-score above 65 and all other scales have one below 65, then the resultant profile is called a "spike-4" profile). Over the past several decades, however, clinicians have found that they are able to increase the accuracy of their interpretations by examining codetypes. The discussion of codetypes that follows is not intended to be exhaustive, but does cover those codetypes which the clinician is most likely to encounter in clinical practice.

Codetypes are typically defined by identifying the two or three highest scales elevated above a T-score of 65. These scales are then coded from highest to lowest. For example, a profile which has scale 9 elevated at 80 and scale 4 elevated at 70, but all other scales below 65, would be described as a "9-4" codetype. However, when the two highest T-scores are within five points of one another, their order is interchangeable and the above profile would be described as 9-4/4-9.

Codetype 1-2/2-1

These clients have a tendency to react to stress with physiological symptoms rather than more useful emotional reactions. These clients often display medical symptoms and vague somatic complaints, such as gastrointestinal problems, abdominal pains, dizziness, headaches, insomnia, fatigue, and decreased sexual drive. They have a tendency to be passive, dependent, whiny, and easily frustrated. Such clients also tend to be passive, introverted, shy, hypersensitive, and insecure. In essence, these clients have a chronic somatizing personality. It is more common for women than men to score for this codetype. Clients with the 1-2/2-1 profile are anxious and depressed about their physiological symptoms and tend to be resistant to psychological explanations for their problems, especially when L and K are both elevated. These clients have typically consulted numerous physicians prior to presenting themselves for treatment with a psychologist, and over time their cluster of symptoms is likely to have been shaped by previous physicians.

This personality may have well have been set in childhood; clients with this profile tend to have been emotionally deprived in childhood, when they learned to express anger and attract attention from others through having multiple somatic problems. Close examination may reveal that the client's symptom presentation is similar or identical to an illness in a family member during childhood, and it is also likely that the client was dominated by his or her siblings during childhood.

Codetype 1-3/3-1

These clients are very similar to 1-2/2-1 clients except their tendency to somatize is more robust and entrenched. When scales 1 and 3 are both elevated, and scale 2 is in the subclinical range, the resultant configuration is referred to as the "conversion V" profile. These clients will present with one or more physical complaints, as they tend to convert emotional distress into physical symptoms. Common presenting symptoms include headaches, back pain, eating problems, fatigue, and sleeping dysfunction. The hallmark of this profile is that the client appears inappropriately content with his or her physical symptoms, described as "la belle indifference." These clients are suggestible and may respond to the traditional doctor-patient relationship by becoming overly dependent and passive. Such clients may be described by others as selfish, immature, insecure, needy, shallow, and superficial. They tend to seek out relationships where they will have their needs met through their expression of physical problems, yet simultaneously are uncomfortable in the dependency role; these clients are difficult to satisfy, and they will hold grudges and unexpressed hostility towards people who reject them. As with the 1-2/2-1 profile, 1-3/3-1 clients tend to be female more often than male.

It is common for these clients to report the death or loss of a parent during childhood. These clients may further report a childhood fraught with deprivation, neglect, and rejection. It is not uncommon for these clients to report having had strong, angry fathers, who withheld love and positive attention. As parents, these clients may adhere to strict parental values with an absence of consistent affections.

Codetype 2-3/3-2

Characteristics of this profile include depression, tension, physical weakness and fatigue, apathy, inadequacy, self-doubt, unexpressed emotions, and general overcontrol. These clients have learned to tolerate unhappiness, and while they are generally uncomfortable, the level of their pathology rarely reaches disabling proportions. Such clients tend to evoke supportive and caring feelings in others. It is much more common for women to obtain this codetype than it is for men, although clients of either gender with this codetype may report sexual dysfunction and feelings of social awkwardness and discomfort, especially in situations with those of the opposite gender. Men are less likely to report physical symptoms, but when they do they tend to be the result of chronic worry (e.g., ulcers). In essence, individuals with this codetype tend to have chronic problems, and so they have learned to tolerate ongoing feelings of dysphoria and lack of fulfillment.

A variation of this codetype is the 2-3-1/2-1-3 codetype. These clients almost invariably present first to a physician and are eventually referred to a mental health professional after no direct medical explanation for their symptoms can be detected. The hallmark of this profile is that the client will only report feeling depressed as a reaction to their physical illness, although they will often clearly evidence signs of depression. These clients may be confused by their own depressive behavior (e.g., "I don't know why I'm crying"). Clients with this profile may show signs of having a "smiling depression," where they present themselves as being in all ways normal and resilient except for feeling stress due to their illness. The key, however, is that the symptoms of the illness are actually psychological manifestations of negative affect. Therefore, these clients may elicit sympathy in others at first, but as their style becomes familiar they elicit increasing resentment. This may lead to the client feeling unappreciated and unloved; in parents, this may take the form of a sacrificing or near martyr-like style in their relationship with their children (e.g., "You'll appreciate me when I'm dead and gone").

These clients often come from disruptive childhood backgrounds. A history of physical abuse, sexual abuse, or both is not uncommon, as is a family history of alcohol problems. These clients learn to respond to internal aggression by using hysterical denial: "If I'm nice to everybody and give them what they want, then nobody will ever leave me." However, underlying this structure is deep-seated resentment and anger, which is being expressed in a passive-aggressive manner.

Codetype 2-4/4-2

This profile is characteristic of clients who present for treatment following problems with the legal system their families, or both. Essentially, this is the profile of someone who has just been "caught." Problems may include being arrested, being fired from a job for inappropriate behavior, having an extramarital relationship exposed, or being caught in a scheme to deceive or manipulate others. These clients are characteristically impulsive, and their inability to delay gratification coupled with their disregard for social conventions puts them at chronic risk for getting into trouble. They may abuse substances, especially alcohol, which further compromises their poor judgment. It is very rare for these clients to be self-referred for treatment. Rather, they are almost invariably ordered into treatment as a result of their reckless behavior. Such clients will typically present as if they are highly motivated for therapy, but they may use their involvement in therapy as proof to the courts or others that they feel guilty for their behavior and that they are making efforts to improve themselves. However, when the threat of punishment passes, the client will typically terminate treatment. When these clients are not in trouble, they tend to present themselves as charming, outgoing, and energetic individuals. Underneath this facade, the client likely feels insecure, inadequate, and incompetent. However, there is a strong tendency to "act out," which may be detected through the abuse of alcohol or drugs, frequent physical altercations, predatory sexual behavior, reckless parasuicidal behaviors, and in some cases actual suicide attempts.

Codetype 2-7/7-2

This is the most common profile encountered in clinical practice; it represents the mixture of depression and anxiety within the client. Manifestations may include nervousness, unhappiness, weakness, lack of initiative, and impoverished self-esteem coupled with poor self-confidence. These clients may present as pessimistic worriers, who are guilt-ridden, excessively self-blaming, and preoccupied with their personal deficiencies. It is not unusual for such clients to present with hypochondriacal tendencies and somatic complaints, especially cardiac symptoms, insomnia, and anorexia. These clients characteristically respond to frustration through self-blame and distorted guilt. They are particularly susceptible to a sudden accumulation of environmental stressors; these clients tend to be able to handle low levels of frustration and stress over time, but they lack the coping mechanisms to adapt to a sudden influx of responsibilities and challenges. In such situations, these clients respond by becoming anxious, depressed, clinging, and helpless.

Type 2-7/7-2 clients tend to be described as hyper-responsible and come from family backgrounds which were success-oriented. Men with this profile tend to overidentify with their fathers, who are perceived as being hard-working, self-controlled, responsible, and as consistent providers. For this reason, the 2-7/7-2 male often is characterized as the "perfect husband." These men also tend to report having significant ambivalence about their relationships with their father, which may be aggravated by the client perceiving his mother as perfectionistic and anxious. Their struggle to be perfect eventually yields flare ups of anxiety and depression.

Codetype 2-8/8-2

These clients are distrustful, keep others at a distance, and are afraid of emotional involvement. They tend towards withdrawal and dissociation and may present as confused, disoriented, and having concentration difficulties. They have very limited problem-solving abilities, which tend to be unoriginal and ineffective. They deny experiencing undesirable impulses, especially those pertaining to anger or sexuality, and may evidence dissociative episodes when these impulses are triggered. These clients are dependent and passive, but are irritable and resentful much of the time, especially when they feel they are not in control of their emotions. These clients are very sensitive to how others react to them and prefer to keep at an emotional distance from others to avoid being hurt. They will typically present with somatic complaints, such as dizziness, nausea, blackouts, and "spells," but will have little to no insight into the psychological nature of these symptoms. They are resistant to treatment, and are typically uncomfortable and suspicious in the therapeutic setting. They may present as having chronic, diffuse, disabling psychopathology, as excessively guilt-ridden, and with impoverished stream of thought and reduced speech. In extreme elevations, the 2-8/8-2 profile suggests psychotic features coupled with depression, consistent with bipolar or schizoaffective disorder. These clients are likely to be preoccupied with suicide and may have a well-constructed plan for carrying this out; special attention to suicidality is warranted.

Codetype 2-9/9-2

This profile may at first seem to be contradictory; the high 9 indicates high levels of energy, and the high 2 indicates depression. However, these clients tend to present with a high level of internal affective pressure, which may erupt as intense emotionality, tension, agitation, and abrupt mood changes. Such clients may be described as egocentric and narcissistic, and they may report feeling inadequate, incompetent, unsuccessful, and worthless. They tend to rapidly shift from topic to topic. They also may be impulsive, have poor judgment, and tend to externalize their depression. This may manifest in binge-drinking behaviors or similar substance use, but it is uncommon for these clients to be chronic substance abusers. Furthermore, it is not unusual for the 2-9 client to become aggressive when intoxicated and get into trouble for their behavior while under the influence of substances.

These clients have presentations which may be consistent with bipolar disorders, such as mania or hypomania. There is also some correspondence between this profile and organic disorders, such as temporal lobe epilepsy. In therapy, it may be revealed that these clients have extremely high expectations for themselves, and it is usually profitable to help the client adopt more realistic expectations that better reflect their situations.

Codetype 3-6/6-3

These clients are most often characterized as hysterical individuals who externalize blame onto others, are self-righteous, defensive, and perhaps paranoid to the point of being psychotic. In the 63 profile, with 6 significantly elevated (T > 80), the client is more likely to have psychotic features, which usually revolve around misinterpretations of other's motives, visual hallucinations, and unusual somatic preoccupations. Where 3 is higher than 6, psychotic features are less likely but the client tends to be overcontrolled, rigid, and demanding of others while being unwilling to recognize personal faults.

These clients tend to have significant difficulty expressing anger, and there is a high incidence of divorce. Temper outbursts usually occur after an accumulation of anger has reached a critical level for the client, and the subsequent eruption is highly self-righteous and rationalized. Type 3-6/6-3 women tend to be preoccupied with their physical appearance and impression management. It is not unusual for these women to have a mixed sexual history, beginning with being "boy-crazy" during adolescence and marrying right out of high school but leading conventional adult lifestyles. Their spouses may act out in some manner as a result of unrelenting pressure applied by the self-righteous 3-6/6-3 partner. Women often report a history of being a cheerleader or beauty pageant contestant. Their outward appearance matters a great deal to them in that it serves to define their social role, which is how they define themselves. These women are people-pleasers who may resort to seduction or flirtation to attract attention to themselves.

In 3-6/6-3 men, there is likely to be a history of an anxious, conflicted, overly controlled mother. These men do not tend to express resentment or criticism towards their mother, because of their considerable pride. However, careful examination may reveal that the father engaged in numerous indiscretions during the client's childhood.

Codetype 3-8/8-3

These clients tend to have peculiar if not bizarre experiences and may exhibit loose or even autistic thinking patterns. Their moods are intense but tend to fluctuate, and their affect is unstable and at times wildly inappropriate. Psychotic episodes may erupt quickly but dissipate when security is achieved; this codetype is the most likely to report visual hallucinations or very unusual illusions. Episodes of acute excitability are also characteristic of this profile, with demanding, agitated, restless, and short-tempered reactions. Cognitive slippage may be evident among these clients, and there is a tendency to "block" when responding to open-ended questions. Their thinking may include bizarre religious or sexual preoccupations; it is not unusual for these clients to have unusual sexual histories and to have sexual identity disturbances. They have unconventional, rigid, stereotyped ways of thinking and tend to emphasize their beliefs in an attempt to cover up their conflicted internal struggles.

These clients are likely to come from family systems that are very tumultuous; this is significant, as they have a poor tolerance for interpersonal conflict. They are seen as highly dependent upon family members, but deeply ambivalent towards them as well. They tend to be chronically conflicted between dependency and independence.

Codetype 4-6/6-4

This profile identifies angry, sullen clients who tend to blame others to excess. They are rigidly argumentative and difficult in social relationships and are frequently seen as obnoxious. Others may describe them as immature, egocentric, and narcissistic. The client may manifest a high degree of rationality while lacking warm and forgiving feelings. Symptoms are characterized by evasiveness, defensiveness about facing conflict, passive resistance, egocentrism, and an exaggerated need for affection. These clients may elicit feelings of annoyance in the clinician; they tend to make attempts to provoke the interviewer into becoming angry, which is a reaction they have come to expect in others. They also may manipulate others by placing high expectations on them, but resent any demands being placed on themselves. These clients may best be described as having a "chip on their shoulder."

There is often a history of considerable bitterness between the client and the same-sex parent. They tend to have romantic relationships which are fraught with conflict, and as with any client with an elevation on Scale 6, temper tantrums are likely.

Codetype 4-7/7-4

This configuration indicates both excessive insensitivity (Scale 4) and excessive concern about the effects of one's behaviors (Scale 7). There may be an extended episode where the client engages in selfish, impulsive, poorly thought-out behavior which causes considerable damage to others. During this period, the client appears to have little concern for social or legal restrictions and violates the feelings and wishes of others with little regard to the consequences. Binging behaviors, particularly those pertaining to alcohol and sexual promiscuity, are not uncommon. However, at the end of this episode clients will express guilt, remorse, and deep regret over their actions and may for a period seem overly controlled and contrite. While their conscious pangs may be severe, and even out of proportion to the actual behavioral deviations, the controls of these individuals do not appear to be effective in preventing further outbreaks.

It is common to find that these clients experienced inconsistent parenting; at times the parents were very indulgent and at other times very depriving. This may instill a sense of "take it when you can get it" in the client, which manifests in adulthood as having a poor ability to delay gratification. These clients tend to experience a constant state of tension and worry, which is only reduced through self-indulgent behaviors suggestive of immediate gratification needs.

Codetype 4-8/8-4

These clients are unpredictable and unusual in action and thought. Distrust is the most central characteristic trait for this profile and is demonstrated through alienation and interpersonal estrangement. These clients are difficult for others to understand and may be described as rapidly changing, hostile, resentful, and irritable. In women, this profile suggests a schizoid, unstable, acting-out client. Pregnancies from casual affairs are not uncommon, although these women do not often raise their own children, probably because of their deficient levels of empathy. Their core problem usually revolves around poor communication skills, low self-concepts, and over-or underreactivity to social situations. This profile is common among prostitutes. They fear emotional involvement and prefer to relate to others only on a sexual level. They tend to prefer being in relationships with men who are inadequate and unsuccessful; when in relationships with adequate partners, they tend to sabotage the relationship.

Men with this profile often break the law and act out in self-destructive ways. They may be seen as the "classic" psychopath who is introverted and leads a nomadic lifestyle. Their crimes or quasi-crimes are typically poorly planned and may be particularly vicious. These men may be sexual offenders, as there is a strong tendency to confuse sexuality with aggression.

The childhood history for these clients tends to be very disturbed and invalidating. In men, the relationship with the mother tends to be both seductive and undermining of self-esteem. The father is described as distant, although there is often a fear of punishment being inflicted by the father. In women, the relationship with the father is also seductive and ambivalent in nature, and it is not unusual for these women to report incest or sexual trauma from childhood. The daughter-mother relationship may be confusing to the client as a child, because the mother is seen as disorganized and avoidant of the client, as if something is wrong with her.

Codetype 4-9/9-4

This is the most common codetype for clients who are described as sociopathic. They are characteristically impulsive, overactive, irresponsible, socially shallow and superficial, have fluctuating morals and poor conscience development. This allows for freedom from anxiety, guilt, insecurity, and self-doubt. They are often very charming and socially acceptable on a superficial level, but over a long period of time they show fundamental unreliability, lack of judgment and control, neglect of obligations, and flagrant excesses in their search for pleasure and self-stimulation. As a result, they typically have few warm human relationships or life-long friendships, except with other 4-9/9-4 personalities. These clients do not seem to learn from past experiences and have profound difficulty delaying gratification. Thus, they tend to have difficulty with any challenge which requires sustained effort. These clients typically present for treatment when they are in trouble for their impulsive, selfish behaviors. This profile is the most likely to divorce, and the client may likely present in an attempt to undo behaviors which contributed to the deterioration of the relationship, although it is unlikely that the client genuinely regrets his or her behavior. It is also common for these clients to be court-ordered for therapy as a result of their behavior, and in such cases, it becomes increasingly likely that the client will attempt to manipulate and deceive the examiner in a self-serving manner. This codetype carries with it the worst prognosis for treatment of any codetype; fundamental changes in the personality structure are unlikely, and these clients are very likely to terminate treatment against clinical advice.

Codetype 6-8/8-6

This profile reflects a clear psychotic pattern in the client. Clients with this profile manifest such symptoms as bizarre paranoid delusions, suspiciousness, florid schizophrenic thought disturbances, auditory hallucinations, confusion, inappropriate and immature behavior, poor memory and concentration, shyness, withdrawal, and a flat, blunted, and inappropriate affect. Expression of anger may erupt suddenly and dissipate just as quickly, but is potentially dangerous; men with this codetype tend to be avid gun collectors who are overly immersed in and fascinated with brute force and violent displays of power.

These clients typically come from broken homes with unstable backgrounds. Sexuality tends to be confusing and deviant within these clients, and their is sometimes a history of incest, particularly with female clients.

Codetype 8-7/7-8

Although the characteristics of the 7-8 and 8-7 profile are similar, there are important differences dependent upon the relative scale elevations. In the 7-8 profile, the client is less likely to be psychotic and is perhaps fighting off psychotic decompensation. These clients tend to be obsessive-compulsive, anxious, and schizoid, but less bizarre than 8-7 clients. In 8-7 clients, psychotic symptoms tend to predominate, and there is greater reality distortion and inappropriate behavior. Other common symptoms include chronic worrying, nervousness, shyness, feelings of inadequacy, social awkwardness, detachment, and estrangement from others. These clients describe a life-long history of feeling as though they "do not fit in."

These clients were often treated as the "baby" in the family, and the family system tends to be described as chaotic and ambivalent towards the client as a child. There is a deep-seated struggle between dependency and independency, and these clients tend to have poor interpersonal relationships as adults.

Codetype 8-9/9-8

The 8-9/9-8 codetype is most commonly associated with clients who are demanding, hostile, hyperactive, circumstantial, and confused. Such clients may appear restless, hyperverbal, evasive, and high-strung. It is not unusual for individuals with this codetype to be religiously preoccupied or to suffer from paranoid and persecutory ideation. The clinician should be alert to the possibility that the client is in the midst of a manic or hypomanic episode, which may include symptoms such as flight of ideas, grandiosity, and boundless energy.

These clients tend to be perfectionistic and set unrealistic goals; when they fail to attain their goals, they may decompensate and subsequently seek treatment. Similarly, the 9-8 profile may indicate an "identity crisis," where the client feels worthless, unfulfilled, and diffusely agitated. Ambivalence surrounding sexual issues is not uncommon with this profile. In general, 8-9/9-8 clients tends to have a background of taking on more than they can handle and experience intense anxiety concerning success at school, work, and in other achievement-oriented environments. Such clients are overreactive to perceived failures and are highly competitive. It is common for these clients to complain of chronic resentment towards their spouse or romantic partner, although this resentment is not dealt with or expressed directly. They have family histories of strong sibling rivalry, and they may perceive one or both of their parents as having favored another sibling.

For high scorers, the 8-9/9-8 codetype is indicative of severe emotional problems. The most common diagnosis associated with this codetype is schizophrenia, and it is common for such clients to have impaired reality testing, difficulty thinking, disturbed consciousness, and psychotic symptomatology. For moderate scorers, this codetype suggests that the client is immature and self-oriented and tends to place high demands on others. They are easily hurt or frustrated by others and tend to be socially avoidant or to react with hostility towards those who disappoint them. Others may describe individuals with this codetype as boastful, loud, and emotionally unstable.

CONTENT INTERPRETATION

Thus far, this chapter has focused on the more traditional, empirical approach toward profile interpretation. Traditional MMPI interpretations do not focus on individual test items, but rather on how clients respond to sets or clusters of items overall. However, the actual content of items also reveals important information about the client, and several MMPI-2 scales have been developed for this purpose. The current trend in MMPI-2 interpretation is to consider responses to specific items as if they are self-reports made by the client. If a client is considered to be responding to the MMPI-2 in an open, frank manner, then the meaning of specific item content would also accurately reflect other areas of client functioning or malfunctioning which the client is willing to share with the examiner.

Harris-Lingoes Scales

The original MMPI scales were developed with little regard to the heterogeneity of test items within the scale. In other words, it is possible for two clients to obtain the same T-score on a given scale, even though they responded quite differently to the items which comprise the scale. Harris and Lingoes developed a set of subscales in an attempt to clarify the meanings of six of the clinical scales. They did not create such subscales for scales 5 and 0 because these scales have been considered to be separate from the standard clinical scales, and no subscales were created for scales 1 and 7 because the item content for these scales was considered to be homogeneous.

A summary of the Harris-Lingoes subscales is presented in Table 8.1. These scales were rationally derived and grouped together according to similarity in item content and theme. These subscales are particularly useful when the T-score on the corresponding "parent" clinical scale is between 65 and 80. The subscales help identify and clarify more specific problem areas pertaining to that scale and give information regarding why that parent scale is elevated. Generally, the Harris-Lingoes subscales should not be given serious weight when the parent scale's T-score is below 65.

Content Scales

The Content scales are a new addition in the MMPI-2, although they have their origins in the scales devised by Wiggins for the original MMPI. Butcher, Graham, Williams, and Ben-Porath developed these scales through a mixture of statistical and rational procedures. Potential content areas were identified based on the item content of the experimental version of the MMPI-2. Items which were found to be highly correlated with the specific content area were used in comprising the content scales; through statistical analyses, these items were found to be homogeneous in terms of their content. A description of the Content scales is presented in Table 8.2.

The T-scores for the Content scales are also uniform T-scores, similar to the standard clinical scales. Uniform T-scores allow meaningful comparisons to be made between these two sets of scales. The Content scales can also help the clinician clarify elevations on the standard scales by focusing on specific areas which represent problems for the client which he or she is willing to admit. Since there is no correction for defensiveness or exaggeration on these scales, they are susceptible to distortion.

Critical Items

Critical items are those items on the MMPI-2 which represent a summary of the patient's present emotional and psychological concerns. In other words, the clinician may benefit from consulting the critical items because they provide both information about client motivations for treatment and important diagnostic information. The critical items are face-valid and are clustered into content areas. When a client endorses a critical item in the deviant direction, the clinician may assume that the client suffers from discomfort in the corresponding content area. For example, a client who answers "False" to "I have never been in trouble with the law," the clinician is alerted to the possibility that the client may have a history of conduct problems or antisocial behavior.

Table 8.1. Harris-Lingoes Subscales

Subscale	Label	Interpretation of Clinical Elevations
D1	Subjective Depression	Feelings of obvious depression; hopelessness, anhedonia, despondency, worrying, unhappiness, fretting. Feels miserable, useless, lacking in self-confidence, inferior, easily hurt and overwhelmed.
D2	Psychomotor Retardation	Feelings of fatigue, lacking in energy, indecisiveness, slowness, lacking in initiative, difficulty making decisions, denial of anger or aggressive impulses.
D3	Physical Malfunctioning	Weakness, loss of appetite, weight fluctuations, GI complaints, overall feeling of being in poor health with little hope that one will ever improve.
D4	Mental Dullness	Feelings of being in a fog, or of losing one's mind; inferiority, easily gives up on tasks, indecisive; lacking in energy, difficulty starting and concentrating on tasks.
D5	Brooding	Feelings of personal worthlessness; ruminates, cries often; hypersensitive.
Hy1	Denial of Social Anxiety	Low scores indicate feelings of social awkwardness and introversion. High scores reflect denial of social inhibition, extroversion, naiveté, inappropriate social ebullience.
Hy2	Need for Affection	Places unearned and unqualified bust into others and denies malevolence in self and others; denies that others may be manipulative or deceptive, and trusts even strangers implicitly.
Hy3	Lassitude-Malaise	Feelings of victimization and of being overwhelmed; externalizes blame, especially through somatization.
Hy4	Somatic Complaints	Conversion symptoms and diffuse somatic complaints.
Hy5	Inhibition of Aggression	Denial of aggressive, assertive impulses. Responds dramatically to such behaviors in others.
Pd1	Familial Discord	Family situation (either past or present) feels antagonistic, loveless, fraught with arguing and criticism.
Pd2	Authority Problems	Opposition towards authority; history of conduct problems in school which are not necessarily indicative of problems in the present.
Pd3	Social Imperturbability	Absence of anxiety in group social settings; able to initiate conversations, although may be too forward, direct, or assertive.
Pd4	Social Alienation	Feels mistreated by others and the world in general; distrustful, somewhat cross, may feel paranoid.
Pd5	Self Alienation	Self-blaming filled with regret and guilt for one's past actions; tends to identify self as own worst enemy.
Pa1	Persecutory Ideas	Fells resentful, unfairly treated, misunderstood, condemned, punished unfairly. May also reflect frank paranoid ideation, such as being talked about, plotted against and so on.
Pa2	Poignancy	Sensitivity to criticism, thin-skinned; feels entitled to sympathy, and may be angry and resentful; usually manipulative in eliciting attention and sympathy from others.
Pa3	Naiveté	Denial of suspiciousness; believes that most people are of good intentions, and do not deliberately harm or take advantage of others. Employs dualistic morality—actions are "all" right or "all" wrong.
SC1	Social Alienation	Feelings of having been mistreated by others; believes that others are trying to sabotage or destroy them; avoids family members, friends, retreats away from social contact.
Sc2	Emotional Alienation	Feels condemned, miserable, with a poor outlook, as if life is a punishment. Has malignant relationships, where client and friend/family member derive pleasure from hurting and being hurt by one another.

(Continued)

Table 8.1. Continued

Subscale	Label	Interpretation of Clinical Elevations
Sc3	Lack of Ego Mastery, Cognitive	Feels that something is wrong with their mind; cognitive slippage may be evident, along with disturbances in memory, concentration, and comprehension.
Sc4	Lack of Ego Mastery, Conative	Feels unmotivated, and may retreat into fantasy because one cannot mobilize their energy.
SC5	Lack of Ego Mastery, Defective Inhibition	Episodes of impulsivity and restlessness, which may at times erupt into shocking and harmful outbursts. May react violently or aggressively with no warning.
Sc6	Bizarre Sensory Experiences	Unexplainable somatic experiences; pseudo-neurological problems; very bizarre conversion symptoms, and/or transient psychotic states.
Ma1	Amorality	Opportunistic, poorly developed morals, appreciates and sanctions behaviors where people take advantage of one another, particularly when such behaviors are clever and gotten away with.
Ma2	Psychomotor Acceleration	Presence of symptoms consistent with mania or hypomania, such restlessness, accelerated thinking impulsivity, thrill-seeking, boundless behaviors.
Ma3	Imperturbability	Socially impulsive in the absence of guilt or regret. May be overly assertive, selfish, outgoing, and unwilling to reciprocate socially appropriate gestures (e.g., returning favors).
Ma4	Ego Inflation	Extreme feelings of self-importance; expansive mood; may react irritably or stubbornly to demands made by others. Needs to feel appreciated.

SUPPLEMENTAL SCALE INTERPRETATION

This chapter has addressed the validity, basic clinical, Harris-Lingoes, and Content scales. However, over the years researchers have developed hundreds of additional scales for use with the MMPI. These scales are calculated without having to administer extra items; in other words, the clinician can derive scores for these scales by using the same answer sheet. These scales have been grouped into a category known as the "Supplemental scales," which as their name suggests, supplement profile interpretation with additional clinical information.

Over the years, and following the restandardization of the MMPI, several supplemental scales have stood out as being particularly useful in profile interpretation. Specific data regarding the construction, reliability, and validity of these scales is beyond the scope of this chapter. However, Table 8.3 summarizes the key elements and interpretive guidelines for several of the most common of the Supplemental scales.

Steps in Interpreting a Profile

The MMPI-2 profile offers the clinician a wide range of interpretive hypotheses which can be integrated with other tests, interview data, and background information. The following steps will assist the new user in understanding the most salient aspects of the profile and assist him or her in organizing the data in a meaningful way. The vast amount of data that the MMPI-2 can provide requires that only the most common interpretive strategies can be reviewed here. Interested readers are encouraged to consult the Suggested Readings list at the end of the chapter for a more complete description of the many strategies, interpretive hypotheses, and scales the MMPI-2 offers.

Table 8.2. Content Scales

Subscale	Label	Interpretation of Clinical Evaluations (T>65)
ANX	Anxiety	Report feelings of anxiety and nervousness; indecisiveness, difficulty making decisions and concentrating, feels tense and overwhelmed. May complain of insomnia or parasomnia, chest pains, shallow breathing. Not hopeful that things will get better.
FRS	Fears	Presence of specific fears which may reach phobic proportions (e.g., fear of heights, animals, etc.). Also, a more generalized tendency to be fearful in day to day life.
OBS	Obsessiveness	Considerable difficulty making decisions; excessive fretting and worrying, where compulsive behaviors may be present; lacks in self-confidence; ruminative, feels overwhelmed, inflexible, frightened by change.
DEP	Depression	General feelings of unhappiness, misery, despondency, hopelessness; anhedonia, unmotivated, lacking in energy, complains of fatigue, cry easily and are self-blaming; feel guilty and worthless; may complain that others are not supportive and appear to others to be demanding and resentful.
HEA	Health Concerns	Complains of multiple and diffuse health problems; feels to be in worse health than others; is preoccupied with their health and bodily functions.
BIZ	Bizarre Mentation	Psychotic symptoms (hallucinations) may be present; recognizes that he or she has unusual or peculiar thoughts; may feel persecuted or plotted against by others; may attribute supernatural powers to others or to self (e.g. mind-reading being on a mission from God, etc.).
ANG	Anger	Temper control problems are evident. Feels angry, hostile, and irritable much of the time. Tends to be easily provoked, and may lash out at others or objects, at times violently. Tends to be stubborn, impatient, and grouchy. May have history of physical assaultiveness.
CYN	Cynicism	Distrust in the motives of others; sees others as manipulative, dishonest, selfish, and insensitive. Looks for hidden agendas in benevolent acts by others; tend to be unfriendly and unpleasant, and overly guarded and defensive in relationships.
ASP	Antisocial Practices	Likely to have had history of conduct problems with the law or at school; shares the perspective on human nature as described in Cynicism; may actively engage in criminal or para-criminal behavior; derives pleasure from getting around rules or laws; tends to be angry, resentful of authority, and unconstrained by social convention.
TPA	Type A	Hard working, competitive, success-driven, ambitious, fast-paced. Easily irritated by others, takes on more tasks than he or she can handle, may be critical and controlling in relationships.
LSE	Low Self-Esteem	Feels worthless, unlikable, incompetent, excessively self-critical and hyper-aware of their perceived faults and shortcomings; tend to be passive, indecisive, and hyper-sensitive to criticism or perceived rejection.
SOD	Social Discomfort	Extremely introverted; prefers to be alone over being with others; reclusive, avoids social situations, has solitary interests and hobbies, not likely to strike up conversations with others.
FAM	Family Problems	View family of origin and/or current family to be a source of considerable stress and discomfort; home life may be fraught with arguments, fighting, demeaning criticism; may feel strong animosity or even hatred towards family member(s) or spouse. May have a history of childhood abuse.
WRK	Work Interference	Reports feelings and problems which are likely to obstruct efficient work performance; may feel unsatisfied at current job, or complain that family is not supportive of their line of work. Feels incompetent or has poor self-confidence, and may complain of concentration difficulties and deficiency in initiative and self-motivation.
TRT	Negative Treatment	Resistant to change; does not feel that doctors can help them, or may feel that he or she doesn't need help; feeling uncomfortable discussing personal problems with others; tend to have poor judgment, little insight, and limited ability to solve problems.

Table 8.3. Supplemental Scales

Scale	Label	Interpretation of Clinical Elevations
A	Anxiety	Uncomfortable, poorly adjusted, nervous, unemotional distant, cold introverted inhibited, overcontrolled, overly compliant with authority and convention.
R	Repression	Passive, submissive, tends to internalize distress, deliberate, conventional.
Es	Ego Strength	Well-defended, good adjustment to stress, tolerant, self-confident, charming; may be manipulative, defiant towards authority, competitive, sarcastic.
MAC-R	MacAndrew Alcoholism-Revised	Likely to have substance abuse problems; sensation and thrill-seeking, assertive, extroverted, excitable, enjoys challenges.
O-H	Overcontrolled Hostility	Low scores indicate chronic tendency to be aggressive. High scores indicate less of a tendency to externalize or act out, although the client may react with inappropriate aggression when buttons are pushed; emotionally well-developed, responsible, high need to achieve.
Do	Dominance	Low scores reflect weakness or passivity during social situations; easily swayed by others, feels incompetent or inadequate in handling stress. High scores suggest the client is confident, resourceful can handle conflict and tension well and is assertive in such situations; feels competent and efficient, good problem solving capacity.
Re	Social Responsibility	Low scores indicate denial of personal culpability, shifty character, loose morals, and irresponsibility. High scores reflect clients who are dependable, accepts negative consequences to own behavior, holds self to high moral and ethical standards.
Mt	College Maladjustment	In college students, likely to have difficulty adapting to structure and expectations of college life. Tends to procrastinate, feels incompetent, somatizes, complains that life is stressful and overwhelming.

1. Assess the test-taking attitude of the examinee and the degree to which their profile is characterized by exaggeration of problems or by defensiveness. Evaluate Scales "?," L, F, K, VRIN, TRIN, and Fb.

2. Identify the 1 or 2 point code type which best summarizes the basic clinical profile. Consider those Clinical scales which are elevated above T-score of 65. A "well-defined" 2-point codetype is one in which both scales are above T-score 65 and the second highest scale is 5 or more T-score points above the third highest scale.

3. Identify all other Clinical scale elevations above T-score 65 which are not part of the 2-point code.

4. To further clarify the meaning of the Clinical scale elevations, assess the Harris-Lingoes subscales for those clinical scales that are above T-score 65. These content-oriented subscales help clarify the meaning of the "parent" Clinical scales most effectively when their elevations are between T-scores of 65 and 80. Do not interpret H-L subscales when the parent scale is below T-score of 65.

5. Interpret the MMPI-2 Content scales which are above T-score of 65. These scales best describe what examinees are freely admitting about themselves and are helpful in describing basic symptoms and problems.

6. Finally, examine the MMPI-2 Supplementary Scales and generate hypotheses which can add to, confirm, or raise questions about other inferences drawn from the data.

7. Integrate all relevant data from MMPI and non-MMPI sources, resolve inconsistencies created by contradictory data, and develop a coherent description of examinees, their difficulties, their diagnostic picture, and treatment implications.

CASE EXAMPLE

Mr. Ledger is a 34-year-old Caucasian, married male who has worked as a certified public accountant for over five years. He was referred for psychological evaluation and treatment by his attorney after he was placed on probation by the state CPA board for unprofessional and unethical conduct . In his initial evaluation, Mr. Ledger reports that he was fired from his accounting firm after he was accused of failing to manage his accounts responsibly and lying to his supervisor to cover up his neglectful behavior. He states that his prior employer also raised the suspicion that he may have been abusing drugs. The client acknowledges that he avoided dealing with problems in the accounts because he did not feel competent to solve the problems and lied to avoid being seen as inadequate and incompetent. He denies substance abuse, however.

Mr. Ledger's wife also interviewed, reported that she felt her husband often handled problems by avoidance and procrastination. She related that after being married for one year she discovered a year's worth of unpaid credit card bills hidden in their closet. Faced with mounting bills and no money, Mr. Ledger decided simply to hide the disturbing reminders. She reported that this type of behavior caused much conflict in their marriage.

The client denied any prior psychiatric or criminal history.

The MMPI-2 was administered to the client as part of a comprehensive clinical assessment and was completed by him in approximately one hour and forty-five minutes (see Figure 81. for results).

Test-Taking Attitude

Mr. Ledger competed the test in an average amount of time and produced an unremarkable validity pattern suggesting that he approached the test openly and honestly. He omitted only one item (?=1) which would have no influence on the validity of the profile. His L score (T=39) suggests that he responded frankly to items, manifesting a willingness to admit to minor faults and the absence of an attempt to present himself as overly virtuous and moral. His F scale (F=51) is average and suggests that he is reporting no deviant thinking or behavior characteristic of clients under stress. Fb (Fb=63) is also within normal limits and reflects the absence of highly deviant responding on the back half of the test. VRIN (VRIN=60) and TRIN (TRIN=64F) T scores suggest that the client responded to test items in a consistent manner and with no response set, respectively. Finally, Mr. Ledger's K score (K=47) is characteristic of clients who manifest a balance between openness and self defense and who are generally feeling positive about themselves and possess good ego strength. In summary, Mr. Ledger appears to be responding to the MMPI-2 in a frank and open manner with no evidence of attempts at defensiveness or exaggeration of problems. His profile appears valid and interpretable.

Clinical Scale Interpretation

Inspection of the clinical profile indicates that the three scales exceed the clinical cutoff of T=65: Scales 7, 4 and 6. Since there is no 7-4-6 three point code available in the MMPI-2 literature, the 7-4/4-7 two point code type is the best way to summarize the profile. Since there are more than 5 T score points separating the second highest (Pd T=74) from the third highest (Pa T=68) scale, we can conclude that this a well defined code type which should yield a reliable and valid description of the client.

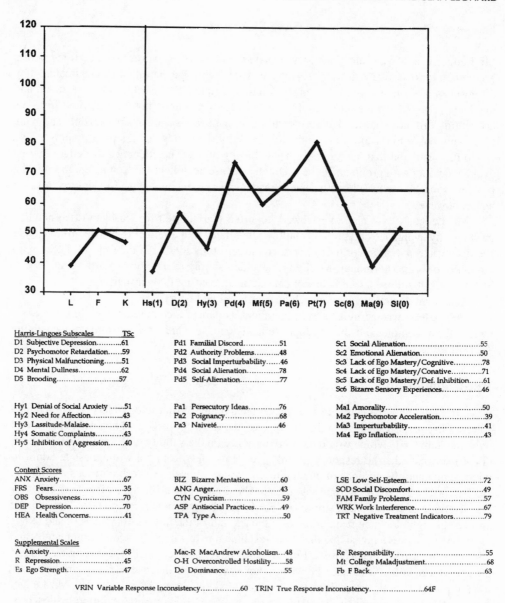

Figure 8.1. MMPI-2 clinical profile of Tom Ledger.

The chart shows the following x-axis labels:

L   F   K   Hs(1)   D(2)   Hy(3)   Pd(4)   Mf(5)   Pa(6)   Pt(7)   Sc(8)   Ma(9)   Sl(0)

Harris-Lingoes Subscales	TSc			
D1 Subjective Depression...........61	Pd1 Familial Discord...............51	Sc1 Social Alienation..............................55
D2 Psychomotor Retardation......59	Pd2 Authority Problems...........48	Sc2 Emotional Alienation........................50
D3 Physical Malfunctioning........51	Pd3 Social Imperturbability......46	Sc3 Lack of Ego Mastery/Cognitive............78
D4 Mental Dullness..................62	Pd4 Social Alienation..............78	Sc4 Lack of Ego Mastery/Conative............71
D5 Brooding...........................57	Pd5 Self-Alienation.................77	Sc5 Lack of Ego Mastery/Def. Inhibition......61
		Sc6 Bizarre Sensory Experiences.................46

Hy1 Denial of Social Anxiety 51	Pa1 Persecutory Ideas.............76	Ma1 Amorality.....................................50
Hy2 Need for Affection...............43	Pa2 Poignancy......................68	Ma2 Psychomotor Acceleration...................39
Hy3 Lassitude-Malaise...............61	Pa3 Naiveté.........................46	Ma3 Imperturbability...............................41
Hy4 Somatic Complaints............43		Ma4 Ego Inflation...................................43
Hy5 Inhibition of Aggression.......40		

Content Scores		
ANX Anxiety...........................67	BIZ Bizarre Mentation.............60	LSE Low Self-Esteem...............................72
FRS Fears..............................35	ANG Anger...........................43	SOD Social Discomfort.............................49
OBS Obsessiveness..................70	CYN Cynicism........................59	FAM Family Problems..............................57
DEP Depression.......................70	ASP Antisocial Practices...........49	WRK Work Interference............................67
HEA Health Concerns...............41	TPA Type A...........................50	TRT Negative Treatment Indicators.............79

Supplemental Scales		
A Anxiety.................................68	Mac-R MacAndrew Alcoholism...48	Re Responsibility.....................................55
R Repression............................45	O-H Overcontrolled Hostility......58	Mt College Maladjustment.........................68
Es Ego Strength........................47	Do Dominance........................55	Fb F Back...63

VRIN Variable Response Inconsistency.................60   TRIN True Response Inconsistency......................64F

7-4/4-7 Codetype

Inferences drawn from this codetype appear quite consistent with Mr. Ledger's self-report . There is evidence that the client experiences two quite contradictory characteristics: insensitivity (Pd) and extreme concern about his behavior (Pt). His profile is similar to that of those clients who are likely to engage in impulsive, self-centered behavior with little regard for others or the consequences of their behavior. Sexual promiscuity and substance abuse are often associated with this profile. Ultimately, however, clients with similar profiles often experience guilt and remorse over their behavior which may inhibit their behavior for a very limited period of time. In short order, their acting out recurs, often after a buildup of tension and worry.

Other Scale Elevations

Scale 6 (T=68) is the most notable elevation beyond the two-point code. It suggests the possibility that Mr. Ledger is feeling suspicious, distrustful, and concerned over what he may perceive as mistreatment by others. We can also infer that he is likely to blame others for his problems, be quite thin-skinned and easily hurt in his relationships, and deal with his anger in indirect ways.

Taken individually, the correlates for Scales 4 and 7 provide some potentially useful inferences regarding the client's personality and behavior. The elevation on Scale 4 (T=74) suggests that the client may be quite rebellious, irresponsible, and given to sensation and thrill-seeking behavior. It is not unusual for clients high on Scale 4 to have many antisocial behaviors and a history of criminal behavior. Unstable family relationships, violent behavior, and substance abuse are common. Scale 7 (T=81) suggests the presence of considerable anxiety, guilt, and tension, often manifested by obsessing and worrying about one's everyday life. It is likely that Mr. Ledger worries excessively over minor problems and tends to be indecisive, perfectionistic, and fearful of failure. Clients with elevated scores on Scale 7 are often seen as immature, unassertive, and insecure. To further clarify the meanings of the elevations on these scales, it will be helpful to examine the Harris-Lingoes subscales as well as the Content scales.

Interpretation of the remaining Clinical scales that fall below T-score=65 must be done very cautiously. However, Scale 5 (T=60) and a low score on Scale 9 (T=39) suggest the possibility that the client is somewhat passive and is currently experiencing low energy and activity levels.

Harris-Lingoes Subscales

These content-oriented subscales assist the clinician in clarifying the meaning of Clinical scales with very heterogeneous content. H-L subscales for Scales 4 and 6 are relevant in this case since both fall above T=65. The Social Alienation score (Pd4, T=78) suggests that the client may feel alienated, misunderstood, and estranged from others. Furthermore, he is likely to be insensitive to others and distrustful of their intentions. Self-Alienation (Pd5, T=77) focuses on the client's reports of guilt and regret and seeing himself as his own worst enemy. These inferences strengthen some of our earlier hypotheses and allow us to place less confidence in others. For instance, Family Discord (Pd1, T=51) and Authority Problems (Pd2, T=48) Scores suggest that family conflict and a history of conduct problems or conflicts with authorities are not prominent in the clinical picture, a hypothesis the parent Scale 4 alone might have suggested.

It appears that the elevation on Scale 6 is significantly related to the scores on subscales Pa1 (T=76) and Pa2 (T=68) reflecting feelings of resentment, unfair treatment and punishment and sensitivity to criticism. Subscale Naiveté (Pa3, T=46) is not significantly elevated indicating that the client does not deny his suspiciousness of others or maintain a naïve view of the world.

Content Scales

Content scales are homogeneous scales which also add information about the client's personality and behavior and clarify the meaning of the Clinical scales, allowing us to strengthen or reject our hypotheses. Six of the fifteen scales scores in this case exceed T=65 and will be interpreted.

The Anxiety score (ANX, T=67) suggests difficulty in making decisions, high levels of nervousness and tension, and feelings of being overwhelmed. The Obsessiveness score (OBS T=70) further confirms difficulty in reaching decisions, constant worrying, absence of self-confidence, and the inflexibility we saw in the Clinical Scale 7. The Depression scale (DEP T=70) reveals feelings of unhappiness, hopelessness, lack of energy, and feelings of guilt. Clients with similar elevations complain of lack of motivation and energy. This elevation is in contrast to a normal Scale 2 in the Clinical scales and may suggest that the subjective feelings of sadness and depression are not prominent in Mr. Ledger. The Low Self-Esteem score (LSE T=72) reflects Mr. Ledger's feelings of incompetence, his awareness of his shortcomings, and his hypersensitivity to criticism from others. Work Interference (WRK T=67) and Negative Treatment Indicators (TRT T=79) scores point to the obvious problems the client has had at work as a result of his behavior, to the resulting feelings of incompetence, as well as to his pessimism about the value of psychological treatment.

Two low scores are helpful in clarifying the meaning of Clinical Scale 4 (Pd). Both Anger (ANG T=43) scores and Antisocial Practices (ASP T=49) help to eliminate the inferences from Scale 4 that the client might have significant temper or aggression problems or have had a significant history of criminal and socially unconventional behavior.

Supplementary Scales

Most Supplementary Scales are considered to be within normal limits or to offer no additional information. However, the average score on the MacAndrew Alcoholism-Revised Scale (MAC-R T=48) helps us to eliminate the inference that substance abuse is likely to be a significant problem, which was suggested by Scale 4 (Pd).

SUMMARY

Mr. Thomas Ledger was administered the MMPI-2 in conjunction with a comprehensive psychological evaluation of his emotional functioning and personality. He appeared to have responded to the test honestly and test results are considered valid. While there is no evidence that the client is suffering from overwhelming turmoil or psychological disorganization at this time, he does appear to be quite anxious, ruminative, and depressed and to be struggling with feelings of inadequacy and low self-esteem. His lack of confidence, constant need for reassurance from others, and demands for perfection in himself seem to have led to his irresponsible behavior at work and home. Rather than face criticism from others or be seen as incompetent, Mr. Ledger is likely to avoid confronting his problems by procrastinating or lying about them, only to feel guilt and remorse later. This is often a cyclical pattern. At the present time, faced with the accusations of his wife and employers, he feels angry, resentful, victimized by others, and perhaps unfairly treated by the system. There is no evidence that Mr. Ledger is overtly aggressive or antisocial. He is likely to express his anger at others indirectly. There is no evidence that he currently suffers from substance abuse.

Diagnostically, Mr. Ledger's MMPI-2 data suggest that he may best be characterized as suffering from a personality disorder with passive-aggressive and obsessive traits. Psychotherapy is likely to be difficult for the client due to his feelings of distrust and his lack of significant emotional discomfort. However, he may respond positively to reassurance and structured interventions aimed at challenging his perfectionism and low self-esteem. Significant changes in personality structure are very unlikely.

SUGGESTED READINGS

Butcher, J. N. (1990). *MMPI-2 in psychological treatment*. New York: Oxford University Press.

Butcher, J. N., & Williams, C. L. (1992). *Essentials of MMPI-2 and MMPI-A interpretation*. Minneapolis: University of Minnesota Press.

Duckworth, J. C., & Anderson, W. P. (1995). *MMPI & MMPI-2 interpretation manual for counselors and clinicians*, (2nd ed.). Bristol, PA: Taylor and Francis.

Graham, J. R. (2000). *MMPI-2: Assessing personality and psychopathology* (3rd ed.). New York: Oxford University Press.

Greene, R. L. (2000). *The MMPI: An interpretive manual* (2nd ed.). Needham Heights, MA: Allyn & Bacon.

Nichols, D. S., & Greene, R. L. (1995). *MMPI-2 structural summary*. Odessa, FL: Psychological Assessment Resources.

9

Millon Clinical Multiaxial Inventory-III (MCMI-III)

Robert J. Craig

INTRODUCTION

The Millon Clinical Multiaxial Inventory (MCMI) is a useful instrument for the assessment of personality disorders and clinical syndromes. A recent survey on psychological test usage indicated that the MCMI is among the 25 most frequently used psychological tests in clinical practice and that the MCMI is ranked third, behind only the MMPI and the Rorschach, in terms of research studies on the test published within the past five years. However, although there is now a substantial clinical and research base with this test, laments continue to be heard concerning the difficulties in interpreting it. Therefore, an objective presentation of interpretive principles is now warranted.

This chapter presents interpretive principles for using the MCMI-III. First, the theory on which the MCMI-III is based will be presented, followed by Millon's domain-oriented approach to understanding personality disorder prototypes. Next, issues of administration and scoring are presented, followed by principles of interpretation which are then illustrated by a detailed case presentation. The chapter concludes with a discussion of computer-based interpretation of this test.

THEORETICAL UNDERPINNINGS

Millon argues that the structure of a clinical science contains four elements: (a) a *theory* to explain and understand the observed phenomena. Theory is then used to test hypotheses derived from the theory, (b) a *taxonomy* which classifies the observed phenomena and which is derived from the theory itself, (c) *instrumentation* which measures, quantifies, or assesses

Robert J. Craig • Bolingbrook, Illinois 60440-1214

Understanding Psychological Assessment, edited by Dorfman and Hersen. Kluwer Academic/Plenum Publishers, New York, 2001.

this phenomena, and (d) *intervention*, which includes techniques and strategies for remediation or amelioration of those phenomena which appear outside the normal range.

All of the Millon inventories (e.g., the *Millon Clinical Multiaxial Inventory [MCMI-III]*, the *Millon Adolescent Clinical Inventory [MACI]*, the *Millon Behavioral Health Inventory [MBHI]*, and the *Millon Index of Personality Styles* emanate from Millon's bioevolutionary theory. This theory posits that three personologic (personology—a phrase originally coined by Harvard psychologist Henry Murray—is the phrase used by Millon to describe the study of personality) polarities exist both in the physical world and in the psychological realm. These polarities are *Survival Aims*, *Adaptive Modes*, and *Replication Strategies*. At the biological level, organisms need to survive, adapt to their surroundings, and reproduce species of their own kind. At the psychological level, our first task also is to survive, but how we choose to survive eventuates into one aspect of our personality functioning, in that we can engage in behaviors that allow us to merely survive (e.g., avoid pain), or we can engage in behaviors that enhance our lives (e.g., seek pleasure). In adapting to an environment, we can do so actively, by changing our environment, or passively, by reacting to our environment. Finally, the psychological extension of the replication strategy can be oriented primarily toward seeking reinforcement from our own achievements (i.e., self-focused) or by seeking reinforcements by nurturing and caring for others (i.e., other-focused).

How we seek reinforcement (an adaptation strategy) is contrasted with where we seek reinforcement (a replication strategy). Millon identified five types of "personality sources of reinforcement": (1) Independent (primarily from self), (2) Dependent (primarily from others), (3) Ambivalent (self-other conflict), (4) Discordant (pain and pleasure is reversed as to reinforcement), and (5) Detached (no pleasure from either self or others). When the five sources of reinforcement are combined with two modes of adaptation, his theory derives ten basic personality patterns or styles and three severe personality disorder variants.

Within the active adaptive mode, the Independent style is called "unruly," the Dependent style is called "sociable," the Ambivalent style is called "sensitive," the Discordant style is called "forceful," and the Detached style is called "inhibited." Within the passive adaptive mode, the Independent style is called "confident," the Dependent style is called "cooperative," the Ambivalent style is called "respectful," the Discordant style is called "defeatist," and the Detached style is called "introversive."

Next, Millon argues that personality exists on a continuum. While normality may be said to reflect a balance of the three polarities (survival, adaptation, and replication), personality disorders are merely extensions of the basic personality style developed in association with compromised biology, learning histories, and environmental stresses. Millon's matrix of personality disorders also derives from his theory. Along the active adaptational mode, the Independent style at the level of disorder is called "antisocial," the Dependent style is called "histrionic," the Ambivalent style is called "negativistic," the Discordant style is called "aggressive" (sadistic), and the Detached style is called "Avoidant." Along the passive adaptational polarity, the Independent Style is called "narcissistic," the Dependent style is called "Dependent," the Ambivalent style is called "compulsive," the Discordant style is called "self-defeating (masochistic)," and the Detached style is called "schizoid."

There are also variations of severe dysfunction that represent the more severe personality disorders. The paranoid disorder can emanate from any of the five basic styles, except the Discordant type; the borderline disorder can emanate any style except from the Detached type; the schizotypal emanates from the Detached style.

Thus at the normal end the Active Dependent type is called "sociable," whereas at the pathological end this type is called "histrionic." At the normal end the Active Independent type is called "unruly," but at the pathological end it is called "antisocial." At the normal end, the Passive Ambivalent type is called "respectful" whereas at the pathological end it is called "Compulsive". If you consider yourself primarily a cooperative person, cordial and compromising in interpersonal relations, agreeable, disinclined to become upset when stressed, and focused primarily on adapting your wishes to conform with the wishes of others, Millon's theory would type you as a Passive Dependent type, whereas if this style lead to interpersonal problems and was more exaggerated in nature, this Passive-Dependent style would be diagnosed as a dependent personality disorder.

Millon's theory-derived personality types and disorders are similar to but not exactly identical to, DSM-IV classification. In fact, Millon has two personality disorder types (aggressive/sadistic and self-defeating) that do not appear in DSM-IV. While he made efforts to bring his classification more in line that in DSM-IV, he was also insistent that his theory need not be isomorphic with the "official" classification of personalty disorders. Believing that his theory derives these personality disorders "in nature," he has elected to retain them in his theory, in his taxonomy, and in his instrumentation.

I have presented Millon's theory in its basic form, but it is far more complex and detailed than is the material provided herein. The interested reader is referred to the Suggested Readings list for more advanced treatments.

PERSONALITY DESCRIPTION

Millon refers to personality prototypes in that his theory discusses a particular style in its purest form. However, in actuality, an individual probably would not be perfectly aligned with only one style and would have both admixtures and patterns associated with two or three of the basic patterns.

In developing a system with which to describe personality prototypes, Millon employed a clinical-domain-criteria approach, emphasizing functional criteria, which are dynamic processes that are used to manage interpersonal relationships, and structural criteria, which are stable internal personality characteristics. There are four essential domains to describe each personality prototype. In the *behavioral domain*, there are expressive acts (a functional attribute), which are observable behaviors of the person, and this is interpersonal conduct (a functional attribute) or style in relating to others. At the *phenomenological domain* there are cognitive styles (a functional attribute) which would describe how a person thinks, perceives, processes information, etc., and object representations (a structural attribute), or the residue imprinted in conscious and unconscious memory which acts as a substrate for how we perceive and relate to others; there is also self-image (a structural attribute), which pertains to how a one thinks about oneself and then displays that perception to others. At the *intrapsychic domain* there are regulatory mechanisms (a functional attribute) which represent unconscious processes, and morphologic organization (a structural attribute), which represents the overall configuration of personality related to psychic boundaries, internal conflicts, the interplay of the id-ego-superego intrapsychic system, etc. Finally, there is the *biophysical domain*, of which mood or temperament is the only structural attribute. This domain pertains to how mood and temperament affect one's functioning.

Each personality disorder can thus be described according to its expressive acts, interpersonal conduct, cognitive style, object representations, self-image, regulatory mechanisms, its morphological organization, and mood or temperament. For a comprehensive report on how the personality disorders are described from this model, the reader is referred to the Suggested

Readings Section. While one can still use the MCMI-III without knowing the theory underlying its development, it is important to recognize that the MCMI-III is a theory-derived test.

The last of Millon's elements of a clinical science pertains to interventions or what is commonly referred to as psychotherapy. Millon is presently at work on a text that will provide his ideas of psychotherapy using domain-oriented techniques, polarity-oriented goals, and personality-oriented integrative strategies, but these are beyond the scope of this chapter.

TEST CONSTRUCTION AND DEVELOPMENT

In developing what eventually became the MCMI (I/II/III), Millon employed a sequential validation strategy originally suggested by Jane Loevinger. In this strategy, test validation proceeds in three phases: theoretical-substantive, internal-structural, and external-criterion.

In the theoretical-substantive phase of test construction and validation, items are evaluated on how well their content conforms to the theory from which they were derived. Millon selected items that represented not only the "official" classification system (i.e., DSM), but also developed items that derived from his theory. For example, the antisocial personality disorder, according to his theoretical model, is referred to as the Active-Independent type. Hence, there is an item on the MCMI-III as follows: " If my family puts pressure on me, I'm likely to feel angry and resist doing what they want." This item taps Millon's theory as to the motivation behind antisocial behavior (e.g., antisocials feel others want to dominate them so they dominate others and actively remain independent in order to resist such influences). Of course, the antisocial scale also contains items that are consistent with DSM-IV notions of antisocial behavior (e.g., "as a teenager I got into lots of trouble because of bad school behavior"). Thus Millon created an initial pool of face-valid items. Some were eliminated due to problems in readability, patient judgment, and sortings by clinicians. The remaining 1100 face-valid items were split into two equivalent forms.

After creating a pool of theoretically-derived items, the next step was to begin the process of internal-structural validation. He administered the two equivalent forms to clinical samples and retained only those items which had the highest item-total scale correlations. He then calculated item-scale intercorrelations as well as item endorsement frequencies and eliminated items with extreme endorsement frequencies using the operational definition of <.15 and >.85. The remaining 440 items were screened to assure an adequate number of items for each scale and to assure that overlapping scales and items were consistent with his theory. For example, there is a high correlation between the antisocial and narcissistic personality pattern scales. This was built in, so to speak, because Millon believes that, in nature, narcissism is part of the personality structure of the antisocial. This final set of items numbered 289.

For the external-criterion validation process, Millon then gave these items to 167 clinicians and asked them to complete a diagnostic form. The items were reduced to a total of 150. At this stage, scales on hypochondriasis, obession-compulsion, and sociopathy were eliminated and three scales were added (hypomania, alcohol abuse, and drug abuse) and the validation process described above was repeated until the final set of 175 items was established. The test was then published as the MCMI.

Because Millon revised his theoretical model somewhat and because DSM-III was also being revised, he also revised the MCMI by adding an aggressive (sadistic) scale and a self-defeating scale and also added three validly scales (Disclosure, Desirability, and Debasement). He also changed 45 items and constructed an item-weighting system, assigning higher weights to "prototype" items (i.e., those items essentially related to the disorder; e.g., "my drug habits have gotten me into a good deal of trouble in the past" from Drug Abuse Scale T, MCMI-II).

Revision of the MCMI-II followed the three-step validation process detailed earlier. Two new scales were added, a depressive personality disorder scale and post-traumatic stress disorder scale. Noteworthy items (i.e., "critical items") now include items pertaining to child abuse and eating disorders, but these are not scored on any scale. The item-weighting system was changed from a three-point to a two-point scale. Prototype items are now given a weight of two rather than three. A total of 95 of the MCMI-II 175 items were changed. Scales that were about 25-items long in the MCMI-II are now about 15-items long in the MCMI-III. Many of these changes were introduced to bring the test into greater conformity with changes in DSM-IV.

In its final form, the MCMI-III consists of four Validity scales (the Validity Index and the three "Modifying indices" consisting of Disclosure (X), Desirability (Y), and Debasement (Z)), 11 Clinical Personality patterns (schizoid (1), avoidant (2A), depressive (2B), dependent (3), histrionic (4), narcissistic (5), antisocial (6A), aggressive/sadistic (6B), compulsive (7), passive-aggressive (8A), and self-defeating (8B), three scales measuring Severe Personality Pathology (schizotypal (S), borderline (C), and paranoid (P)), seven clinical syndromes (anxiety disorder (A), somatoform disorder (H), bipolar: manic disorder (N), dysthymic disorder (D), alcohol dependence (B), drug dependence (T), and post-traumatic stress (R)), and three severe clinical syndromes (thought disorder (SS), major depression (CC), and delusional disorder (PP)).

ADMINISTRATION AND SCORING

The MCMI-III was designed to be used with patients who are being evaluated or treated in a clinical/psychiatric setting when personality pathology is suspected as part of the clinical presentation. The test is not meant for nonclinical patients and use of this instrument with normals will distort the description of their personality and hence should not be done.

The MCMI-III is a 175-item self-report inventory, with items presented in a true-false dichotomy. The test can be administered to small groups or, more commonly, in an individual format. The respondents are asked to answer as honestly as possible and to express their true feelings and attitudes. The instructions are written in language requiring a sixth-grade reading ability.

Millon argues that, while abilities and traits are probably normally distributed and hence raw scores from ability and personality tests can be transformed to a normalized distribution, personality disorders are quite skewed in the general population. This means that normal distributions, such as z scores or T-scores, are inappropriate in such cases. Instead, MCMI-III raw scores are converted to Base Rate (BR) scores, which Millon describes as a transformed score which ensures that the proportion of patients scoring above each scale's cut-off point is equal to the actual prevalence among a representative population of patients who possess each scale's corresponding disorder. Millon arbitrarily selected a BR score of 60 as the mean BR score for all psychiatric patients who took the test in the standardization sample. A BR score of 30 was the mean score for testees without personality or clinical pathology. A BR score of 85 and above signifies the "most prominent" disorder (i.e., severe), a BR score of 75 to 84 reflects the "presence of characteristics" of the disorder (i.e., moderate), scores between 65 and 74 suggest the patient has some of the traits defined by the scale (i.e., mild), and scores between 0 and 64 are considered clinically nonsignificant. Different BR transformation tables are used for males and females for all scales except Scale X (disclosure).

Validity Indices: The MCMI-III has four scales that assess validity, e.g., test-taking attitude or the manner in which a person responded to the items. The first of these is the Validity Index, which consists of three items of an improbable nature. An answer of "true" to one of the items makes the accuracy of the test questionable. Two such answers result in profile invalidity and hence the test should not be interpreted. These items pertain to scenarios such as claiming to never have seen a car, being on the front cover of several magazines and flying across the ocean 30 times in one year. These items are likely to detect patients who are confused, dyslexic, or responding randomly to the items. The scores on the Validity Index do not appear on the profile sheet and are not converted to BR scores. The examiner is expected to consult answers to these items prior to scoring the test to ensure honest responses to these items.

My preference in orienting the person to take the MCMI-III is to tell the patient that "there are some 'trick' items on the test to see if you're paying attention—so pay attention." I have found this to be helpful in maximizing the probability of obtaining an interpretable profile.

The next validity scale, the Disclosure (X), was designed to detect patients who are self-revealing or highly defensive. It is not a scale with item composition. Rather it is an index that is based on the degree of positive or negative deviation from the midrange of an adjusted composite raw score total for the 11 Clinical Personality Patterns scales. A test protocol is considered invalid if the raw score on this scale is below 34 (e.g., excessive nondisclosure and denial of problems) or above 178 (e.g., gross exaggeration of problems and symptoms).

The Desirability Index (Y) is a 21-item scale that assesses the degree to which one patient is attempting to show oneself in a highly favorable light, as excessively virtuous, as emotionally stable, and as socially "together." BR scores above 74 on Scale Y suggest a possibly "faking good" response set. The mean score on this scale was 81, while the mean score of respondents instructed to "fake good" was BR96.

The *Debasement Index (Z)* is a 33-item scale which assesses the degree to which a respondent is "faking bad" or feigning symptoms or problems that are either exaggerated or do not exist at all. The mean BR score for patients was 87 whereas the mean BR score for respondents instructed to "fake bad" was BR108.

BR SCORE ADJUSTMENTS

After the raw scores have been converted to BR scores, these, in turn, may be adjusted based on one or more of the following considerations:

The *disclosure adjustment* adjusts scores on Scales 1 through PP. Scores on these scales are increased if scores on Scale X are <61 and decreased if scores on Scale X are >123. The exact amount of the adjustment depends on the value of Scale X. Note that it is impossible to invalidate scores on the personality disorder scales based on Scale X scores because adjustments are made to offset either a secretive or overly frank response set.

Scores are also adjusted by the *high anxiety/high depression adjustment*. If patients present in acute emotional turmoil characterized by acute anxiety or depression at the time of testing, these emotional states could distort the individual's true personality pattern. Millon determined which MCMI-III scales are most affected by such manifestations of psychological pain (i.e., avoidant [2B], depressive [2B], self-defeating [8B], schizotypal [S], and borderline [C]) and adjusts scores on those scales based on the final adjusted BR score on scales A (anxiety) and D (dysthymia), providing that BR scores on scales A and/or D are >74.

The *denial versus complaint adjustment* increases scores on scales 1 through 8B, provided the patient's BR scores are highest on the histrionic (4), narcissistic (5), or compulsive

(7) among scales 1 through 8B. In such cases, scores are increased on that scale by 8 BR points.

Scores are also adjusted if the patient is tested while an inpatient. This is done to counteract the tendency among hospitalized patients to not accurately report the severity of their psychological state. The *inpatient adjustment* increases scores on thought disorder (SS), major depression (CC), and delusional disorder (PP) provided that patient is an inpatient and the disorder has lasted four weeks or less.

Finally, no adjustments can decrease a score to below 1 or increase a score above 115.

This test is extremely difficult and quite cumbersome to score by hand. It is estimated that hand-scoring takes approximately 45 minutes, and there are serious doubts as to the accuracy and reliability of scores done by hand due to the possibility of multiple scorer error. Therefore, most psychologists prefer to have the test computer-scored by the test's publisher, National Computer Systems. However, this is somewhat costly, particularly for low volume operations. The difficulty of hand-scoring and the necessity of computer-scoring has been one of the complaints about this test.

INTERPRETIVE GUIDELINES

I recommend the following steps in interpreting the MCMI-III:

1. *Consider the context of testing.* Patients undergoing psychological evaluation for child custody are likely to respond to tests by denying symptoms or problems, whereas patients who are tested as part of an evaluation to determine sanity associated with a "not guilty by reason of insanity" plea to escape murder charges may respond to the test by exaggerating their symptoms and problems. Take into account the context of the evaluation and how this may affect a person's approach to testing.

2. *Examine the Validity Indices.*
   a. Make sure the patient has not omitted more than 10 items. If possible, have the patient go back and complete as many unanswered items as possible. Do not interpret the test if the number of unanswered items is >10.
   b. Make sure the Validity Index is <2 and preferably 0.
   c. Look at the Disclosure scale (X) and make sure BR>35 and <85. This is the only scale where both ends of the base rate distribution need to be interpreted. Low (but valid) scores reflect tendencies to deny psychological problems while scores >BR74 but <BR85 suggest unusual willingness to report problems.
   d. Look at the Desirability Scale (Y). If the BR scores are >74 suggest a response set to understate pathology, to deny problems and symptoms, and to place oneself in a positive light.
   e. If scores on the Debasement scale (Z) are >BR75, the patient may be exaggerating the extent of his or her problems.

3. *Examine the Clinical Personality Patterns and the Severe Personality Disorders.*
   a. Any scales with BR scores >84 mandate interpretation. Such scores indicate that the patient has the traits and characteristics associated with the disorder at diagnosable levels.
   b. Scores between BR>74 and BR<85 suggests the presence of traits associated with the content of the scale but at non-diagnosable levels.
   c. In general, if more than three scales reflect clinically significant elevations on the

      clinical personality pattern scales and/or severe personality scales, interpret the
more severe disorders.

    d. Also, elevations on the severe personality disorder scales (S, C, P) normally are be
given preference in interpretation over scales 1 through 8B, unless there is clinical
justification not to do so.

    e. Configural interpretation will result in more refined and more accurate interpreta-
tions. By configural interpretation I mean the combination of two or three clinical
scales in a combined interpretation.

  4. *Examine the Clinical Syndrome scales.*

    a. Scores above BR84 indicate the presence of the syndrome at a diagnosable level,
whereas scores between BR>74 and <85 suggest the presence of some but not all
of the symptoms associated with the syndrome.

    b. It is important not merely to diagnose a clinical syndrome but also to interpret it in
the light of the context of the evaluation and to understand the meaning of the
symptoms in the personality style/disorder in which it is embedded. For example,
if a patient has clinically significant elevations on antisocial (6A), alcohol dependence (B), and anxiety disorder (A), then one possible interpretation is that the
elevation on B may be residual effects of alcohol withdrawal and not truly an
"anxiety reaction." However, if this same patient has significant elevations on 6A
and A, the elevation on A would be unusual for someone with a purely antisocial
personality and may suggest the individual is faced with some external problem
(court case?) which is inducing a temporary level of stress that would not normally
be a part of the personality structure.

  5. *Review noteworthy responses.* Check any noteworthy responses that are highlighted in
the endorsed direction.

  6. Consider Extra-test information. Review patient background information, relevant
history, and other available records and test results.

  7. Establish a DSM-IV Diagnosis (using all relevant information).

  8. Make treatment recommendations. Consider not only the likelihood of response to
treatment for the clinical syndromes but, more importantly, how a patient is likely to behave
and what barriers there might be to psychological treatment given the underlying personality
structure.

CASE EXAMPLES

Case Example 1

    Table 9.1 presents MCMI-III scores for a 44-year-old, divorced, unemployed, African-
American male with 12 years of education. The patient's presenting problem was substance
abuse, but he also reported a history of seizures for which he takes phenobarbital and low back
pain for which he takes Motrin as needed.

    He alleged daily alcohol use, heroin use twice a day through insufflation (snorting) at a
cost of $100–$150 per day, and cocaine abuse (free-basing) by history. He had one prior
inpatient treatment episode for alcohol abuse but relapsed about two months after discharge.
He has never been in outpatient treatment. His stated motivation for requesting treatment was
"I want to get over being depressed and my habit (heroin) is getting worse and I don't have
much to live for". He wanted to be placed on methadone maintenance. He reported two prior

Table 9.1. MCMI-III Scores for Case Example 1

Scale	BR Score
Disclosure (X)	89
Desirability (Y)	39
Debasement (Z)	95
Schizoid (1)	69
Avoidant (2A)	79
Depressive (2B)	90
Dependent (3)	78
Histrionic (4)	28
Narcissistic (5)	32
Antisocial (6A)	77
Aggressive/Sadistic (6B)	49
Compulsive (7)	25
Passive-Aggressive (8A)	69
Self-Defeating (8B)	61
Schizotypal (S)	79
Borderline (C)	86
Paranoid (P)	74
Anxiety Disorder (A)	102
Somatoform Disorder (H)	87
Bipolar: Manic Disorder (N)	97
Dysthymic Disorder (D)	107
Alcohol Dependence (B)	97
Drug Dependence (T)	90
Post-Traumatic Stress (R)	97
Thought Disorder (SS)	77
Major Depression (CC)	107
Delusional Disorder (PP)	75

psychiatric treatments associated with attempted suicides via overdoses of barbiturates. He was hospitalized once at a VA psychiatric treatment unit and once at a State Mental Hospital. He alleges he is hearing voices telling him to steal and claims to see spots before his eyes that are not there.

He also reported a history of childhood physical abuse from his father, admitted to being a street fighter in a gang in his youth, and involved in homicidal behavior, but would not elaborate. He also admitted to repeated episodes of domestic abuse with his former wife and went to jail twice on battery convictions. He said he still routinely carries weapons on his person.

Notes from the clinical interview described this patient as lonely, introverted, and dysthymic, yet also aggressive and antisocial with borderline traits. He related in a somewhat deferential, respectful, and perhaps dependent manner. Mild auditory and visual hallucinations needed to be ruled out. His cognitions centered mostly on where he was going to live, how he would support himself, and how he would overcome his addiction. He dressed in neat but somewhat dirty clothing. He was not considered suicidal.

Interpretation

The patient's validity scales indicates that he was quite self-revealing (X) but what he had to say about himself was essentially negative (Z). Note that essentially all clinical syndrome scales are elevated in the clinically significant ranges but there is much more individuation in scores among the personality disorder scales. I suspect this patient was rather honest in responding to questions pertaining to his personality style but tended to endorse an item as "true" whenever he came across an item pertaining to a symptom. Perhaps he responded in this way in the mistaken belief that this would increase his chances of being prescribed methadone, a narcotic drug.

This patient has essentially an introverted and detached personality style (2B2A) with a core of depressive personality traits (3) and antisocial traits complicating the clinical picture. Such patients have difficulty maintaining relationships and seem to prefer to be alone. They are generally bland and apathetic and tend to behave in a submissive and compliant manner. Yet he also has quixotic emotionality (C) that can erupt in antisocial ways (6A). Also, his detached and unemotional personality allows him to engage in antisocial behavior without the emotions of guilt, remorse, or empathy.

A few other comments are warranted. First, because of this patient's history of major depression with suicidal attempts, I am reluctant to describe him in terms of a depressive personality style, even though Scale 2B is his most elevated personality disorder scale. I attribute this elevation to his probable depressive disorder and suspect that scores on Scale 2B will abate as his clinical condition improves. Second, his introverted and antisocial style is consistent with his history and with the way he related to the interviewer during a mental status examination. Third, his past problems with domestic violence seem more attributable to his tendency to erupt with uncontrolled emotions when stressed (6A, C) than to a truly aggressive personality style (6B). Fourth, because of his exaggerated response set to clinical syndrome items, I am reluctant to include them in a report but would address his substance abuse and his clinical depression since those have been confirmed. We might speculate that anger is the major emotion driving this patient and that anger has been both turned in against himself (in depression and later suicide) and turned against others (in street fighting, murder, and domestic violence). Substance abuse may soothe him and quell this emotion for a time, but represents only a temporary solution. Millon would describe this personality style as a "restive depressive" and speculates that their behavior is designed to elicit sympathy, support, nurturance, and reassurance from significant others.

Computer-Generated Interpretive Report

While it is essential for an assessment psychologist to interpret an MCMI profile, many psychologists have relied on computer-assisted interpreted reports, which are now available on most major objective, self-report personality instruments. There are two computer narrative reports available for interpreting the MCMI-III. One is published by the test's publishers, National Computer Systems, and was written by Ted Millon. The other is published by Psychological Assessment Resources (PAR) and was written by this author. Below is an edited version of the PAR computer report generated for this patient's MCMI profile.

Sample Report

The following is a sample report:

The MCMI (as revised) was normed on individuals being evaluated or treated in mental health settings. Thus, the test should only be used with individuals who are in similar clinical settings for problems that are defined as psychological/psychiatric. Administering this test to people without clinical symptoms is inappropriate and will result in inaccurate descriptions of their functioning. Because this test is focused on personality disorders and clinical symptoms, the report is necessarily focused on these problematic behaviors and cannot describe a person's strengths and competencies.

The interpretive information contained in this report should be viewed as only one source of hypotheses about the individual being evaluated. No decisions should be based solely on the information contained in this report. This material should be integrated with all other sources of information in reaching professional decisions about this individual.

This report is confidential and intended for use by qualified professionals only. It should not be released to the individual being evaluated.

Modifier Indices

Configuration: This patient may have a tendency toward self-abasement as a characterological trait or may have endorsed more problems and symptoms that would be determined by an objective review. The patient may have responded to the test items as a "cry for help," by endorsing so many problems to ensure that he would come to the clinician's attention. On the other hand, it is possible that the patient is seriously disturbed by many characterological problems. MCMI-III scoring adjustments have been made to correct for the "cry for help" tendency by decreasing scores on scales known to be affected by such a response strategy. However, the individual clinician must personally evaluate the extent to which such adjustments have made the necessary correction to improve profile validity. This patient also exhibits a high degree of self-disclosure. It is not unusual for high self-disclosing patients to also receive elevated scores on the Debasement Index.

Personality Style

This patient may be described as generally gloomy, pessimistic, overly serious, quiet, passive, and preoccupied with negative events. Such patients often feel inadequate and have low self-esteem. They tend to unnecessarily brood and worry and, though they are usually responsible and conscientious, they are also self-reproaching and self-critical, regardless of their level of accomplishment. They seem to be "down" all the time and are quite hard to please. They tend to find fault in even the most joyous experience. These people are often described negatively rather than positively. They feel it is futile to try to make improvements in themselves, in their relationships, or in any significant aspect of their lives because their incessant pessimism leads them toward a defeatist outlook. Their depressive demeanor often makes others around them feel guilty, since these patients are overly dependent on others for support and acceptance. They have difficulty expressing anger and aggression and perhaps displace it onto themselves. Interestingly, while their mood is often one of dejection and while their cognitions are often dominated by negative thoughts, they do not consider themselves depressed.

This personality style is present, even in the absence of a clinical depression. Their melancholic, sober demeanor, combined with their passivity and self-doubts, puts them at risk for occupational and marital problems. They are also at risk for dysthymia, if stressed with loss.

The patient may also be quite narcissistic, fearless, pugnacious, daring, blunt, aggressive, assertive, irresponsible, impulsive, ruthless, victimizing, intimidating, dominating, often energetic and competitive, but quite determined and independent. He is argumentative, self-reliant, revengeful and vindictive. He is chronically dissatisfied and harbors resentments against people who challenge, criticize, or express disapproval about his behavior.

He is characteristically touchy and jealous, broods over perceived slights and wrongs, and provokes fear in those around him through his intimidating social demeanor. He tends to present with angry and hostile affect. He is suspicious and skeptical of the motives of other people, plans revenge for past grievances, and views others as untrustworthy. He avoids experiences of warmth, gentleness, closeness, and intimacy, viewing such involvements as a sign of weakness. These types of patients often ascribe their own malicious tendencies onto the motives of others. They feel comfortable only when they have power and control over others. They are continually on guard against anticipated ridicule and act out in a socially intimidating manner, desiring to provoke fear in others and to exploit them for self-gain. Such patients are driven by power, by malevolent projections, and by an expectation to anticipate suffering from others, so they react to maintain their autonomy and independence. Millon believes that their behavior is motivated by an expectancy that people will be rejecting and that other people are malicious, devious, and vengeful, thus justifying a forceful counteraction to maintain their own autonomy. They are alert for signs of ridicule and contempt, and they react with impulsive hostility in response to felt resentments. They are prone toward substance abuse, relationship difficulties, vocational deficits, and legal problems.

NOTE: It is possible to have an antisocial character style without engaging in antisocial (criminal) behavior.

While this patient may not meet all of the criteria to warrant a diagnosis of antisocial personality disorder, antisocial traits are present.

Clinical Syndromes

Dysthymic Disorder/Major Depression: The patient is reporting many problems and symptoms associated with dysthymia. These problems and symptoms include apathy, social withdrawal, guilt, pessimism, low self-esteem, feelings of inadequacy and worthlessness, self-doubts, and a diminished sense of pleasure. Generally such patients can't meet their day-to-day responsibilities but continue to experience chronic dysphoria. A diagnosis of depression is usually associated with scores at this level, with major depression or dysthymic disorder the most prevalent diagnoses. A more thorough clinical evaluation is recommended to determine if there are vegetative signs of depression, psychotic symptoms, and/or suicidal ideation.

Alcohol Dependence: This patient has reported symptoms and traits commonly associated with alcohol abuse and/or alcohol dependence. It is also possible that the patient has endorsed personality traits often seen in patients who subsequently develop problematic drinking. It is also possible that the patient has had problems with alcohol and is in recovery. A more thorough clinical evaluation should be conducted to determine the presence of any specific problems that may be associated with this condition (e.g., medical, social, legal, psychological, psychiatric, vocational, spiritual). Scores at this level almost always reflect a diagnosis associated with alcohol.

Drug Dependence: This patient has reported symptoms and traits commonly associated with alcohol and drug abuse and/or dependence. A more thorough clinical evaluation of the patient's drug and alcohol abuse history, pattern, and problems is recommended to determine the nature and extent of problems that may be associated with polysubstance abuse. Scores at this level almost always reflect a diagnosis associated with drug dependence. Additional scrutiny is necessary to determine if medical referral is necessary to deal with possible syndromes associated with drug and/or alcohol withdrawal.

Delusional Disorder: This patient is reporting many symptoms associated with paranoia. The patient's mood may be hostile, and the patient may be hypervigilant to perceived
threat. Ideas of reference, thought control, or thought influence may be presence. Given this
patient's apparent substance abuse, a drug-induced paranoia may also be present. A more
thorough clinical evaluation is recommended to determine which specific symptoms are present,
their cause, and what kind of clinical intervention is necessary. On the other hand, there is a
high correlation between scales PP and B and T. Thus the patient's primary diagnosis may be
substance abuse and traits and behaviors, such as hypervigilance, defensive scanning of the
environment, a feeling that people are out to get him, etc., are really associated with the drug
lifestyle rather than with clinical paranoia. A clinical evaluation is necessary to determine
which diagnosis is the case.

Research: There is no published research on a codetype similar to the one obtained
from this patient.

Computer-Derived Diagnoses

A computer-generated report follows.

I. Alcohol Abuse/Dependence
    Drug Abuse/Dependence
    r/o Drug-Induced Paranoia
    r/o Dysthymia and/or Major depression
    r/o Anxiety Disorder
II. Personality Disorder NOS, Antisocial and depressive traits.
End of report (Note: The original report was 11 pages, too lengthy for inclusion here).

Comment

This case illustrates some of the difficulties associated with computer-generated reports,
particularly as they pertains to scale interactions. By scale interaction, we mean that elevations
on one or more scales may attenuate or make more salient interpretations on another scale.

Note some inconsistencies in the personality description. One paragraph, describing the
depressive aspect, reports that these patients are often responsible, whereas another paragraph, describing the antisocial aspect, reports that these patients are often irresponsible. The
computer program cannot determine if a depression is superimposed over an antisocial personality or whether they exist independently of one another. Thus, the clinician must review
and accurately interpret the test (e.g. not simply rely on computer interpretations), integrating
this with other clinical information for final a decision. Remember, APA ethics stipulate that
psychologists should be qualified to administer, score, and interpret the tests for which they
are using computerized interpretations.

SUMMARY

The MCMI-III has become a mainstream clinical instrument to assess personality disorders and some clinical syndromes. Interpretation requires knowledge and understanding of
base rate scores signs and symptoms of the major personality disorders, personality disorder

prototypes, and of psychodynamics, clinical syndromes, and how these fit into some type of theoretical foundation.

SUGGESTED READINGS

American Psychological Association Committee on Professional Standards (COPS) and Committee on Psychological Tests and Assessments (CPTA). *Guidelines for computer-based tests and interpretations.* Washington, DC: American Psychological Association.

Choca, J. P. & VanDenburg, E. (1994). *Interpretive guide to the Millon Clinical Multiaxial Inventory.* Washington, DC: American Psychological Association.

Craig, R. J. (Ed.). (1993a). *The Millon Clinical Multiaxial Inventory: A clinical research information synthesis.* Hillsdale, NJ: Lawrence Erlbaum Associates.

Craig, R. J. (1993b). *MCMI-II/III interpretive system.* Odessa, FL: Psychological Assessment Resources.

Craig, R. J. (1997). A selected review of the MCMI empirical literature. In T. Millon (Ed.), *The Millon inventories* (pp. 303–336). New York: Guilford Publications.

Millon, T. (1990). *Toward a new personology: An evolutionary model.* New York: Wiley-Interscience.

Millon, T. (1994). *Millon Clinical Multiaxial Inventory-III: manual.* Minneapolis, MN: National Computer Systems

Millon, T., & Davis, R. D. (1995). *Disorders of personality: DSM-IV and beyond.* New York: Wiley-Interscience.

Retzlaff, P. D. (Ed.). (1995). *Tactical psychotherapy of the personality disorders: An MCMI-III-based approach.* Needham Heights, MA: Allyn & Bacon.

10

The Sixteen Personality Factor (16PF) Questionnaire

Heather E. P. Cattell

INTRODUCTION

The Sixteen Personality Factor Questionnaire is a comprehensive measure of normal range personality. Although it was not developed to identify psychopathology, it has been used extensively and productively in clinical settings due to its ability to give a deep, integrated picture of the whole person, including both personal strengths *and* weaknesses. The 16PF questionnaire can be used to identify patterns of behavior in a wide variety of real-life circumstances. For example, it can be used to understand a person's self-esteem, coping patterns, capacity for empathy, interpersonal needs, likely attitude toward power and authority, cognitive processing style, internalization of societal rules or standards, and likely occupational preferences. Because of this comprehensive scope, 16PF results are useful in a wide variety of settings, including clinical, counseling, industrial, career development, and research.

The 16PF questionnaire can be particularly effective in managed care environments, where the therapist simply doesn't have time to gradually develop an understanding of the client's underlying personality structure. In time-limited settings, it is particularly important for clinicians to "hit the ground running" by developing a picture of the whole person, so that the presenting problems can be placed in the context of the total personality. The 16PF questionnaire can also help in developing a therapeutic plan by shedding light on which modes of treatment or therapeutic interventions might best suit the client.

The easy administration of the 16PF measure makes it a very effective source of comprehensive information for the professional. Typically the test is administered at the end of the first session, after the client has met with the professional and developed an understanding of the purpose of the testing. The second session may include a discussion of the test results and their implications for clarifying and elaborating the meaning of the presenting problem.

Heather E. P. Cattell • Institute for Personality and Ability Testing, Inc., Walnut Creek, California 94595-2611.

Understanding Psychological Assessment, edited by Dorfman and Hersen. Kluwer Academic/Plenum Publishers, New York, 2001.

16PF results can also facilitate the therapeutic dialogue between the clinician and client. Unlike tests measuring psychopathology, 16PF scales represent relatively common areas of everyday experience that can be easily discussed with clients. Sharing 16PF results can facilitate the client's sense of being fully understood and of being a part of the assessment and treatment planning process, in addition to generally increasing self-awareness. Even if not shared, the deep understanding of clients gained through 16PF results can contribute to empathy, rapport, and the client's respect for the clinician.

Finally, although 16PF results can be useful in both long-term and short-term therapy in treating individuals, couples, or families, it does not provide all the information needed for psychological evaluation. Other information, such as life history interviews, mental status exams, measures of psychopathological dimensions, and measures of cognitive and neurological functioning, is also needed, depending on the professional's assessment of the individual case. The 16PF findings cannot replace, but rather can augment, the clinician's interview and evaluation process.

HISTORICAL AND THEORETICAL PERSPECTIVE

History

The history of the 16PF questionnaire spans almost the whole history of objective personality measurement. First published in 1949, the measure has seen four major revisions, with the most recent release being the 16PF Fifth Edition in 1993. The development of this recent edition is described later in this chapter.

The 16PF questionnaire was developed from a unique perspective. Rather than measuring preconceived dimensions of interest to a particular author, the test was developed from the perspective of trying first to discover all the basic structural elements of personality and then to construct scales to measure these fundamental dimensions. To do this, Raymond Cattell decided to apply to personality the then recently-developed method of factor analysis—a powerful tool that is used especially for discovering and mapping the important influences that underlie a vast array of observable, experimental variables. Further, Cattell hypothesized that "Over the centuries, by the pressure of urgent necessity, every aspect of one human being's behavior that is likely to affect another has come to be handled by some verbal symbol". This idea, that all important aspects of human personality have over time become encoded in our language, has come to be called the "lexical hypothesis." It is the basis for the recent "Big-Five" theories, and has been supported by a wide range of influential psychologists.

Thus, in seeking to include all important concepts of personality in his search, Cattell started with a list (compiled by Allport and Odbert) of all the English-language adjectives that describe "personal traits." Additionally, he reviewed all theoretical models of personality traits and types for further descriptors. After years of careful factor-analytic study of ratings, questionnaire data, and objective behavioral measures, Cattell arrived at his list of underlying traits—the fundamental building blocks of personality, which he called "primary factors." Table 10.1 lists and describes these scales, which reflect the traits identified through the factor analyses.

Origins of the Big-Five

Cattell's early research also included the original discovery of the broad dimensions currently called the "Big-Five." He found that when he factor analyzed the sixteen primary

Table 10.1: *16PF Fifth Edition* Primary Factor Scales[5]

Low Scores	High Scores

Warmth (A)

Low A: Reserved, impersonal, distant, formal. They tend to be reserved and cautious about involvement and attachment. They tend to like solitude, often focusing attention on mechanical, intellectual or artistic pursuits, where they can be quite effective. Low scorers can be uncomfortable in situations that call for emotional closeness or extensive interaction.

High A: Warm, caring, soft-hearted, generous. They tend to have an intrinsic interest in people and they often seek situations that call for closeness with other people. Their friends describe them as comforting. Extreme scorers may be seen as dependent or gullible, and may be uncomfortable in situations where close relationships are inaccessible.

Reasoning (B)

Low B: Less able to solve verbal and numerical problems of an academic nature. This can indicate lower intellectual ability, but it is also related to educational level. Low scores can also result from a range of problems affecting concentration and motivation.

High B: More able to solve verbal and numerical problems of an academic nature. This is often indicative of intellectual ability, but is also related to educational level. This index should not replace full-length measures of mental ability.

Emotional Stability (C)

Low C: Reactive, easily upset, temperamental. They tend to feel a lack of control over life's challenges and to react to life rather than making adaptive or proactive choices. For some test-takers, reactivity can reflect current life stressors; for others, it may characterize their way of life.

High C: Calm, stable, mature, unruffled. They tend to take life in stride and to cope with day-to-day life and its challenges in a balanced, adaptive way. Extreme scorers may tend to avoid "negative" feelings or use strong defenses like denial.

Dominance (E)

Low E: Deferential, modest, submissive. They tend to accommodate others' wishes, and are cooperative and agreeable. They are likely to avoid conflict by acquiescing to the wishes of others, and they are willing to set aside their own wishes and feelings. Extreme deference can disappoint those who wish for a more forceful or participating response.

High E: Assertive, forceful, competitive. They tend to be vocal in expressing their opinions and wishes. While dominance can create a commanding, take-charge social presence, extreme dominance can be seen as overbearing, stubborn or argumentative, and can alienate people.

Liveliness (F)

Low F: Serious, quiet, cautious, reflective. The quiet attentiveness of low scorers can make them reliable and mature, though they may not be the life of the party or the most entertaining person in a group. At the extreme, they can inhibit their spontaneity, sometimes to the point of appearing constricted.

High F: Carefree, enthusiastic, spontaneous, energetic. They are high spirited and stimulating and drawn to lively social situations. Extreme scores may reflect an impulsive, unreliable, or immature quality. They may find it hard to rein in their enthusiasm in situations that call for restraint or decorum.

Rule Consciousness (G)

Low G: Expedient, non-conforming, weak superego. They tend to eschew rules and regulations, either because they lack internalized standards or simply because they follow unconventional values.

High G: Rule-conscious, dutiful, scrupulous, strong superego. They tend to conform to conventional cultural standards. At the extreme, they can be perceived as inflexible, moralistic, or high-minded.

Social Boldness (H)

Low H: Shy, socially timid, threat-sensitive, easily embarrassed. They find speaking in front of groups to be difficult, and may feel intimidated when facing stressful situations of an interpersonal nature.

High H: Socially bold, outgoing, gregarious, adventuresome. They tend to initiate social contacts and be fearless in the face of new or intimidating social settings. Extreme scorers may be thick-skinned or attention seeking.

Table 10.1. Continued

Low Scores	High Scores

Sensitivity (I)

Low I: Tough, realistic, logical, unsentimental. They attend more to how things work than to aesthetics or refined sensibilities, and may be so concerned with utility and objectivity that they exclude feelings from consideration. Because they don't tend to indulge vulnerability, extreme low scorers may have trouble in situations that demand awareness of feelings.

High I: Emotionally sensitive, intuitive, cultured, sentimental. They tend to be refined in their interests and tastes, and to be empathic and more attuned to emotions than their low-scoring counterparts. Extreme scorers may be so focused on subjective aspects of situations that they overlook more functional aspects.

Vigilance (L)

Low L: Trusting, unsuspecting, forgiving, accepting. They tend to expect fair treatment and good intentions from others, and to have trusting relationships. However, extremely low scorers may be taken advantage of because they do not give enough thought to others' motivations.

High L: Vigilant, suspicious, distrustful, wary. They tend to be suspicious about others' motives and intentions, expecting to be misunderstood or taken advantage of. They may be unable to relax their vigilance, and at the extreme their mistrust may have an aspect of animosity.

Abstractedness (M)

Low M: Grounded, practical, down-to-earth. They tend to focus on practical, observable data and outer realities of their environment and may be better at implementing a specific solution than at generating possible solutions. Extreme scorers may be so concrete, prosaic in their focus or literal that they "miss the forest for the trees."

High M: Abstracted, imaginative, idea-oriented, contemplative. They are more oriented to abstract internal mental processes than to external facts and practicalities. Being preoccupied with thinking, imagination and fantasy, high scorers generate many ideas and theories and are often creative. At the extreme, they can be so absorbed in thought that they can be absentminded and impractical.

Privateness (N)

Low N: Forthright, self-revealing, transparent. They tend to be open and willing to talk about themselves readily. They tend to "put all their cards on the table," and to be genuine and unguarded. At the extreme, they may be forthright in situations where it might be more astute to be circumspect or tactful.

High N: Private, discreet, nondisclosing. They tend to be reluctant to disclose personal information, and "play their hand close to their chest." They may be tactful, diplomatic and insightful regarding others' motives. At the extreme, they maintain their privacy at the expense of developing few close relationships with others.

Apprehension (O)

Low O: Self-assured, unworried, complacent. They tend to be self-confident and untroubled by self-doubt. While this may make them more resilient in stressful situations, at the extreme, the person's confidence may be unshaken, even in situations that call for self-evaluation and self-improvement. The low score may reflect a blocking from awareness of anything negative about the self.

High O: Apprehensive, self-doubting, guilt-prone. They tend to worry about things and to feel anxious and insecure. These feelings may be in response to current life events or they may be characteristic. While worrying can help the person anticipate dangers and anticipate consequences of actions, it can also be painful and make a poor social impression on others.

Openness to Change (Q1)

Low Q1: Traditional, attached to familiar, resistant to change. They tend to stick to traditional ways of doing things. They prefer what's predictable and routine, and so they don't tend to challenge the status quo. At the extreme, they may not initiate or be open to change, even when the situation calls for it.

High Q1: Open to change, experimenting, free-thinking. They tend to be open-minded and innovative, and see ways to improve the status quo. They enjoy experimenting, and tend to think critically or question authority. They may find it hard to "leave well enough alone."

Table 10.1. Continued

Low Scores	High Scores
Self Reliance (Q2)	
Low Q2: Group-oriented, affiliative, group-dependent. They tend to prefer being around others people, and enjoy social groups, and working in teams. At the extreme, they may not be effective in situations where they need to function independently or where others are giving poor direction or advice.	**High Q2:** Self-reliant, solitary, individualistic. They enjoy spending time alone and prefer to rely on their own thinking and judgment. While self-reliant people are autonomous in their thoughts and actions, extreme scorers may have trouble working collaboratively or neglect interpersonal consequences of their actions.
Perfectionism (Q3)	
Low Q3: Tolerates disorder, unexacting, casual, lax. They tend to be comfortable leaving things to chance, tending to "go with the flow" rather than to be planful and structured. While they can seem flexible and spontaneous, they may also seem unorganized, unprepared, or undisciplined.	**High Q3:** Perfectionistic, self-disciplined, goal-oriented. They tend to be organized, plan ahead, persevere, and work conscientiously. They are most comfortable in organized and structured situations, and may find it hard to deal with unpredictability. At the extreme, they may be seen as inflexible or compulsive.
Tension (Q4)	
Low Q4: Relaxed, placid, tranquil, patient. They are laid back, composed, and slow to become frustrated. At the extreme, their low level of arousal can make them unmotivated. That is, because they are comfortable, they may be disinclined to change or push themselves.	**High Q4:** Tense, driven, high energy, impatient. They tend to have a lot of drive, to be high strung, and to be fidgety when made to wait. While a certain amount of tension can be focused effectively and can motivate action, extremely high tension can lead to impatience and irritability. The source of tension should be explored when scores are extremely high.

[5]Modified from the *16PF Fifth Edition Administrator's Manual*, Copyright ©1994 the Institute for Personality and Ability Testing, Champaign, IL.

scales, five "second-order" or global factors emerged, which represented broad patterns of influence at a higher level of personality structure. The 16PF model, then, is a hierarchical one: The Big-Five, global factor scales describe personality at the most general level, but each of these five factors can then be broken down into the primary factors that reveal the nuances and particulars that make each personality unique. Table 10.2 describes the 16PF's five global factor scales, and Table 10.3 describes which primary factor scales make up each global factor scale.

As will be discussed in the interpretive guidelines, it is important to know both an individual's global scale scores and their scores on the primary scales that make up each global dimension. For example, two individuals may both have the same elevated scores on global Extraversion, but their constellation of scores on the primary scales within Extraversion may show them to have rather different styles. For example, their primary scores may indicate that one individual is warm, sensitive, and self-revealing, while the other is bold, flashy, and attention-seeking. That is, while each would move toward social interaction, they do so for very different reasons and with a very different impact on their social environment.

Research

The 16PF questionnaire has an extensive body of research that stretches back a half century and provides information about its usefulness in clinical, counseling, industrial/organizational, educational, and research settings. This rich data base of several thousand publica-

Table 10.2. *16PF Fifth Edition* Global Factor Scales[5]

Low Scorers	High Scorers
Introversion	Extraversion
Low Scorers tend to value time spent alone or in solitary pursuits, being generally less inclined to seek out interaction with others. The introvert can have one or several of these qualities: personal aloofness and a tendency to make few close connections; caution, restraint and a tendency to take life seriously; an inclination to be shy or fearful about reaching out to others; discomfort about revealing personal information; and/or a preference for working alone and functioning autonomously.	**High Scorers** tend to be people-oriented, to seek interaction with others, and to value time spent with others, in social pursuits. The extravert can have one or several of these qualities: warmth and a wish to feel close connections with people, a lively social energy and seeking of social stimulation; comfort in the company of others; bold gregariousness; and/or an interest in being forthright and self-disclosing. A high EX score, however, doesn't guarantee the relationship quality.
Low Anxiety	High Anxiety
Low Scorers tend to be unperturbed by most events and less easily upset than most people. They can be: emotionally stable, facing life's challenges with calm and stability; trusting of others; unworried and self-assured; and/or relaxed and placid. Extremely low scorers may minimize the ways that life or personal limitations can pose stress or challenges, or may be so comfortable that they are not motivated to change.	**High Scorers** tend to be more easily upset by events; they are more perturbed, both by internal thoughts and feelings as well as by external events. This may be characteristic or may be due to current life stress. Anxious people can experience one or more of the following: feeling overwhelmed and unable to cope with day-to-day living; being suspicious or doubting of others; worrying and self-doubting; feeling tense, driven, or frustrated.
Receptivity	Tough-Mindedness
Low Scorers tend to be open to people, feelings, imagination, and new ideas. Their focus is on: emotional and aesthetic sensibilities; ideas and thoughts, especially imaginative ones; caring connections with people; or experimenting and trying new approaches. They may overlook the need to be practical, objective, or realistic in dealing with the world.	**High Scorers** tend to prefer known, concrete, familiar territory. They focus on: objectivity (as opposed to sentimentality); practical, concrete things rather than abstract ideas or theories; keeping things on an impersonal level; or valuing methods and traditions that are tried-and-true. Extreme tough-mindedness may result in resolute entrenchment and avoidance of new or imaginative approaches.
Accommodation	Independence
Low Scorers tend to be accommodating to other people and external influences rather than being self-determining. They may be uncomfortable in situations that call for independence or assertiveness. Low scorers have varying degrees of deference, cooperation, shyness, trust, and satisfaction with the status quo. Their ability to accommodate others' wishes often comes at their own expense, and may alienate others who desire more active participation.	**High Scorers** tend to be "take-charge" people who influence rather than being influenced. Their active stance on life can include these elements: dominance and an unwillingness to acquiesce; social boldness and fearlessness; being skeptical of others, especially about being controlled; and willingness to question and improve on the status quo. High scorers can be seen as disagreeable by others who feel controlled or dominated. They may find it hard to accommodate others when it is important to do so.

tions has been equaled by few other instruments. Because the 16PF questionnaire has been used in diverse settings, research has generated a wide range of profiles and prediction equations for criteria such as psychological and marital adjustment, self-esteem, interpersonal skills, creativity, and leadership, plus dozens of occupational profiles. Indeed, many of these studies

Table 10.2. Continued

Low Scorers	High Scorers
Lack of Restraint	Self-Control
Low Scorers are unrestrained and tend to have fewer resources for controlling their behavior. They may find it hard to place limits on their own urges or to focus their attention. They may be spontaneous, carefree or impulsive; nonconforming, or inattentive to rules and regulations; so caught up in internal mental processes that they don't focus on practicalities; or so undisciplined that they "go with the flow" and do not plan. While perceived as flexible, playful and casual, low scorers can also be seen as unreliable, expedient, or careless.	**High Scorers** have resources upon which they can call for controlling their behavior and meeting their responsibilities. These resources include being cautious, restrained and taking matters seriously; placing importance on following rules and meeting expectations; being grounded, practical, and realistic; being self-disciplined and organized. While they tend to be seen as conscientious and reliable, high scorers can also be seen as overly controlled—that is, *too* serious or moralistic or compulsive.

[5]Modified from the *16PF Fifth Edition Administrator's Manual*, Copyright ©1994 the Institute for Personality and Ability Testing, Champaign, IL.

have been carried out cross-culturally, and the measure has been translated into more than 40 languages and dialects.

TEST CONSTRUCTION AND DEVELOPMENT

The development of the 16PF Fifth Edition (1993) began by finding the best items (those that showed strong relationships with the scale they measure) from all existing 16PF forms. These items were updated and combined with new items, which were written with the goals of (a) being highly related to their scale and not to other scales; (b) being short, simple and unambiguous; (c) avoiding content that might lead to gender, race, or disability bias; (d) being easily translatable into other languages or cultures; (e) avoiding material that might be considered invasive, offensive, or otherwise unacceptable in an industrial/organizational setting; and (f) avoiding socially desirable content that might lead to motivational distortion.

Item selection was carried out over four experimental stages based on test results from large, diverse national samples of 1,204, 646, 872, and 3,498 subjects, respectively. Inclusion of an item in the final form was based on factor analytic loadings, item-scale correlations, and coefficient alpha internal consistency reliabilities, with an eye to creating solid metric properties in the resulting scales. The final normative sample of 2,500 people was stratified on the basis of age, sex, race, and educational level to match the 1990 U.S. Census figures as closely as possible.

The features of the 16PF Fifth Edition include the following:

- Overall length is 185 items, with 10–15 items per scale.
- Sixteen primary factor scales, one of which (Factor B) is a brief measure of general ability.
- Five global (or "second-order") factor scales—the original big-five factors.
- Three response style or validity indices: a bipolar Impression Management (IM) scale, an Infrequency (INF) scale, and an Acquiescence (ACQ) scale.
- Administration time is 30–50 minutes for paper-and-pencil administration and 25–35 minutes for computer administration.

Table 10.3. The Global Factors and Their Contributing Primary Scales[5]

Factors	Primary Scales	Factors
Introversion	vs.	Extraversion
Reserved, Impersonal, Distant	Warmth (A)	Warm, Outgoing, Attentive to Others
Serious, Restrained, Careful	Liveliness (F)	Lively, Animated, Spontaneous
Shy, Threat–Sensitive, Timid	Social Boldness (H)	Bold, Venturesome, Thick–Skinned
Private, Discreet, Non–Disclosing	Privateness (N)	Forthright, Genuine, Artless
Self–Reliant, Solitary, Individualistic	Self-Reliance (Q2)	Group–Oriented, Affiliative
Low Anxiety	vs.	High Anxiety
Emotionally Stable, Adaptive, Mature	Emotional Stability (C)	Reactive, Emotionally Changeable
Trusting, Unsuspecting, Accepting	Vigilance (L)	Vigilant, Suspicious, Skeptical, Wary
Self–Assured, Unworried, Complacent	Apprehension (O)	Apprehensive, Self–Doubting, Worried
Relaxed, Placid, Patient	Tension (Q4)	Tense, High Energy, Impatient, Driven
Receptivity	vs.	Tough–Mindedness
Warm, Outgoing, Attentive to Others	Warmth (A)	Reserved, Impersonal, Distant
Sensitive, Aesthetic, Sentimental	Sensitivity (I)	Utilitarian, Objective, Unsentimental
Abstracted, Imaginative, Idea–oriented	Abstractedness (M)	Grounded, Practical, Solution–Oriented
Open to Change, Experimenting	Openness to Change (Q1)	Traditional, Attached to Familiar
Accommodation	vs.	Independence
Deferential, Cooperative, Avoids Conflict	Dominance (E)	Dominant, Forceful, Assertive
Shy, Threat–Sensitive, Timid	Social Boldness (H)	Bold, Venturesome, Thick-Skinned
Trusting, Unsuspecting, Accepting	Vigilance (L)	Vigilant, Suspicious, Skeptical, Wary
Traditional, Attached to Familiar	Openness to Change (Q1)	Open to Change, Experimenting
Lack of Restraint	vs.	Self–Control
Lively, Animated, Spontaneous	Liveliness (F)	Serious, Restrained, Careful
Expedient, Nonconforming	Rule-Consciousness (G)	Rule–Conscious, Dutiful
Abstracted, Imaginative, Idea–oriented	Abstractedness (M)	Grounded, Practical, Solution–Oriented
Tolerates Disorder, Unexacting, Flexible	Perfectionism (Q3)	Perfectionist, Organized, Self–Disciplined

Note. Primary scales can contribute to globals in either a positive or a negative direction. For example, Liveliness (F) contributes positively to Extraversion (a high score on F contributes to a high score on Extraversion), but negatively to Self-Control (a high score on F lowers the individual's Self-Control score). Primary factors that contribute negatively to a global have been marked with a "a".

[5]Modified from the *16PF Fifth Edition Administrator's Manual*, Copyright ©1994 the Institute for Personality and Ability Testing, Champaign, IL.

- Designed for ages 16 years and older with at least a fifth-grade reading level.
- Coefficient alpha reliabilities for the primary scales average .74 (with a range from .64 to .85). Test-retest reliabilities for a two-week interval average .80 (with a range from .69 to .87).
- Scoring options include hand-scoring, fax or mail-in services, and the OnSite computer administration and scoring program for PCs. A range of computer-generated interpretive reports are available.

ADMINISTRATION AND SCORING

Although the 16PF Fifth Edition is virtually self-administrable, the test administrator is advised to take time to establish a comfortable rapport with examinees, since the creation of a positive test-taking attitude is essential in acquiring accurate data. Examinees should under-stand that it is in their own self interest to be frank and honest in their self-descriptions. The test should be completed in a quiet, well-lit location, and the administrator should be available to answer any questions.

The test can be administered using paper-and-pencil materials or using IPAT's OnSite computer software system. Paper-and-pencil materials include the test booklet and a single-page answer sheet, which may be hand-scored or computer scored. In both cases, the questionnaire itself provides clear, simple instructions for examinees, which the administrator may either read aloud or let examinees read silently. Note that all items except Factor B have a three-choice response format (a, b, or c), with the middle answer (b) being a question mark "?". The test-taker chooses (b) when neither the (a) nor the (c) choice is true for them.

When using the answer sheet, examinees are asked to enter their name and sex in the grids on the answer sheet, *which requires the use of a No. 2 or softer pencil if it is to be computer-scored.* During testing, the administrator may want to check that examinees are marking responses appropriately. Completed answer sheets should be reviewed for missing or multiple answers, which examinees should be asked to correct before scoring.

Scoring

Hand-Scoring: Materials needed for hand-scoring include a set of four scoring keys (templates), the norm table, and an Individual Record Form. Instructions are written on the scoring keys, and the process simply involves obtaining the test-taker's raw scores for each scale by counting marks through each template and using the norm table to convert the raw scores to standardized (sten) scores. The Individual Record Form allows graphing of the 16PF profile on one side and, on the back side, offers a simple worksheet for calculating the global factor scores from the primary factor scale sten scores.

Computer Scoring: Answer sheets can be mailed or faxed to IPAT for computer scoring, or scored on location with IPAT's OnSite software system. (Note: On computer-scored answer sheets, the sex of the examinee must be indicated for appropriate pronouns to appear in the interpretive report.) Numerous computer-generated interpretive reports are available to aid in interpretation of scores in clinical, counseling, industrial, or research settings.

Norm Choices: For both hand-scoring and computer-scoring, the test administrator must decide which of two norm groups to use. When "combined-sex" norms are chosen, the examinee's scores are compared to the total normative group, containing both men and women. When "sex-specific" norms are selected, the norm table provides separate comparison tables for men and women (only three factor scales showed gender differences in the raw score distributions—Warmth [Factor A], Dominance [Factor E], and Sensitivity [Factor I]).

INTERPRETIVE GUIDELINES

Background

Empirical Foundations

Underlying the use of the 16PF questionnaire in counseling and clinical settings is the assumption that the test is valid. The validity of a test is not easily summed up in a single number, such as a "validity coefficient," or in one reference or book. Rather, there are many different kinds of validity evidence that together build a body of evidence about the test's effectiveness. Thus, a wide range of studies using the 16PF questionnaire and linking it to important behaviors or outcomes adds to what is known about the questionnaire's validity.

Our purpose here is not to summarize all of the relevant literature; the resource books listed at the end of this chapter are excellent references that contain different types of validity evidence important to counseling- and clinically-focused uses of the 16PF measure. One example of useful 16PF research has been the study of the effects of personality similarities and differences on couples' relationships. Other research has supported the use of normal range personality data in clinical assessment by identifying potential areas of personal concern for the client (such as quality of attachments, passive-aggression), or issues relevant to the counseling process (such as capacity for insight, power dynamics, or resistance to change). Other research has centered around career guidance and employee development and the implications of personality style for career and world-of-work issues. And, of course, studies linking other personality measures with the 16PF help to establish its construct validity. Previous 16PF versions have sometimes been used to distinguish between different types of clinically-diagnosed groups, or to evaluate how a given clinically-diagnosed group differs from the general population. While the 16PF was not designed for the purpose of making diagnostic distinctions, the relationships between 16PF profiles and diagnostic groupings can be useful in formulating hypotheses about the clinical relevance of certain 16PF scores.

Expert Opinion

All practitioner-scientists can observe the relationship between clients' 16PF scores and behaviors and can formulate hypotheses to be tested, based upon such observations. In fact, the systematic collection and reporting of clinicians' findings serves as a significant contribution to our understanding about the clinical relevance of the 16PF scales. Samuel Karson, Ph.D. and Jerry O'Dell, Ph.D., in their 1976 book, *A Guide to the Clinical Use of the 16PF,* described the 16PF scales in terms of their clinical importance. In 1997, Dr. Michael Karson co-wrote an expanded, updated guide with these same authors: *16PF Interpretation in Clinical Practice: A Guide to the Fifth Edition.*

In 1989, Dr. Heather Birkett Cattell authored *The 16PF: Personality in Depth.* This book summarizes 10 years of research that the author conducted in her clinical practice using the 16PF questionnaire. In her work with three databases of clients who took the 16PF measure, she carefully recorded clients' 16PF scores and then noted her direct observations of their behavior. She also listened to and recorded any insights, self-disclosures, and remarks that clients volunteered in response to 16PF test result feedback. Cattell also drew on other sources of information such as mental status exams, clinical assessments, and psycho-social histories; whenever possible, she observed interactions with family members, group therapy members, and co-workers. She found that certain patterns of thinking, feeling and behaving were associated with individual factor scale scores and with certain score combinations.

Of course, many other authors and researchers have also contributed to the 16PF knowledge base. Additional resources that are especially relevant for clinicians and counselors are listed in the suggested readings at the end of this chapter.

16PF Profile Interpretation Sequence

A 16PF profile can seem complex, especially to a beginning interpreter. However, there are strategies for interpreting a profile that can help reduce the complexity into smaller, manageable components. A common interpretive strategy is presented below. First, though, the interpreter should be aware of some basic facts relevant to interpreting 16PF profiles.

Sten Scores

The 16PF personality scales use a sten ("standardized ten") distribution. Sten scores range from 1–10, with a mean of 5.5 and a standard deviation of 2. The scores fall farther from the mean in either the high or the low direction, are the more extreme they are more likely they are to reflect traits that will be salient in the examinee's behavior. A rule-of-thumb convention is to consider stens of 5–6 to be average while stens of 4–7 fall within a broader average range (which includes those between the 16th percentile and the 84th percentile), stens of 1–3 to fall in the low range, and stens of 8–10 to fall in the high range (representing the top and bottom 16% of the population). This convention reflects the sten distribution, in which about 68% of the population obtains a score within plus-or-minus one standard deviation from the mean, while about 16% have low scores and 16% have high scores. Within these broad categories of scores, of course, finer distinctions are important. For example, stens of 4 are termed "low-average" and represent the 16th to 31st percentile, while stens of 7 are termed "high-average" and cover the 69th to 84th percentiles. Stens of 8, 9 or 10 might be termed high, very high and extremely high, respectively; at the opposite pole of the distribution, stens of 3, 2 and 1 might be termed low, very low and extremely low.

As with all test scores, 16PF scores are in fact an estimate of a person's true score on any given personality factor. Because most 16PF scales have a standard error of measurement (SE_M) that is close to 1 sten score point (SE_M's range from .79 to 1.17 for primary factor scales), the person's true score usually would be in a range of plus-or-minus 1 sten score point around his or her obtained score. For example, the true score range for a sten score of 4 would be expected to fall, 68% of the time, within a sten score range of 3–5. Given this fact, the low/average/high rule of thumb expressed above must be used judiciously; that is, the interpreter should recognize that for a sten score of 4 ("low-average") the true score could possibly be a sten of 3 ("low") or a sten of 5 ("average").

Bipolar Scales

The 16PF scales are bipolar; that is, both high and low scores have a well-defined meaning. The right-side pole, or high-score range, of a factor scale is described as the plus (+) pole. The left-side pole, or low-score range, is the minus (-) pole. For example, high scorers on Warmth (Factor A) are described as warm-hearted (A+), whereas low-scorers are described as reserved (A-). However, interpreters should not assume that high scores are "good" and that low scores are "bad." While to some people warm may seem to be "good" and reserved "bad," the fact is that being reserved can serve quite well in some situations (for example, in occupations or situations that require solitude or a focus on solving objective problems or managing functional operations). On the other hand, warmth might serve better for roles that involve being helpful or nurturing when interacting with others.

Some 16PF scales, especially those related to the Anxiety global factor scale, do have a pole that seems more socially desirable (again, though, the desirable pole may not be the high pole). However, even on such scales, an extreme score in either direction may have undesirable ramifications. For example, an extremely low score on Apprehensiveness (Factor O) can suggest that the test-taker is defended against admitting any self-doubt or personal insecurity.

Such an extreme score could also mean that the test-taker's confidence may be unshakable, even in situations where realistic self-evaluation and self-improvement are desirable.

 Interpretive Sequence

Although the individual interpreter's approach to interpreting a profile may vary depending on the interpreter's level of experience, a common strategy is described here:

- **Review the Response Style (Validity) Indices:** Check for atypical test-response styles.
- **Review the Global Factor Scores:** These scales give a "big picture view" of five broad themes that represent fundamental organizing influences among the sixteen primary scales.
- **Review the Primary Factor Scales:** (a) Identify the extreme scores. (b) Review the primary factor scales within the context of each global factor scale (to fill in the details of the big picture).
- **Put It All Together:** Look at how all the scales fit together and interact—global scales, including contributing primaries, are reviewed and combined to give a comprehensive picture, particular primary score combinations are examined, and predicted scores and computer-generated report content are reviewed.

In the next section, each step in the interpretive sequence is described. The profile presented in Figure 10.1, will be used in each step to give the reader a clearer idea of the process performed and information gleaned at each step.

Validity Indices

	Raw Score	Percentiles	
Impression Management	17	88%	within expected range
Infrequency	2	68%	within expected range
Acquiescence	53	33%	within expected range

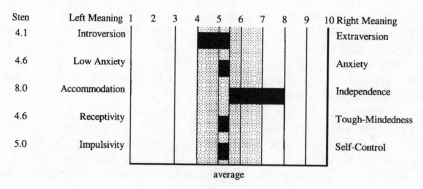

Global Scores

Sten	Left Meaning	1 2 3 4 5 6 7 8 9 10	Right Meaning
4.1	Introversion		Extraversion
4.6	Low Anxiety		Anxiety
8.0	Accommodation		Independence
4.6	Receptivity		Tough-Mindedness
5.0	Impulsivity		Self-Control

average

Figure 10.1a. Mr. Jones' 16PF scores.

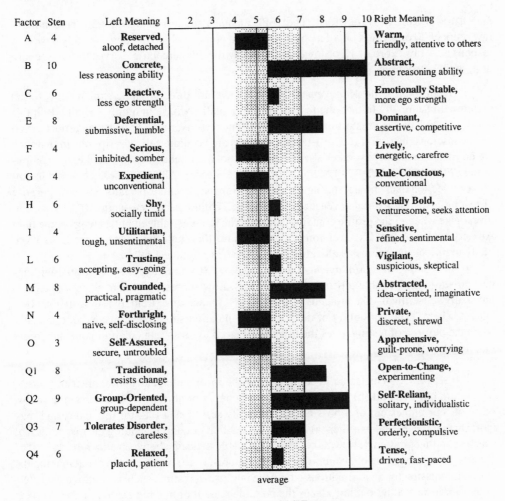

Factor	Sten	Left Meaning	1	2	3	4	5	6	7	8	9	10	Right Meaning
A	4	**Reserved,** aloof, detached											**Warm,** friendly, attentive to others
B	10	**Concrete,** less reasoning ability											**Abstract,** more reasoning ability
C	6	**Reactive,** less ego strength											**Emotionally Stable,** more ego strength
E	8	**Deferential,** submissive, humble											**Dominant,** assertive, competitive
F	4	**Serious,** inhibited, somber											**Lively,** energetic, carefree
G	4	**Expedient,** unconventional											**Rule-Conscious,** conventional
H	6	**Shy,** socially timid											**Socially Bold,** venturesome, seeks attention
I	4	**Utilitarian,** tough, unsentimental											**Sensitive,** refined, sentimental
L	6	**Trusting,** accepting, easy-going											**Vigilant,** suspicious, skeptical
M	8	**Grounded,** practical, pragmatic											**Abstracted,** idea-oriented, imaginative
N	4	**Forthright,** naive, self-disclosing											**Private,** discreet, shrewd
O	3	**Self-Assured,** secure, untroubled											**Apprehensive,** guilt-prone, worrying
Q1	8	**Traditional,** resists change											**Open-to-Change,** experimenting
Q2	9	**Group-Oriented,** group-dependent											**Self-Reliant,** solitary, individualistic
Q3	7	**Tolerates Disorder,** careless											**Perfectionistic,** orderly, compulsive
Q4	6	**Relaxed,** placid, patient											**Tense,** driven, fast-paced

average

Figure 10.1b. Mr. Jones' 16PF scores.

Sample Profile: Mr. Jones was a 28-year-old computer scientist who sought consultation when he failed to gain promotion to Manager of Research and Development at the computer software company where he worked. He sought counseling only at the suggestion of his boss and only in the circumscribed area of achieving his career goals.

1. Review the Response Style (Validity) Indices

There are three response style or validity indices: Impression Management (IM), Infrequency (INF), and Acquiescence (ACQ). These indices are presented as a raw score or percentile, rather than as a sten score. Extreme percentiles are used to "flag" the possibility of a response set. If any of the indices is extreme, the interpreter should evaluate whether the test-taker's response sets might be affecting the validity of the profile, as discussed below.

Impression Management: The 16PF manuals suggest using the 95th percentile (a raw score of 20 or greater, out of a possible 24) as a point at which to "flag" socially desirable responses. A raw score of 12 or lower (at or below the 5th percentile) serves to flag socially undesirable responses.

a. *High Impression Management Scores:* There are three possible explanations for an extreme IM score. (1) In fact, the test-taker may actually behave in highly socially desirable ways, in which case no distortion is at work. (2) The test-taker's responses may reflect a kind of unconscious distortion (the test-taker's answers are accurate self-descriptions in that they are consistent with the test-taker's self-image, but not their behavior). (3) Deliberate manipulation of the answers may also account for a high IM score. Although more common in employee selection than clinical settings, such distortion may occur, especially when the purpose of testing gives the test-taker reason to do so (e.g., child custody evaluations). It is wise to investigate whether the profile contains at least some less-desirable qualities (e. g., some high Anxiety scales or low Extraversion scales), because this indicates that the profile is more likely to reflect some honest self-reflection on the part of the test-taker.

b. *Low Impression Management Scores:* A low IM score suggests an unusual willingness to admit undesirable attributes or behaviors. Low scores can occur when a person is unusually self-critical, discouraged, or under stress. In fact, an extremely low score may be a "plea for help." The possibility of deliberate manipulation should be considered, especially when the purpose of testing gives the test-taker reason to do so (e.g., claiming mental duress in a litigation).

Infrequency: This scale is comprised of the most statistically infrequent responses, which turn out to be all (b) responses. Again, a score at or above the 95th percentile (a raw score of 8 or higher out of a possible 32) typically serves as a flag for this index and may indicate that the test-taker either (a) had trouble reading or comprehending the questions; (b) was responding randomly; (c) was consistently unable to decide between either the "a" or "c" choice (perhaps because of an ambiguous self-picture); or (d) was trying to avoid making the wrong impression (e. g., in situations where the purpose of testing, such as employment selection or forensic evaluation, introduces the possible benefit of making a good impression).

Acquiescence: This new scale serves to raise a flag about the possibility that the person tended to agree to items regardless of what was being asked. A high score results when the test-taker repeatedly chooses the agreeable ("a. true") response to true-false items (doing so 71 times or more exceeds the 95th percentile for this index). A high score might indicate that the test taker (a) misunderstood the item content; (b) was responding randomly; (c) had an unclear self-image; or (d) had a "yea-saying" response style. The latter two causes might also mean that the test-taker will tend to agree with or defer to the professional or to be highly sensitive to cues of approval or self-definition from others.

Sample Profile: Mr. Jones' IM score is at the 88th percentile, but this probably does not indicate that the validity of the profile is in doubt. In job-related settings, the IM scale is commonly above average and may indicate something positive—that the individual has a good understanding of social expectations and has the ability to put his or her best foot forward when appropriate. This conclusion is further supported by the fact that most of Mr. Jones' Extraversion scores are average or introverted (Factors A, F, H, and Q2) and most of his Anxiety scores are average (Factors C, L, and Q4), indicating that he did not try to present a uniformly positive picture of himself. The professional will want to confirm this finding with data from other sources.

The average scores on the INF and ACQ indices suggest that Mr. Jones had no problem reading and understanding the test questions and answering them in a meaningful way.

2. Review the Global Factor Scores

Identify Extreme Global Factor Scores: As mentioned in describing the sten distribution above, scores that fall outside the average range are more noteworthy. In the normative sample, the percentage of the population receiving different numbers of extreme global scores (that is, scores either in the sten range 1–3 or 8–10) is as follows:

0–2 extreme scores are received by 79%
3 extreme scores are received by 15%
4 extreme scores are received by 5%
5 extreme scores are received by 1%

Overview: In her book, Heather Birkett Cattell recommends reviewing the global factor scores before looking at the primary factor scales. She suggests that the information provided by the global factor scales

is analogous to the first broad outline created by an artist's brush before the canvas is filled in with the details, contrasts, and highlights that give the picture its final form. This outline, though rough, foreshadows the particulars to come. The outline also provides a general framework for organizing pieces of information as they are gleaned from each primary factor interpretation.[1]

The 16PF global factor scales (which were developed in the 1950s and 1960s) represent the original Big-Five scales which are so popular in the current personality literature. Developing a picture of the individual's global profile can be helpful in getting a "bird's-eye view" of the test-taker. Table 10.2 describes the meaning of extreme scores on the five global factor scales. Once the interpreter has developed a sense of the big picture painted by the test-taker's global factor scores, the next step is to review the primary factor scores to fill in the "fine-grain" specifics of the individual's personality.

Sample Profile: First, since Mr. Jones' profile shows only one elevated global score and one low-average score, he is in the average range for overall number of elevated scores. His below-average Extraversion score indicates that people and social activities do not play as big a role in his life as in the average person's life. In the next step, investigating the Extraversion primary scales will reveal the particular style and motivation of his social reserve.

Mr. Jones' high score on Independence suggests that he is a self-directed individual who tends to act autonomously and to have a significant impact on his environment (rather than accommodating to it). High-Independence individuals such as Mr. Jones tend to be willful and individualistic and are often seen as "a force unto themselves." The Independence primary scale scores will reveal the particular style of his impact on his environment.

Although Mr. Jones' other three global scores are in the average range, it is important to remember that an average global score may be attained by having extreme but opposite scores on contributing primary scales—which is the case for both Mr. Jones' Tough-Mindedness and Self-Control globals.

3. Review the Primary Factor Scales

A. Identify the Extreme Primary Factor Scores: The greater the number of extreme scores found within a profile, the more the person is likely to have a well-defined, individualistic personality style that stands out from others'. In fact, an extreme score results when the person chooses item responses that describe one distinct kind of behavior consistently. In the normative sample, the percentage of the population earning different numbers of extreme primary scores are as follows:

1–2 extreme scores are received by 14%
3–7 extreme scores are received by 69%
8+ extreme scores are received by 17%

Extreme scale scores suggest that the test-taker may find it difficult to shift his or her behavior, even in situations where his or her predominant style may not be ideal or appropriate. When a profile contains few extreme scores, it may be because the person's behavior is not extreme in either direction (is average), or it could be that the person has a rather unclear self-picture on certain traits. Also, in some cases, people who wish to avoid making a poor impression can achieve a fairly "flat" profile either by answering similar items in inconsistent directions, or by choosing a relatively high number of "b" responses.

Sample Profile: Mr. Jones shows six extreme primary scales, which is within the average range, although above average. Thus, although Mr. Jones appears to have a good deal of distinctive features in his personality, he is not extreme in this way.

B. Review the Primary Scales in the Context of the Global Factor Scales: As with the global factor scales, primary factor scale scores that fall outside the average range are more definitive and likely to describe the test-takers' strongest traits. The interpreter should review each scale that is extreme and begin to form an overall picture of the person's strongest features. Table 10.1 describes the meaning of the primary factor scales; full descriptions can be found in the 16PF resource books listed at the end of this chapter.

Next, the primary scales that make up each global factor are usually reviewed together, in order to gain a thorough picture of the individual's functioning in each domain. Table 10.3 shows which primary factor scales contribute to each of the five global factor scales. In most profiles, there will be a few primary scores in each global factor that are elevated, and these will shed light on how the global quality will be expressed. Note that primary scales may contribute in a positive direction or in a negative direction to a global scale, depending on the meaning of the factor. For each global factor scale, the interpreter should identify which of the individual primary factor scales are *raising* the overall global factor score, and which are *lowering* it. High scores on Extraversion, for example, come from high scores on Warmth (Factor A), Liveliness (Factor F), and Social Boldness (Factor H), and low scores on Privateness (Factor N) and Self Reliance (Factor Q2). Furthermore, while Liveliness (Factor F) thus contributes positively to Extraversion, it also contributes in a negative direction to Self-Control, indicating that this uninhibited, spontaneous quality may limit a person's ability to be conscientious.

In some cases, one primary factor score is *inconsistent with* the rest of the primary scores in a global factor score (e.g., a high score on Extraversion, but a low score on Warmth [A]) and these scores are particularly noteworthy as a contradiction to the general trend. Alternatively, a person may get an average global factor score by combining extreme but opposite scores on some of the relevant primary factor scales.

This kind of disparate mix of qualities is especially noteworthy and useful in building a picture of the individual's unique needs and style. For example, disparate primary scores within Extraversion may help to identify what particular needs or motivations lead the client to seek social contact or avoid social contact. In a similar way, the subfactors of Self-Control may elucidate some sources of internal controls but reveal other contributors to impulsivity. Disparate patterns of primary factors may also be explored with the test-taker, to ascertain the impact or meaning of these unique combinations. For example, the counselor might ask, "On the one hand, you tend to be X, but you also describe yourself as Y. How do these disparate qualities make a 'fit' for you? Do you find that it is sometimes hard to express (or accommodate) both styles?"

Sample Profile: *Extraversion:* Among the primary scales that make up Extraversion, Mr. Jones shows signs of Introversion on Factors A, F, and especially Q2—a powerful combination. First, since Mr. Jones tends to be reserved (A–), he is not very interested in people or their feelings, and his attention is more likely focused on facts, ideas, or other objective matters. Furthermore, his low-average score on Liveliness (F–) suggests a serious, subdued individual who does not have a lot of energy for interpersonal interaction or playful activities. Most importantly, his high score on Self-Reliance (Q2+) indicates a solitary, autonomous style. Thus, Mr. Jones probably prefers to rely only on his own thinking and judgment and to spend time by himself, working on his own projects. He does not welcome advice or opinions from others and may view these rather as intrusions or attempts to control him. Finally, these qualities may be exacerbated by his one Extraverted score—Forthrightness (N–). Although some will enjoy this straightforward, transparent quality, at times he may seem naive or tactless in his interactions with people, and this will also tend to make his general trait make-up more apparent to others. These Extraversion traits taken together suggest a solemn, reserved, loner style.

Independence: Mr. Jones' Independence primaries further build on this interpersonal style to describe someone who is a forceful, individualistic loner. First of all, his high score on Dominance (E+) indicates that he is likely to be assertive, competitive, and opinionated in social situations. His average score on Social Boldness (H) suggests that he is not shy, inhibited or insecure in group settings. Finally, Mr. Jones' high score on Q1 indicates that he is an open-minded, experimenting individual who may question established ways of doing things. Taken together, Mr. Jones' Independence primaries describe someone who is forceful, individualistic, and not afraid of rocking the boat in advancing his own ideas.

Tough-Mindedness: On the traits that make up global Tough-Mindedness (often thought of as describing cognitive processing style), Mr. Jones' scores indicate a strong creative potential. His below average scores on Warmth (A–) and Sensitivity (I–) denote an aloof individual who is not very interested in people, feelings, or artistic values but who tends to focus on logical, objective aspects of situations. However, Mr. Jones shows a strong interest in abstract ideas and theoretical thinking, and he tends to focus on the underlying reasons and meaning behind things (M+). This imaginative quality is complemented by his openmindedness and tendency to seek new and original solutions to problems (Q1+). When these Tough-Mindedness scales are combined with his superior reasoning ability (B+), a strong potential for innovative and creative functioning is revealed. However, being so attuned to abstract thoughts and ideas, he may at times be absent-minded, be inattentive to practical details, or become bored when he has to follow established routines. Thus, while Mr. Jones' creative qualities from Tough-Mindedness have probably led to great success in his scientific endeavors, they may sometimes present limitations in the practical aspects of being a manager—such as attending to details and schedules or following established policy.

Self-Control: Mr. Jones' average-range score on global Self-Control results from combining scores that are in opposite directions on the contributing primary scales. His low-average score on Rule-Consciousness (G–) suggests that he does not feel a strong need to follow rules, nor does he judge himself by conventional standards of right and wrong. This quality is fairly common in creative occupations, where individuals often need to think beyond conventional viewpoints. However, it could sometimes be a liability in a management position that requires following and defending rules and regulations. On the other hand, Mr. Jones' high-average score on Perfectionism (Q3+) suggests that he is a self-disciplined individual who tends to be organized and planful in achieving his goals. These two Self-Control factors may compensate for each other to some degree in a management role, just as Mr. Jones' serious, restrained quality (F–) may compensate for the distracted, impractical trends inherent in his imaginative style (M+).

Anxiety: Most of Mr. Jones' Anxiety primaries are in the average range, indicating that, overall, he is experiencing about the same level of distress or tension right now as most people. However, his low score on Apprehension (O–) reveals a tendency to be unworried, self-assured, and not prone to self-doubt. Thus, he is probably quite self-confident, but may be complacent or insensitive even to appropriate criticism.

4. Putting It All Together (Integrate all primary scales, consider the meaning of particular multiple score combinations, predicted scores, and report content)

The interpreter can begin to build a comprehensive picture of the individual's functioning, including strengths and weaknesses, in a broad range of life situations by putting together the scales in the following steps:

a. In trying to put together the whole personality, combining primaries from the different globals, clinicians often start by combining global Extraversion and Independence scales. Since these both tend to focus on interpersonal behavior, they can be used to build a picture of the individual's interpersonal style, both in terms of making connections with others and influencing others.

b. Then Self-Control and Tough-Mindedness scales elucidate areas of internal functioning, particularly ways of controlling impulses and openness to experiencing emotions, fantasy, and new viewpoints.

c. Last, Anxiety factors may indicate the individual's style of dealing with conflict or unpleasant feelings, whether they originate in the interpersonal domain or the internal one.

In addition, sophisticated users of the 16PF questionnaire will learn to look at the primary factor scales, not just one at a time, but in particular combinations that have been identified as significant. Resource books on the 16PF scales help users learn about these combinations; also, using the test over time will help interpreters to develop their own insights about important combinations to evaluate. An easy way for 16PF test users to capitalize on the wealth of information available is to use the wide variety of interpretive reports that summarize important relationships between the 16PF and other criteria of interest. Computer interpretations often incorporate findings from research that are not available elsewhere, and *interpretive report manuals often summarize relevant research conducted by the report's author and include a bibliography of related research studies.*

Information from the following interpretive reports appears in the cases in this chapter :

- BIR—Basic Interpretive Report
- CCPI—Cattell Comprehensive Personality Interpretation
- HRDR—Human Resource Development Report
- KCR—Karson Clinical Report
- PCDP—Personal Career Development Profile

Sample Profile: Mr. Jones' Extraversion primaries suggest a subdued loner style, someone who prefers to work by himself on most projects. These traits indicate strengths as well as weaknesses for a management role. The CCPI states, "While this may make him autonomous in his decision-making, he may be seen as uncompromising or close-minded at times."[2]

Mr. Jones' scores on the Independence scales, particularly Dominance (E+) and Openness-to-Change (Q1+), further elaborate a picture of a person who is a forceful, individualistic loner rather than, *alternatively*, a shy, inhibited type of introvert. The KCR elaborates on this: "His drive to get his way is rarely subordinated to concerns about how he is coming across. He can get so caught up in his point of view that he loses track of his interpersonal impact."[3] A more fine-grained analysis from the CCPI states:

He is often so intent on convincing others to accept his views that he gives little consideration to theirs. For example, he may be so busy rehearsing what he is going to say next to get his point across that he does not really hear what others are saying.[2]

This picture of an "extrapunitive" rather than an "intropunitive" loner style is further supported by scores from other primaries. Mr. Jones' low score on Apprehension (O–) points to a self-assured, even self-satisfied, quality. This well-defended style may leave him untroubled by self-doubt and resilient under stress, but it suggests that he feels little need to explain his actions to others and may not take his share of responsibility when things go wrong. Mr. Jones' detached, forceful style may also be exacerbated by his tendency to focus on objective aspects of situations rather than on social or emotional issues (I–). The KCR points out the advantages of this style: "He is the kind

---

[2]Excerpted from Cattell Comprehensive Personality Inventory copyright © 1997 Institute for Personality and Ability Testing, Inc., Champaign, IL.
[3]Excerpted from Karson Clinical Report copyright © 1995 Institute for Personality and Ability Testing, Inc., Champaign, IL.

of person who tends to keep his poise under duress, and he generally copes well when the going gets tough, partly because it is a source of pride to him to stand up to adversity."[3] However, this tough, forceful style may make it difficult for him to empathize with others' feelings and needs or to provide emotional support to others, and it may contribute to his lack of awareness of his impact on others. Finally, his forthrightness (N–) may serve to make these traits more evident to others because of his transparent, unpolished style. The KCR states, "He tends to be very blunt when he does speak up, and others may come to resent his outspokenness."[3]

The forceful, confident loner style revealed in Mr. Jones' Extraversion, Independence, and Anxiety primaries suggest that he probably presents well in social settings and is decisive and resilient in most situations. The CCPI reports one of the ways in which these qualities would be an asset in leadership roles: "Since he is independent and self-reliant, he has the potential to be a self-starter. He may be able to use these qualities to demonstrate great initiative and enterprise in the workplace or to branch out on his own."[2] However, as mentioned, these strengths also involve some inherent drawbacks. Being tough, aloof and self-reliant, Mr. Jones will probably show a limited interest in others and their feelings or concerns. It will be hard for him to listen to others' opinions, accept others' ideas, or work collaboratively toward a common goal. Overall, these combined scores indicate that Mr. Jones is probably not very savvy socially and undoubtedly tunes out all kinds of feedback from others—qualities that were probably influential in his failure to gain promotion.

The strong creative potential found in Mr. Jones' Tough-Mindedness primaries is supported by his high score on the PCDP creativity equation (8.9). The CCPI states:

He has a talent for innovative work that requires thinking outside the usual cultural paradigms. In addition to being open-minded and original, he is also imaginative. Stepping back to see the 'big picture' and envisioning the possibilities therein are among his strongest attributes, and so his intelligence would be best used in work that involves putting ideas together creatively. . . . Mr Jones' innovative temperament is unlikely to be a good match with a large, authoritarian institution or one that is set in its ways. He would fit better in a newly emerging industry or an organization where the lines of authority are not highly structured and policies and procedures are flexible. He also is well suited to an environment where individual enterprise and resourcefulness are valued rather than teamwork or conformity.[2]

Mr. Jones' overall configuration of scores shows an extremely good fit with the Investigative Holland career theme (these scores appear in both the BIR and the PCDP), a theme that involves analytic and conceptual problem-solving in fields such as the physical, biological, or social sciences, engineering, or mathematics. Comparatively, the Enterprising Holland theme (which represents management and marketing roles, involving skills of convincing, directing or persuading others to attain organizational goals) ranks only third or fourth among Mr. Jones' career theme scores.

Overall, these 16PF scores suggest that Mr. Jones has both some strengths and weaknesses for a management position, which could profitably be explored by the consulting professional with particular suggestions for training and development.

---

[2]Excerpted from Cattell Comprehensive Personality Inventory copyright © 1997 Institute for Personality and Ability Testing, Inc., Champaign, IL.
[3]Excerpted from Karson Clinical Report copyright © 1995 Institute for Personality and Ability Testing, Inc., Champaign, IL.

THE CASE STUDY

Figure 10.2 presents a 16PF profile that will be interpreted in its entirety, using the interpretive strategy outlined above. The case study gives insights that would be available from a hand-scoring interpretation of the 16PF, and also incorporates content from various interpretive reports.

John Smith, age 23 years, was the youngest of three sons in an educated, upper-middle class family, in which both parents had professional careers. He was still living at home and unemployed when he sought therapy. He presented as a pleasant, cheerful individual, but was unconvincing in his assertion that he wanted psychotherapy to help him develop goals and to guide him in choosing a career. Later, it became clear that his parents had made participation in therapy a condition for his remaining in the family home and that his girlfriend was threatening to end their relationship if he did not find a decent job.

Though of at least average intelligence, he had dropped out of high school at age 16. He was encouraged by his parents to obtain a G.E.D. and to enroll in junior college, but he dropped out before completing the first semester. His parents then accepted that he was not academically inclined and attempted to interest him in a variety of careers. Despite his early enthusiasm for several, he never stayed in any one job or training program for more than four months. He cited boredom as his reason for quitting.

John spent most of his time with a group of young men who seemed bonded together by their similar lifestyle. Most of their group activities involved hanging out, partying, working

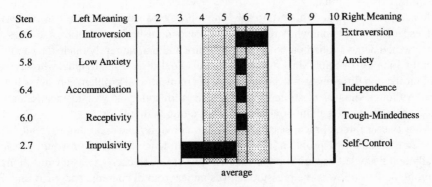

Figure 10.2a. John Smith's 16PF scores.

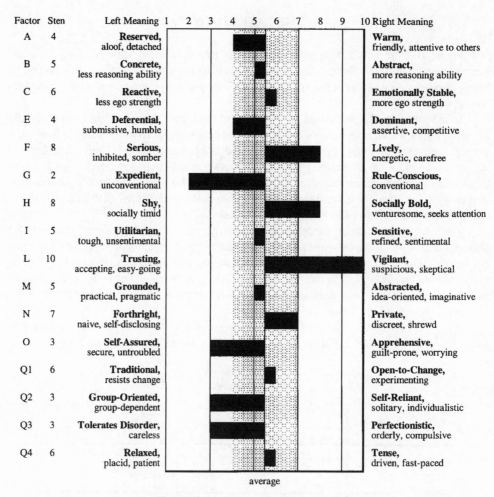

Factor	Sten	Left Meaning	1	2	3	4	5	6	7	8	9	10	Right Meaning
A	4	**Reserved,** aloof, detached											**Warm,** friendly, attentive to others
B	5	**Concrete,** less reasoning ability											**Abstract,** more reasoning ability
C	6	**Reactive,** less ego strength											**Emotionally Stable,** more ego strength
E	4	**Deferential,** submissive, humble											**Dominant,** assertive, competitive
F	8	**Serious,** inhibited, somber											**Lively,** energetic, carefree
G	2	**Expedient,** unconventional											**Rule-Conscious,** conventional
H	8	**Shy,** socially timid											**Socially Bold,** venturesome, seeks attention
I	5	**Utilitarian,** tough, unsentimental											**Sensitive,** refined, sentimental
L	10	**Trusting,** accepting, easy-going											**Vigilant,** suspicious, skeptical
M	5	**Grounded,** practical, pragmatic											**Abstracted,** idea-oriented, imaginative
N	7	**Forthright,** naive, self-disclosing											**Private,** discreet, shrewd
O	3	**Self-Assured,** secure, untroubled											**Apprehensive,** guilt-prone, worrying
Q1	6	**Traditional,** resists change											**Open-to-Change,** experimenting
Q2	3	**Group-Oriented,** group-dependent											**Self-Reliant,** solitary, individualistic
Q3	3	**Tolerates Disorder,** careless											**Perfectionistic,** orderly, compulsive
Q4	6	**Relaxed,** placid, patient											**Tense,** driven, fast-paced

average

Figure 10.2b. John Smith's 16PF scores.

on one another's cars, as well as some drag racing and surfing. Some of these young men had had minor brushes with the law. Even within this group, John had obtained a reputation for being quite a "party animal."

John's parents blamed this group for John's problems saying that he was easily influenced, especially by people who offered steady companionship and exciting activities. They felt that he had always relied on others to guide him and that he rarely made decisions independently. John's girlfriend, Mary, was an extremely goal-directed individual who saw John's lack of motivation differently. She believed that his motivational problems lay in his low self-esteem. Although she was frustrated by his goal-less lifestyle, she was hesitant to leave him because she was worried about how he would get along without her.

After two or three clinical sessions, it became obvious that John did not really see his lack of career goals as a problem. He expressed confidence that his life would just unfold naturally and that what was most important was just enjoying each day as it came along. His only problem, he said, was the pressure he was under from his parents and girlfriend. However, he was formulating a plan to deal with this. Since he was attracted to Mary's serious, responsible style, he was planning to look for a replacement who was similar but more relaxed and accepting of him and whom he could move in with, thus relieving himself of his need to rely on his parents.

16PF Interpretation

1. Review Validity Indices

Since all of the validity indices are within expected limits, Mr. Smith apparently did not present a particularly positive or negative picture of himself, and he appeared to understand the questions and respond in a meaningful way to them.

2. Review Global Factors

Since Mr. Smith has only one extreme global factor (Self-Control) and one high-average global factor (Extraversion), his overall number of elevated global scores is within the average range and is not unusual.

Since Mr. Smith's Extraversion score is high-average, it appears that social interaction plays a somewhat more important role in his life than in the average person's life.

Mr. Smith's score on Self-Control is quite low, indicating that his level of internalized standards and controls is very low. While he may be perceived as easy-going and flexible by some, he probably shows a significant lack of self-restraint and follows his own urges without the usual consideration for others' needs or for his own responsibilities.

Although global Anxiety, Independence, and Tough-Mindedness are all within the average range, Anxiety and Independence show some extreme but opposite scores among their contributing primary scales.

3. Review Primary Scales

Mr. Smith's profile shows 7 elevated primary scales, which is in the high-average range for number of elevated scores. This suggests that his personality does contain some strongly defined characteristics and behavior patterns but not an extreme number.

Extraversion: Mr. Smith's high-average score on global Extraversion is made up of three high scores plus two below-average scores on the contributing primary scales—an unusual combination. Beginning with the low Extraversion scores, Mr. Smith's below-average score on Warmth (A–) suggests that he is somewhat reserved or detached and tends to keep some emotional distance between himself and others. His above-average score on Privateness (N+) denotes a similar tendency to be cautious and guarded about revealing personal information. These results are consistent with the clinician's experience of Mr. Smith in that he did not originally reveal his true motivation for seeking therapy, often did not reveal his real intentions to his parents or girlfriend, and generally tended to view people from the standpoint of what he could get from them.

On the other hand, Mr. Smith's high score on Liveliness (F+) indicates that he brings a lot of energy and high spirits to his interactions and that he may be enthusiastic and carefree but also impulsive and changeable. His high score on Social Boldness (H+) further denotes someone who is sociable, talkative, and gregarious but probably thick-skinned and attention-seeking. These two scores taken together suggest someone whose social manner is enthusiastic and entertaining, but who is often not sensitive to others' feelings and reactions and may be perceived as self-centered. Mr. Smith's low score on Self-Reliance (Q2–) further indicates that he feels a strong need for companionship and prefers to do most things with others rather than by himself.

Thus, overall Mr. Smith's Extraversion scores suggest someone who feels a strong need to socialize, be among others, and interact in a superficial, stimulating, attention-seeking way rather than to develop deeper, more mutual relationships. These scores are consistent with the clinician's experience of Mr. Smith as a lively, sociable person who spends most of his time as part of a small group of peers pursuing stimulating activities together.

Independence: Mr. Smith's scores on the Independence subfactors further elaborate this picture of someone whose underlying social needs tend to be expressed superficially and passively. Although his global Independence score is in the average range, the contributing primary scores are in opposite directions. Although his Social Boldness (H+) indicates that he is talkative and risk taking, Mr. Smith's high Vigilance (L+) score denotes mistrust of others and his below average scores on Dominance (E–) plus Self-Reliance (Q2–) suggest that some general, underlying dependency needs may be present. Although no signs of suspiciousness were evident in the clinical sessions or life history, his apparent tendency to be easily influenced by friends and to depend on his parents and girlfriend are consistent with the rest of these scores.

Self-Control: Mr. Smith's scores on the Self-Control primaries are consistently low; three out of four are strongly in the poorly controlled direction. Mr. Smith's high score on Liveliness (F+) suggests a carefree, spontaneous style that usually involves impulsivity and a lack of inhibition. Thus, he may be unreliable in following through on tasks and interests and flighty in his focus. His very low score on Rule-Consciousness (G–) suggests that he has not internalized conventional standards of right and wrong and tends to be expedient rather than following established rules. Additionally, his low score on Perfectionism (Q3–) indicates a tendency to be disorganized and lacking in self-discipline. It suggests that he probably feels little compulsion to complete tasks conscientiously, to follow through on commitments, or to work toward long-term goals for himself. Overall, these Self-Control primaries suggest that Mr. Smith is substantially lacking in internalized controls and standards and probably follows his own urges regardless of others' needs or his own responsibilities. These results are consistent with many aspects of Mr. Smith's life history including his lack of development of career goals, his lack of follow-through with previous jobs, and his general attitude about life.

Anxiety: In the area of global Anxiety, Mr. Smith's average score is the result of combining extreme but opposite scores on two contributing primaries. His low score on Apprehension (O–) indicates that Mr. Smith experiences little worry or anxiety and strongly maintains an attitude of untroubled self-assurance. While this probably makes him resilient in stressful situations, he may seem self-satisfied or complacent to others and may not accept responsibility or blame, even when it is appropriate. Although his high score on Vigilance (L+) indicates a tendency to be suspicious and guarded, this score was not supported by other clinical information, indicating a need for further assessment in this area. Taken together, these Anxiety factors suggest that Mr. Smith tends to use strong defenses like denial, which is consistent with his cheerful, thick-skinned interpersonal style. It is also consistent with his unworried, self-satisfied attitude about his current life situation.

Tough-Mindedness: All of Mr. Smith's Tough-Mindedness scores are in the average range, except for his below-average score on Warmth (A-), which has already been discussed under Extraversion. These average scores in the areas of Sensitivity (I), Imaginative Abstractedness (M), and Openness to Change (Q1), plus his average-range score on the Reasoning ability factor (B), are consistent with his self-presentation in the sessions and with his life history information, which showed no signs of particular aesthetic sensitivity, creative imagination, or intellectual curiosity. However, given Mr. Smith's tendency to not apply himself or put forth his best effort, especially academically, his actual reasoning ability may well be higher than measured here.

4. Putting It All Together

Mr. Smith's mixed scores on the Extraversion primaries present an interesting picture of his social needs. In his 1976 book, Sam Karson describes low scores on Warmth (A–) as indicating a classic "burnt child" syndrome where unrewarding, frustrating, or austere early relationships lead the individual to avoid close human relationships. While Mr. Smith's score on Warmth is not extremely low, the general meaning here seems applicable. His above-average score on Privateness (N+) further develops a picture of an individual who is fearful about how others' might use personal information that he reveals. The CCPI states: "He tends to keep his reactions to himself and to carefully consider how much to say before speaking. Thus, overall, others may find him elusive or hard to really get to know." [2]

Mr. Smith's high scores on Social Boldness (H+) and Liveliness (F+) further create a picture of someone whose social behavior is quite stimulating and entertaining but is superficial and attention-seeking in nature. The CCPI states:

> Once the initial novelty of meeting someone new has worn off, he tends to lose interest in them. He is less emotionally attached to others than his engaging conversational manner would suggest. . . . He may be attention-seeking and may particularly enjoy the company of people who allow him to do more than his share of the talking. [2]

These scores create a picture of someone whose frustrating early experience left him reserved and cautious about close social relationships and also left him with strong unmet needs for attention from others and for dependable companionship. This picture is further supported by his low score on Self-Reliance (Q2–), which indicates some dependent features. The KCR states:

> When confronted with a situation that requires independent action, he often finds himself unable to act alone. His desire to do things with others may easily lead him to defer his personal agenda in favor of the group's. . . . His group orientation may be motivated by a desire to avoid weaknesses in areas of self-esteem and self-discipline. [3]

This picture of someone whose unmet social needs leave him dependent on others is further supported by Mr. Smith's scores on the Independence primaries. His below-average score on Dominance (E–), especially in combination with his low score on Self-Reliance (Q2-), indicates a general tendency toward being compliant, passive, and dependent on others. The CCPI states, "Since Mr. Smith relies heavily on other people's ideas and support, he may be easily

---

[2]Excerpted from Cattell Comprehensive Personality Inventory copyright © 1997 Institute for Personality and Ability Testing, Inc., Champaign, IL.

[3]Excerpted from Karson Clinical Report copyright © 1995 Institute for Personality and Ability Testing, Inc., Champaign, IL.

swayed by others. . . . He may give in to others' wishes rather than have a disagreement."[2] The CCPI discusses the application of this score combination to intimate relationships:

> This suggests that his fear of abandonment may lead him to be yielding and conciliatory when he sees signs that his partner is pulling away . . . Because of the high value he places on togetherness, he may gloss over problems or deny that certain disagreements exists, thus promoting enmeshment between him and his partner. [2]

The KCR states, "He does not always speak up when his needs and his point of view are ignored. This can lead to pockets of resentment, and he may express this resentment indirectly."[3] The CCPI makes suggestions for the treating professional: "Because he tries to avoid conflict, he most likely expresses his hostile feelings covertly. Overlooking appointments, procrastinating, sulking, 'forgetting' to perform a task, and other annoying but seemingly 'accidental' behaviors should be examined from this perspective."[2] The CCPI focuses on therapeutic goals for this individual: "Therapeutic goals for Mr. Smith include developing a more assertive, independent style. Working toward this goal will include overcoming his fear that if he expresses disagreement or makes demands, he will lose the support and companionship on which he depends."[2]

Mr. Smith's low scores on the Self-Control primaries are also consistent with the picture of underdevelopment seen in his interpersonal scores. Individuals whose early relationships are unsatisfying and frustrating generally do not tend to identify closely with others, especially authority figures, and thus do not tend to internalize the usual standards and controls. Regarding Mr. Smith's low score on Rule-Consciousness (G–), the CCPI states, "He feels little compulsion to conform to societal rules and standards. . . . Nor is he inclined to experience guilt or self-reproach when he breaks rules or conventions."[2] The KCR states:

> He shows so little regard for the rules of conduct associated with conventional standards of behavior that conforming to societal expectations may be difficult for him. Many of the tasks of living usually taken for granted may become optional in his mind. Other people, especially authority figures, may see him as unresponsive to their expectations. Activities that require a willingness to follow rules may make him feel too constricted to participate effectively. [3]

Regarding Mr. Smith's low score on Perfectionism (Q3), the CCPI states, "He has low personal standards of achievement and probably is undisciplined and disorganized at times. He may not take pride in doing well or feel shame when he falls short of these standards."[2] The KCR states, "His relative paucity of good habits to fall back on when necessary can leave him vulnerable to emotional distress."[3] Mr. Smith's high score on Liveliness (F+) denotes a fast-paced, spontaneous, think-on-your-feet style which also involves some impulsivity and unreliability. As the KCR states, "Circumspection and reflection are not typical characteristics of his thinking. . . . He may jump to conclusions before considering all the facts."[3]

Thus, Mr. Smith's overall behavior probably shows a lack of conscientiousness in meeting obligations and responsibilities, a lack of consideration for other people and their needs, and a lack of development of long-term goals for himself. Furthermore, Mr. Smith's lack of self-control may affect his ability to get his dependency needs met; people are less likely to affiliate with and support those who are irresponsible, disrespectful, or unreliable.

Mr. Smith's scores on the Anxiety primaries indicate something about his defenses. The

---

[2]Excerpted from Cattell Comprehensive Personality Inventory copyright © 1997 Institute for Personality and Ability Testing, Inc., Champaign, IL.
[3]Excerpted from Karson Clinical Report copyright © 1995 Institute for Personality and Ability Testing, Inc., Champaign, IL.

untroubled, self-assured style indicated by his low Apprehension (O–) score may make him confident and resilient in stressful situations, but it also may be defensive in nature. The CCPI states, "His self-esteem at present is above the optimal level for fairly appraising both his strengths and weaknesses. He may be defended against recognizing his own shortcomings."[2] The PCDP adds, "He appears to have little need to explain his actions to himself or to other people."[4] The CCPI reflects on the effect this trait has in relationships: "Mr. Smith does not take his fair share of responsibility and blame when things go wrong. Any problems between him and his partner may be exacerbated by his tendency to deny his role in them."[2] The CCPI makes the following suggestions for the therapeutic process:

> Even constructive negative feedback is rarely used by Mr. Smith to gain self-understanding since it often exacerbates his defensiveness or triggers a flood of upsetting emotions. Thus, helping professionals should resist confronting his defense mechanisms prematurely or abruptly since they probably serve as protection for the low level of personal acceptance that underlies his confident veneer. Projecting blame onto others may be his standard way of guarding himself from recognizing his own faults and mistakes. Although it may be tempting to correct these projective distortions, they cannot be corrected simply by logical argument because they have a defensive role in guarding him against perceptions that might cause strong self-doubt.[2]

Mr. Smith's high score on Vigilance (L+) usually indicates a strong tendency to be distrustful and suspicious of others' intentions. However, since this trait was noticeably absent from the clinical interviews, further assessment in this area is indicated.

These Anxiety factors suggest that Mr. Smith tends to use strong defenses like denial. This is consistent with his interpersonal profile depicting a cheerful, carefree, thick-skinned style with underlying dependency needs. These interpersonal needs plus his very low level of self-discipline, internalized standards, or goals for himself may present too many challenges to his defenses. The KCR states:

> On a whole, his current average emotional adjustment seems to depend somewhat on his having found circumstances that do not overly challenge his defenses. Although his ego strength is adequate, he may not possess a reliable degree of self-control in difficult situations. To maintain his positive emotional adjustment, he will need to keep coming up with unique solutions to the demands made on him.[3]

Case Follow-Up

No excessive suspiciousness or other signs of John's extremely high Vigilance (L+) score were detected in his self-presentation or in his life history. This extreme Vigilance score was thus a signal to the clinician that there was more to John's story than was currently apparent. Although high Vigilance scores most often indicate a tendency to be suspicious and distrustful of others' motives and to dwell on these suspicions of imagined danger, the other possible meaning of high Vigilance scores is the presence of a wary, hyper-vigilant orientation that is based on some real, present danger. Given John's lack of internalized social values and his peers' less-than-sterling pasts, the clinician thought it quite possible that something was going

---

[2]Excerpted from Cattell Comprehensive Personality Inventory copyright © 1997 Institute for Personality and Ability Testing, Inc., Champaign, IL.

[3]Excerpted from Karson Clinical Report copyright © 1995 Institute for Personality and Ability Testing, Inc., Champaign, IL.

[4]Excerpted from Personal Career Development Profile copyright © 1995 Institute for Personality and Ability Testing, Inc., Champaign, IL.

on in John's life about which he needed to be hyper-vigilant and defensive.

After several sessions in which attempts to discover suspiciousness in John's behavior were unsuccessful, the clinician confronted him with the conjecture about some kind of illegal activity. John was taken aback, thinking that the therapist had somehow learned his carefully guarded secret, and admitted that he and his friends had been growing and dealing marijuana for several years. He expressed no guilt or shame about this and said that in addition to earning easy money, he enjoyed the adrenaline rush associated with growing marijuana in the hills behind his parents' home and the need to be constantly on guard against discovery in his dealing activities. Like most marijuana dealers, John smoked on a daily basis, and this frequent and prolonged use probably contributed further to his motivational problems.

Soon, John's girlfriend left him and his parents told him he could no longer remain in their home. Because he had no place to live, he reluctantly agreed to follow the clinician's suggestion to enter a residential drug treatment program. Many aspects of this program meshed very well with John's dynamics—the emphasis on participation in regular group meetings, fellowship with others recovering from chemical dependency, mentoring through sponsorship, and following a clear 12-step program. John's needs for companionship, for external structure and direction from others, and for supportive figures to rely on were uniquely met in this environment and he easily gave up his ties with his former friends. The values and beliefs of the 12-step program gave him a set of external standards and values around which to structure his life, making up for his lack of development of his own internal ones.

Although John did not have the motivation to pursue long-term therapy, he functioned fairly well within the Narcotics Anonymous community. Follow-up indicated that he was attending meetings several times a week, talking almost daily with his sponsor, and had adopted the higher-order values from Narcotics Anonymous 12-step philosophy. However, he was still unemployed and receiving assistance from his parents while he lived with people from Narcotics Anonymous. In fact, his animated, uninhibited style made him in great demand as a speaker at Narcotics Anonymous meetings, where he clearly enjoyed the limelight.

While some may see John as merely transferring his dependency to Narcotics' Anonymous, this represented a substantial improvement in his overall quality of life. It moved him away from dependency on drugs, involvement in criminal behavior, dependency and conflict with his family, and limited relationships with others.

This case indicates how 16PF results can be useful in identifying aspects of the individual's functioning that would otherwise come to light only over an extended period of time (or not at all). In giving a comprehensive picture of John's personality, the 16PF results allowed the clinician to accurately assess his strengths and weaknesses and work towards realistic options.

SUMMARY

This chapter describes the development, administartion, scoring, and interpretation of the 16PF questionnaire. This normal range measure of personality can be used to comprehensively assess an individual's enduring personality make-up, rather than merely provide fragmentary information about symptomatology. The 16PF test has been used extensively in clinical settings becaue of its ability to give a deep and integrated picture of the whole person, both strengths and weaknesses, including such areas as self-esteem, coping style, internalization of rules and standards, capacity for empathy, quality of attachments, interpersonal needs, power dynamics, cognitive style, and compatible occupations.

The first section of the chapter briefly describes the development of the 16PF test from basic research onto the structure of personality, including the discovery of the original Big-Five factors. Next, the simple administration and scoring of the test are described. The rest of the chapter focuses on providing a sequence of interpretive steps to aid in 16PF interpretation. A case study illustrates how the test can be used to provide a comprehensive understanding of an individual from the beginning of the therapeutic process. It demonstrates how, particularly in a managed care setting, this information can be very effective in helping the clinician to place the presenting problem in context, develop empathy and rapport, and develop a treatment plan and appropriate therapeutic interventions.

SUGGESTED READINGS

Clinical/Counseling:

Cattell, H. B. (1989). *The 16PF: Personality in depth.* Champaign, IL: Institute for Personality and Ability Testing, Inc.

Karson, M., Karson, S., & O'Dell, J. (1997). *16PF interpretation in clinical practice: A guide to the Fifth Edition.* Champaign, IL: Institute for Personality & Ability Testing, Inc.

Karson, S., & O'Dell, J. W. (1976). *A guide to the clinical use of the 16PF.* Champaign, IL: Institute for Personality and Ability Testing.

Krug, S. E., & Johns, E. F. (1990). The 16 Personality Factor Questionnaire. In E. E. Watkins and V. L. Campbell (Eds.), *Testing in counseling practice.* Hillsdale, NJ: Lawrence Erlbaum Associates.

Meyer, R. G., & Deitsch, S. E. (1995). *The clinician's handbook* (4th ed). Boston, MA: Allyn and Bacon.

Russell, M. T. (1995). *16PF Couple's Counseling Report user's guide.* Champaign, IL: Institute for Personality and Ability Testing, Inc.

Schuerger, J., & Watterson, D. W. (1977). *Using tests and other information in counseling.* Champaign, IL: Institute for Personality and Ability Testing.

Career Counseling:

Karol, D. L. (1994). Holland occupational typology. In S. R. Conn & M. L. Rieke (Eds.), *The 16PF Fifth Edition technical manual.* Champaign, IL: Institute for Personality and Ability Testing, Inc.

Schuerger, J. W. (1995). Career assessment and the Sixteen Personality Factor Questionnaire. *Journal of Career Assessment,* (3)2 Spring, 157–175.

Walter, V. (1995) *16PF Personal Career Development Profile technical and interpretive manual.* Champaign, IL: Institute for Personality and Ability Testing, Inc.

Manuals and Technical References:

Cattell, R. B. (1957). *Personality and motivation structure and measurement.* New York: World Book.

Cattell, R. B., Eber, H. W., & Tatsuoka, M. M. (1970). *The handbook for the Sixteen Personality Factor Questionnaire.* Champaign, IL: Institute for Personality and Ability Testing, Inc.

Conn, S. R., & Rieke, M. L. (1994). *The 16PF Fifth Edition technical manual.* Champaign, IL: Institute for Personality and Ablity Testing, Inc.

Russell, M. T., & Karol, D. (1994). *16PF Fifth Edition administrator's manual.* Champaign, IL: Institute for Personality and Ability Testing, Inc.

II

Child/Adolescent

11

Wechsler Intelligence Scale for Children-Third Edition (WISC-III)

Christi Woolger

INTRODUCTION

Intelligence can manifest itself in many forms and has been defined and measured in various ways. Although this chapter will not delve into the theories, it will define intelligence according to David Wechsler's conception that intelligence is not a particular ability, but "the aggregate or global capacity of the individual to act purposefully, to think rationally, and to deal effectively with his or her environment." Intelligence is closely intertwined with aspects of one's personality and overall adaptive functioning.

In development of IQ tests, Wechsler was guided by his focus on the global nature of intelligence—being a part of the whole personality. Although he selected items and scales to measure specific functions, he took into account factors that contribute to the total intelligence of the individual. Thus, the overall IQ obtained represents an index of general mental ability.

The WISC-III is one of the most widely used tests of cognitive ability. It is useful and appropriate for psychoeducational assessment, as part of educational planning and placement, neuropsychological assessment, and clinical assessment. Although WISC-III scores are correlated with academic achievement more so than with actual school grades, as a measure of intellectual functioning, they can provide an estimate of a child's ability to demonstrate the kind of learning expected in a classroom setting

TEST CONSTRUCTION AND DEVELOPMENT

The WISC-III is the latest version of the Wechsler scales for children ages 6 through 16 years. The original version of this test, the WISC, was developed by Wechsler in 1949 as a

Christi Woolger • Kissimmee, Florida 34744

Understanding Psychological Assessment, edited by Dorfman and Hersen. Kluwer Academic/Plenum Publishers, New York, 2001.

downward extension of the adult intelligence test, the Wechsler-Bellevue Intelligence Scale. Easier items were added to the beginnings of the subtests to make the original adult scale more suitable for children.

The second version of the WISC developed in 1974, was called the Wechsler Intelligence Scale for Children—Revised (WISC-R). Individual subtest reliability was improved, as many of the ambiguous, obsolete, or unfair WISC items were discarded. In addition, more up-to-date items were added or created through revision, such as more pictures of women and African-Americans being included on the Picture Completion subtest.

The WISC-III was developed in 1991 with several goals in mind. The primary goal was to update norms. Research indicates that average performance on intelligence tests increases over time. Updated norms are therefore necessary in order to compensate for such gradual increase. Without updated norms, a child's IQ will appear higher than should be the case if compared to current norms. An important norm offered in the WISC-III is with regard to base rate information. Tables now provide information as to frequency with which a given difference between two scores is found to occur in the standardization sample as representative of the total population. This change recognizes that statistical significance does not necessarily imply diagnostic significance unless the base rate (occurrence rate) is low.

A second goal of the revision was to maintain the basic structure and content of the WISC-R to help maintain longitudinal stability and to maintain the theoretical underpinnings of the Wechsler scales. In addition, by retaining a large number of items from the WISC-R (73%), continuity was maintained. Item familiarity may increase the ease of transition for test users.

A third goal was the further investigation and enhancement of the underlying factor structure of the WISC-R. This structure includes the two major factors, Verbal and Performance, which have been repeatedly identified over years of research. A third factor, Freedom from Distractibility, had been identified in studies. Wechsler added a new subtest, Symbol Search, to better distinguish this third factor, but analysis resulted in the emergence of a fourth factor. The factor structure will be discussed more thoroughly in the Interpretive Guidelines section of this chapter.

The final goal of WISC-III development was improvement of subtest content, administration, and scoring rules. Bias of content was minimized through empirical analysis and psychologist review. Artwork was refined and updated. New items were created in order to extend accurate measurement both downward and upward in age groups. In addition, minor changes in administration procedures and scoring rules were made.

The WISC-III was standardized on 2200 children; 100 boys and 100 girls in each of 11 age groups from 6 through 16 years. The birth month for each age group was the 6th month. The sample was stratified on age, race/ethnicity, geographic region, and parent education. Within each age group, children were selected to match as closely as possible the proportions found in the 1988 U.S. Census Data. This sampling procedure is better than the one used on the WISC-R, where stratification was less detailed (only white versus non-white).

The WISC-III overlaps with the Wechsler Preschool and Primary Scale of Intelligence—Revised (WPPSI-R) for ages 6–0–0 to 7–3–15, and with the Wechsler Adult Intelligence Scale—Revised (WISC-R) for ages 16–0–0 to 16–11–30. Although the overlap in ages can be helpful in retest situations, the tests are not truly independent and caution should be exercised. Based on internal psychometric data, it is recommended that the WPPSI-R be used for children ages 6–0 to 6–11 of below-average ability, and the WISC-III be used for all other ability levels at this age range and for ages 7–0 to 7–3. The WISC-III is recommended rather than the WISC-R for all ability levels at ages 16–0 to 16–11.

Reliability on the WISC-III is quite good. The three scales have internal reliability coefficients of .89 or above over the entire age range covered by the test. Although there is less research on its validity, substantial correlations and item overlap between the WISC-R and the WISC-III suggest similar validity data. In fact, studies indicate adequate construct, concurrent, predictive, and discriminant validity for the WISC-III.

The WISC-III contains 13 subtests: 6 in the Verbal Scale and 7 in the Performance Scale. Five subtests in each scale are designated as standard subtests. These two scales measure two separate factors or underlying cognitive abilities. Below is a list of the subtests according to order of administration. The Verbal and Performance tests are given in alternating order to help maintain the child's interest during testing.

WISC-III Subtests

Verbal	Performance
2. Information	1. Picture Completion
4. Similarities	3. Coding
6. Arithmetic	5. Picture Arrangement
8. Vocabulary	7. Block Design
10. Comprehension	9. Object Assembly
12. Digit Span	11. Symbol Search
	13. Mazes

Note that while Symbol Search, Digit Span, and Mazes are all supplementary subtests, Mazes can substitute only for Coding.

For a complete discussion of the comparison between the WISC-III and WISC-R, the reader is referred to the WISC-III manual and other suggested readings listed at the end of this chapter for more thorough reviews of similarities and differences between the two versions of the test.

ADMINISTRATION AND SCORING

There are various guidelines and procedures that should be followed when administering psychological tests. Articles, chapters, and even books have been written on the subject of testing children. Detailed descriptions will not be given here; rather, more general guidelines will be discussed to assist the examiner in administering the WISC-III as part of the overall assessment process. The reader is referred to the WISC-III manual and other texts for discussions of administration techniques for special populations.

There are a number of factors that should be considered when administering the WISC-III. It is important for the examiner to be aware of such factors and take them into consideration both when administering the test and interpreting results. Examiner variables include professional role and status, training and experience, personal and professional identity, gender, race, test administration style, and expectations for the child. A competent examiner should genuinely enjoy working with children and be flexible, vigilant, and self-aware. Child or examinee variables include the child's perception of being the "client," developmental status, child expectations, gender, race, and situational variables such as mood, affect, fatigue, and hunger. Aspects of the test situation include the physical surroundings (e.g., room, lighting, seating arrangement) and time allowed for testing. In addition, the examiner/examinee relationship can significantly impact the overall results of the testing. Especially important is building and maintaining of rapport.

It is essential that the examiner master the special procedures developed specifically for the WISC-III. Beginning examiners tend to make more administrative errors, including failing to follow scoring rules, to complete the form properly, to adhere to directions, to probe ambiguous responses, and to follow the starting and stopping rules. It is important to avoid confusing procedures from the various Wechsler scales, as they do differ. Changes in seemingly minor administrative features, such as phrasing or presentation of a test item could significantly reduce the validity of test results. When standard procedures are not followed, the obtained scores may not be appropriately compared to the test norms.

Administration of the regular battery of 10 subtests, according to the manual, requires approximately 50–70 minutes. The three supplementary subtests may add an additional 10–15 minutes. Variations in examinees' test-taking styles and in the examiner's administration style may affect overall time. It is recommended that the entire test be administered in a single session to prevent flaws in the data. However, if a child's motivation wanes or fatigue degrades interfere performance, it is better to stop the session and resume within the week than to continue and obtain a nonvalid result.

The abilities measured and factors influencing performance are offered to assist the examiner in establishing hypotheses about the child's performance. The examiner is cautioned to avoid relying on such information in the absence of other background information, observations, and test data. A description of the individual subtests in order of administration follows.

Picture Completion Subtest

The Picture Completion subtest requires the child to name or point to the most important missing detail in each of 30 drawings of common objects, animals, or people. There is a 20–second time limit, and pictures are shown one at a time. All children start with the sample item, and then depending on age, are given the next item. The subtest is discontinued after five consecutive failures.

Picture Completion is a measure of visual discrimination—the ability to differentiate essential from nonessential details. It is also a measure of perceptual organization and conceptual abilities involved in the visual recognition and identification of familiar objects from the child's long-term memory. Performance on this subtest can be influenced by a child's alertness to the environment, ability to respond when uncertain, concentration and ability to work under pressure, and negativism ("nothing's missing"). Performance on this subtest is minimally affected by brain damage and therefore can be a good indicator of premorbid intelligence.

Information Subtest

This subtest requires the child to answer a broad range of questions dealing with factual information. The child responds orally to 30 questions that address general knowledge about names of objects, common events, people, and places. The child's age determines the starting point. All items are scored 1 or 0 (pass-fail). The subtest is not timed and is discontinued after five consecutive failures.

In general, the Information subtest measures a child's general fund of information and long-term memory, as influenced by his or her alertness to the environment, social and cultural background, and knowledge of school-like tasks. Intellectual drive and curiosity, as well as a foreign language background, often influence performance on this subtest. The information subtest is a good measure of overall intellectual functioning and is one of the most stable subtests on the WISC-III.

Coding Subtest

The Coding subtest requires a child to copy symbols paired with geometric shapes (Coding A) or with numbers (Coding B). Coding A is given to children under 8 years of age and Coding B to children 8 years and older. In Coding A, the child draws a symbol in its corresponding shape; in Coding B the child draws a symbol under its corresponding number. The total score is measured by the number of symbols correctly drawn within the 2-minute time limit.

Coding taps the child's ability to hold attention and flexibility in learning an unfamiliar task that involves attentional skills, visual scanning and focusing, sequential processing, short-term memory, and psychomotor speed. Visual-motor dexterity and fine motor skills are also assessed with this paper-and-pencil measure. This subtest is often influenced by anxiety, distractibility, concern for accuracy and detail, the ability to work under time pressure, persistence, and motivation. Coding is sensitive to the effects of brain damage or emotional dysfunction.

Similarities Subtest

For the Similarities subtest, the child is presented with two words and is asked to describe how these words which represent common objects or concepts, are alike. All children start with the sample item and are then given the first item. The first five are scored 1 or 0 (pass-fail), and then items 6 through 19 are scored 2, 1, or 0, depending on the conceptual quality of the response. The subtest is not timed and is discontinued after four consecutive failures.

Similarities is postulated to measure a child's abstract and concrete reasoning abilities. Verbal concept formation and logical abstract thinking are assessed by measuring the child's ability to recognize relationships between apparently diverse objects or events. Performance on this subtest is often influenced by the availability of cultural opportunities, flexibility in thinking, interest patterns, and outside reading experiences. In addition, a negativistic style ("they're not alike") may also influence performance.

Picture Arrangement Subtest

This subtest requires placement of a series of pictures in logical order. Each item is a set of picture cards that, when arranged correctly, describe a story in a comic-strip format. The cards are presented in a specified mixed-up order, and the child is asked to rearrange the pictures into the "right" order, so that the story will make sense. The number of pictures ranges from 3 to 6. All children start with the sample item and then go on to start an item specific to their age. Scoring depends on the completion time and accuracy of the story arrangement. The subtest is discontinued after three consecutive failures.

Picture Arrangement measures the child's ability to anticipate consequences and to comprehend and evaluate a situation by logically and sequentially organizing visual or pictorial information that is socially meaningful. Nonverbal reasoning, planning ability, visual organization, and temporal sequencing are used for this subtest. Influential factors include creativity, cultural opportunities, ability to work under pressure, and exposure to comic strips.

Arithmetic Subtest

For Arithmetic, the child is asked to solve a series of arithmetic problems, ranging from the simple to complex. The child must solve each problem mentally, without-paper-and pencil and respond orally within a time limit. Some problems are read aloud to the child, but the more difficult ones are presented on cards that the child must read. The starting point depends on the child's age. Scores range from 2, 1 or 0 depending on the completion time. The subtest is discontinued after three consecutive failures.

Arithmetic tests various skills, dependent upon the child's age. It taps the child's ability to visually or auditorally process information and use numerical operations, as well as mathematical reasoning operations, long-term memory, and attentional skills. Performance on this subtest is influenced by a child's anxiety level, distractibility, attention span, and concentration. The ability to work under time pressure, educational experiences, interests, and transient emotional reactions have also been suggested as influential factors.

Block Design Subtest

For Block Design, the child uses blocks to reproduce a two-color design. While viewing a model or picture, the child must use a specified number of blocks to replicate the design within a time limit. The blocks are three dimensional with a red surface, a white surface, and a surface that is cut diagonally into half red and half white. There are 12 items in all. Starting points depend on the child's age, and the patterns are arranged in order of increasing difficulty. All items are timed and scored according to the corrected completion time. The subtest is discontinued after two consecutive failures.

Block Design assesses a variety of functions, including visual analysis of a whole into its component parts and synthesis or reintegration of those parts into the identical design. Nonverbal reasoning, abstract conceptualization, spatial visualization and orientation, and perceptual-motor coordination are also measured. The ability to discriminate block designs may be intact even though the ability to reproduce them is impaired. Performance on Block Design is influenced by the rate of motor activity and vision, the ability to work under time pressure, and visual-perceptual skills. The examiner should be aware of the child's response style, as it can provide information about the child's underlying personality traits.

Vocabulary Subtest

For Vocabulary subtest, a test of word knowledge, the examiner reads words aloud and then asks the child to define the words. Thirty words are arranged in order of increasing difficulty. The starting point varies with age. All items are scored 2, 1, or 0 depending on the quality of the response. There is no time limit, and the test is discontinued after four consecutive failures.

The Vocabulary subtest reflects the child's fund of information, learning ability, long-term memory, concept formation, and language development. Other influences include a foreign language background and intellectual curiosity and striving. Vocabulary is the best indicator of the child's overall intellectual functioning and is the most stable of all the subtests. Because of this, it is often used as an indicator of premorbid functioning.

Object Assembly Subtest

The Object Assembly subtest requires the child to put jigsaw pieces together to form common objects. For each puzzle item, there is a time limit to assemble the pieces, which are presented in the specified disarranged pattern. Every item is given to each child. Scores are based on completion time and the accuracy of assembled items.

Object Assembly measures visual organization, synthesis and integration of components to form familiar objects, simultaneous processing, planning ability, and visual-motor coordination. Performance is influenced by the rate and precision of motor activity, the ability to respond when uncertain, previous experience with puzzles, flexibility, persistence, and the ability to work under time pressure. As with Block Design, the examiner should observe the child's problem-solving approach, as it can provide important clinical information.

Comprehension Subtest

The Comprehension subtest requires the child to respond orally to a series of questions that require solutions to familiar problems or an understanding of social rules and concepts. Several content areas are covered, including knowledge of one's body, interpersonal relations, and social mores. All children start with the first item. Items are scored 2, 1, or 0, depending on the quality of the response or the degree of understanding expressed. The subtest is not timed and is discontinued after three consecutive failures.

Comprehension has often been called a measure of social intelligence and requires common ability to recognize cause-and-effect relationships, knowledge of conventional social expectations, verbal reasoning, practical information, and social maturity and judgment. Influential factors include the cultural opportunities in the home and a negativistic thinking style.

Symbol Search Subtest

This is a supplementary subtest, that requires the child to look at a symbol and then decide whether the symbol is present in an array of symbols. It is not used in computation of IQ when the five standard Performance Scale subtests are administered. However, it is recommended that it be administered at all times. If Coding is omitted or "spoiled" because of improper administration or disruption. Symbol Search may be substituted when calculating the IQ. Some authors recommended that it be used in place of Coding because correlations with other scales and with factor loadings are higher for Symbol Search than for Coding. Symbol Search measures mental process speed, whereas Coding measures psychomotor speed.

There are two separate parts: Part A is administered to children aged 6 to 7 and Part B to children of ages 8 to 16.

In Part A, there is one target symbol and three symbols in the array. The child is asked to indicate by marking the appropriate box whether or not the target symbol appears in the array. Part B contains two target symbols and five symbols in the array. Similar to Part A, the child is asked to indicate whether either one of the target symbols is in the array. Each part has a time limit of 120 seconds. The score is the number of correct items minus the number of incorrect items. There are no time bonus points.

The Symbol Search task measures the child's visual discrimination and visual-perceptual scanning, as well as attention and concentration, short-term memory, cognitive flexibility, and speed and accuracy. Fine-motor skills are also assessed with this paper-and-pencil measure. Performance on this subtest is influenced by anxiety, distractibility, motivation, persistence, the ability to work under time pressure, and visual-perceptual skills. It is likely that this subtest is sensitive to neurological dysfunction.

Digit Span Subtest

The Digit Span subtest is a supplementary Verbal subtest. It requires the child to repeat a series of digits given orally by the examiner. There are two parts: Digits Forward, where the child repeats the numbers in the same order as spoken; and Digits Backward, where the child must repeat the series in reverse order. All items are scored 2, 1, or 0, and the subtest is discontinued after the child fails two consecutive trials.

Digit Span is a measure of a child's short-term auditory memory and attention. The task involves sequencing and the ability to concentrate, rote learning (Digits Forward), and more complex internal mental operations, such as reversibility in thinking (Digits Backward). Performance is influenced by attention span, anxiety, distractibility, flexibility in thinking, and negativism where there may be a refusal to try such a task. Emotional and neurological impairments can affect performance.

Mazes Subtest

The Mazes subtest is a supplementary subtest that requires the child to solve paper-and-pencil mazes that differ in complexity. Mazes is not used in the computation of the IQ when the five standard Performance Scale subtests are administered. Mazes is not highly reviewed in the literature, either from a theoretical interpretive level or from a clinical practical level.

The child is asked to draw a line from the center of the maze to the outside without crossing any of the lines that indicate walls. Each maze is presented separately. The starting point varies according to age. All items are timed, and the time limit increases with difficulty. The subtest is discontinued after two consecutive failures.

Mazes appears to measure the child's ability to follow a visual pattern, planning ability, nonverbal reasoning, visual-motor coordination, perceptual organization, speed, and accuracy.

Scoring of IQ

After each subtest is scored, raw scores are converted to standard scores or scaled scores (mean = 10, standard deviation = 3) within the child's own age group through the use of tables in the WISC-III manual. Standard scores allow for the same distributional characteristics across all ages. Age groups are divided into four-month intervals between the ages 6-0-0 (years, months, days) and 16-11-30.

The Verbal score is the sum of scaled scores on the five regularly administered Verbal subtests, while the Performance score is the sum of the scaled scores on the five regularly administered Performance subtests. The Full Scale score is the sum of the Verbal and Performance scores. These scaled scores are then converted into IQs by use of another table in the manual, resulting in a Verbal IQ, a Performance IQ, and a Full Scale IQ. The WISC-III, like the other Wechsler scales, uses the Deviation IQ (mean = 100, standard deviation = 15) for the Verbal, Performance, and Full Scale IQs. A score of 100 on any scales suggests average performance for that age on that scale.

It is also possible to calculate four factor-based Index scores, including Verbal Comprehension, Perceptual Organization, Freedom from Distractibility, and Processing Speed. These scores (mean = 100, standard deviation = 15) are the result of previous analyses with the WISC-R and factor analysis of the standardization data of the WISC-III.

The subtests of Digit Span and Mazes are supplementary and are not used in the calculation of the child's IQs, although they may be administered to obtain additional information about the child's intellectual functioning and are recommended for use to determine the factor scores. Digit Span may substitute for any Verbal subtest, and Mazes may substitute for any

Performance subtest if one of the standard subtests has been invalidated or cannot be administered.

Care should be taken when using the WISC-III for repeated evaluation as there appears to be practice effects, especially with the Performance scale. If the results are used for placement, eligibility, or diagnostic decisions, this is especially true.

INTERPRETIVE GUIDELINES

When interpreting results of the WISC-III, a number of approaches or frameworks can be used. An attempt will be made to briefly discuss some of them, and then to more thoroughly examine an interpretive approach that integrates aspects of other approaches to form a "level" approach. These approaches include the following: the fluid-crystallized model, the ACID profile, the recategorization approach, the factor-analytic approach, and the information processing model. The framework chosen will depend on the examiner's or clinician's belief system. The chosen method becomes the framework on which to base clinical interpretation, to conceptualize performance, and to develop the clinical report.

The fluid-crystallized approach is based on the same-named model of intelligence, which views intelligence as consisting of two broad constructs: fluid—referring to the ability to solve new problems regardless of level of schooling or acculturation, and crystallized—referring to factual learning and problem-solving that is dependent on formal schooling and acculturation. Interestingly, the subtests that reflect fluid intelligence (Picture Completion, Picture Arrangement, Block Design, Object Assembly, Similarities, and Arithmetic or Digit Span) and those that support crystallized intelligence (Information, Similarities, Vocabulary, and Comprehension) closely match the factor-analytic approach in terms of the Verbal Comprehension and Perceptual Organization factors. Authors differ on whether Arithmetic or Digit Span is included in the Fluid calculation.

In addition, this model proposes a second level of organization of human abilities. These abilities, as measured by subtests in the WISC-III, include broad visualization (Picture Completion, Block Design, and Object Assembly), short-term acquisition and retrieval (Arithmetic and Digit Span), and speed in dealing with intellectual problems (Coding, Object Assembly, and Symbol Search).

The so-called ACID profile was developed in an attempt to identify particular patterns of subtest performance that are characteristic of specific populations. This profile refers to a pattern of low scores on Arithmetic, Coding, Information, and Digit Span that often suggests learning problems, such as reading disabilities. However, studies also indicate that children diagnosed with behavioral difficulties display the same patterns as LD children. Although the ACID profile can provide useful information for the clinician and educator, using such a profile solely for diagnostic purposes is not recommended.

Another model of interpretation is often referred to as the recategorization approach. In this approach, scaled subtest scores are grouped based on the following categories: Conceptual, which involves language functioning and manipulation of spatial images conceptually (Vocabulary, Similarities, and Comprehension); Sequential, which taps the ability to remember auditorially and visually presented information (Arithmetic, Digit Span, and Coding); Spatial, which requires manipulation of objects either directly or symbolically (Picture Completion, Block Design, and Object Assembly); and Acquired Knowledge reflects educational factors (Information, Arithmetic, and Vocabulary).

Some studies have shown that learning-disabled children will often show the following pattern: Spatial > Conceptual > Sequencing > Acquired Knowledge. However, these findings are not consistent, especially with various minority and cultural subgroupings. If a pattern is obtained, it can provide helpful information about the child's style of learning and processing, but should not be the sole source of diagnosing a learning disability. Additional tests and further investigation should be done for a complete diagnostic picture.

The factor-analytic approach is based on the assumption that intercorrelations among a group of scores are explained by an underlying factor or set of factors. Although this approach has been the primary tool for investigating the structure of intelligence, there is controversy regarding the fact that results depend upon the factoring method used. The WISC-III manual states that a number of methods were applied to standardized data yielding a four-factor solution. Verbal Comprehension (Information, Similarities, Vocabulary, and Comprehension) and Perceptual Organization (Picture Completion, Picture Arrangement, Block Design, and Object Assembly) have been found in past analyses of the WISC-R to be the two major factors and are often considered the "purer" versions of the verbal and nonverbal dimensions. The two smaller supplementary factors are Freedom from Distractibility (Arithmetic and Digit Span) from the Verbal scale and Processing Speed (Coding and Symbol Search) from the Performance scale. Having four factors can allow the examiner to subdivide each scale into two meaningful components.

There are differing points of view as to the most appropriate factor structures for the WISC-III. Some authors agree with the four-factor approach, while others believe that a three-factor model best characterizes the WISC-III: Verbal Comprehension (Information, Similarities, Vocabulary, and Comprehension), Perceptual Organization (Picture Completion, Block Design, and Object Assembly), and Processing Speed (Coding and Symbol Search). In the three-factor model, it is proposed that evidence is lacking in support for the existence of the Freedom from Distractibility factor, especially at certain ages (6, 8, 10, and 16 years). Whatever factor structure is used, it is important to exercise discretion and then to report findings with the chosen model in mind.

The information-processing model is another interpretive approach to the WISC-III. Such a model attempts to identify processes involved in learning. It has four components: 1) input—how information is received and enters the brain; 2) integration—interpreting and processing the information; 3) storage—memory for storing the information for use; 4) output—expressing the information. This model provides a conceptual framework for interpreting data from the WISC-III, including the IQs, Factor Index scores, and scaled scores. All four components are considered when interpreting a child's cognitive functioning.

Regarding input, the Verbal and Performance subtests can be separated into auditory and visual input, although unique aspects of intake/input are apparent (e.g., long versus short questions, concrete versus abstract stimuli). Integration focuses on how the different tasks often require different cognitive processes for success. Reasoning/problem-solving and imitation of a model are two examples of integration. Storage requirements range from the more immediate short-term memory to long-term storage. Output is basically vocal for Verbal subtests and motor for Performance subtests, although tasks differ in the amount of output required. The following table summarizes the four components with sample subtests:

Channel	Input (Reception)	Integration (Processing)	Storage (Memory)	Output (Expression)
Auditory	Information	Similarities	Digit Span	Vocabulary
Visual	Picture Completion	Picture Arrangement	Symbol Search	Coding

authors' prefered method

The final approach, to be discussed in more detail, combines facets of the previously [COMBINATION] discussed frameworks. This approach emphasizes successive levels of interpretation, beginning with the more general and working to the more specific. This approach requires a synthesis of the actual test scores, background information, and observations/interpretations of the child's behavior during the administration of the test. The goal is not to classify a child, as with other approaches, such as the ACID profile, but to better understand the child's abilities, which will in turn assist the examiner in making clinical recommendations for treatment or educational purposes. Interpretation comes from both a normative perspective and an individual perspective.

The Full Scale IQ provides a starting point for evaluating other scores. It is first inter-preted within the ability level or classification, which ranges from Intellectually Deficient to Very Superior, as the corresponding percentile rank in order to see how the child ranks at a particular time against the standardization sample. The confidence interval gives the band of error associated with the score, thereby putting the IQ in better perspective. The Full Scale IQ is considered representative of a child's general intellectual functioning only if there is not a significant difference between the Verbal and Performance scale IQs.

The Verbal-Performance discrepancy is then assessed for clinical significance. Table (B.1) in the manual provides values for statistically significant differences between IQ scores and Factor Index scores (see below) at various age levels and confidence intervals.

The Factor Index scores are also investigated to more thoroughly assess the child's abili-ties. Verbal Comprehension and Freedom from Distractibility comprise the Verbal scale, and Perceptual Organization and Processing Speed comprise the Performance scale. These factors can be discussed in terms of their relationship to the standardization sample (i.e., percentile and confidence interval), as well as to each other. Comparisons between the Factor Index scores are assessed for clinical significance.

Because most children will demonstrate variability in their performance, it is important to be aware of the values for statistical significance as well as the base rates in the population. Just because a Verbal-Performance discrepancy or a Factor Index score discrepancy is statis-tically significant does not necessarily mean that is "unusual" in the normal population. Table B.2 in the manual provides information regarding the cumulative percentages of the standard-ization sample that obtained various differences in their scores and can be useful when inter-preting and describing the findings. Some authors indicate that clinically significant values in the standardization sample are 15% or less. This would indicate that such a value occurred in the extreme 15% (or less) of children assessed.

The examiner can also assess the scatter among the subtests in the Verbal scale, Perfor-mance scale, Verbal Comprehension factor, and Perceptual Organization factor. Scatter can be defined as the highest standard score minus the lowest standard score. By examining subtest scatter, the examiner can determine how consistently the child performed on the various tasks constituting each score. If there is significant subtest scatter within the scale or factor, then the particular scale or factor is likely not unitary in what it is supposed to measure, and this may indicate variability in the child's development of the abilities measured. The manual provides a table (B.5) that gives base rate information as measured by cumulative percentages regard-ing the intersubtest scatter found in the standardization sample.

Individual strengths and weaknesses can then be interpreted by investigating the indi-vidual subtests. Two options are possible: to compare the child's score on a particular subtest in relation to the normative sample (interindividual comparison) or to compare the score to the child's own unique profile (intraindividual comparison or ipsative approach). In the first option, if a scaled score is 13 or above, it is considered to be a strength. If a scaled score is 7 or below, it is considered to be a weakness.

In the second instance, the performance of a child may be evaluated to determine relative strengths and weaknesses in cognitive ability. The examiner calculates a subtest mean based on the most uniform scale: if Verbal-Performance IQ discrepancy is less than 19 points, then a mean of all given subtests is calculated; if the Verbal-Performance IQ discrepancy is 19 or more points, then a mean of all administered Verbal subtests is computed separate from a mean of all administered Performance subtests. The child's individual subtest scaled score is then compared to the most appropriate mean score to determine his or her relative strengths and weaknesses. Tables in the manual (B.3) provide specific values regarding differences for statistical significance and base rate differences for the population.

Because combined subtests are statistically more reliable than a subtest by itself, it is important to determine if those subtests that reveal individual strengths or weaknesses for the child can be clustered in some meaningful way.

The "level" approach described above can be taken even further to discuss the particular comparisons between pairs of individual subtests (see Table B.4 in the manual) and patterns of response within a particular subtest. Tables in the manual provide more specific information regarding the Digit Span subtest, including cumulative percentages of the longest digit spans forward and backward (Table B.6), and the differences between the longest digit spans forward and backward (Table B.7). Item-by-item analyses would include investigating the content of responses, actual response times, responses to types of questions grouped by knowledge areas, and the style of response (e.g., impulsive, methodical). The reader is referred to the suggested readings list for a more detailed description of these comparisons.

CASE EXAMPLE

The front page of a WISC-III scoring table with all scores entered is given in the appendix.

Reason for Referral

John Doe is an 11-year-old male who was referred for a psychological evaluation by his therapist for diagnostic purposes and to assist with treatment planning. The results of this evaluation will be made available to the therapist in her treatment with the client and family and should be made available to the client's school for educational and placement purposes.

Behavioral Observations

John approached the evaluation sessions with a pleasant and cooperative attitude. However, he would frequently change the subject and go off task to discuss topics that he was more comfortable with, such as computer games. He responded well to redirection. Eye contact was good.

John approached each task initially with interest and effort. He seemed concerned about getting things right and would often ask if he answered correctly. He tended to talk his way through tasks, taking a methodical approach. He moved frequently during both interviews, fidgeting with his hands and often grabbing test materials from this examiner. As tasks became more difficult or required more effort, John visibly lost interest and would often give up. At times he would refuse to progress, and continued praise and encouragement from this examiner did not seem to motivate John to continue with such tasks.

Test Results

On the Wechsler Intelligence Scale for Children—III (WISC-III), John achieved a Verbal IQ of 104 (61st percentile) and a Performance IQ of 103 (58th percentile), resulting in a Full Scale IQ score of 104 ± 5. This score places him in the overall Average range of intellectual functioning and ranked in the 61st percentile. The chances that the range of scores from 98 to 109 includes his true IQ are about 95 out of 100. Current test results suggest that this is a valid measure of his intellectual functioning.

There was no significant difference between John's Verbal and Performance IQs, suggesting that his verbal and nonverbal reasoning abilities are generally consistent. He is likely to be functioning at about the same level on tasks that require him to understand verbal concepts and express his ideas verbally as on visual-motor tasks that assess nonverbal thinking.

In reviewing the Factor Index scores, it is apparent that John demonstrates an overall weakness in Freedom from Distractibility and Processing Speed, as compared to the other two factors. This suggests that he has difficulties in sustaining attention, concentrating, processing information quickly, exerting mental control, and visual-motor dexterity.

Within the Verbal domain, a strength was indicated in John's abstract and concrete reasoning abilities where he was asked to select and verbalize appropriate relationships between two objects or concepts (Similarities). Such strengths are often associated with flexibility in thinking and available cultural experiences. A weakness was indicated in his short-term auditory memory for number sequences (Digit Span). Such deficits are often associated with poor attention span, distractibility, and refusal to try more difficult tasks.

Within the Performance domain, John demonstrated a strength in his ability to visually analyze a whole into its component parts and then synthesize those parts into an identical design (Block Design). Strengths in this area indicate good spatial visualization and orientation, perceptual motor coordination, and visual-perceptual skills. Within this domain, weaknesses were found in John's ability to hold attention and demonstrate flexibility in new learning situations requiring visual-motor dexterity (Coding), and in his visual discrimination and visual scanning where he was asked to determine if a symbol is present in an array of symbols (Symbol Search). Weaknesses in these areas suggest visual scanning difficulties and delays in mental and psychomotor processes. Influential factors include distractibility, poor motivation, lack of persistence at the task, and inattention.

Conclusion

Results of this evaluation revealed that John is of Average intellectual functioning. Although his verbal and nonverbal reasoning abilities are relatively consistent, he demonstrated difficulties in sustaining attention, concentrating, processing information quickly, exerting mental control, and visual-motor dexterity. He lacked motivation and persistence on more difficult tasks.

When the above findings were incorporated with the results from additional achievement and personality testing, further information was provided regarding factors that might be influencing John's ability to pay attention, concentrate, and process information more efficiently. In fact, a potential learning disability, underlying depression and anxiety, thinking errors, and poor coping skills were suggested.

SUMMARY

The WISC-III is a well-standardized test, with good overall psychometric properties. It is widely used and accepted as sound test of cognitive abilities. Caution should be exercised when using the WISC-III, especially with regard to testing severely retarded or gifted children, when substituting a supplementary subtest for a regular subtest, when testing repeatedly which may produce practice effects on the Performance Scale, and when testing children who are not fast workers. In spite of these cautions, the WISC-III is a valuable instrument in the assessment of a child's cognitive abilities.

It is important to remember that interpretation of a child's performance on the WISC-III involves not only taking into account differences between various parts of the test, but also integrating findings with clinical observations, background information, and other test data. The interpretive approach offered in this chapter attempts to offer a framework based not only on normative data, but also on the individualized information provided by such an assessment. Intellectual assessment can provide important information about a child, especially regarding his or her cognitive abilities within the context of the overall personality and interactional style. In the overall assessment of a child, it is crucial to use a variety of techniques or tests (e.g., formal tests, the clinical interview, observation, and reports from significant others), rather than base decisions on one sample of behavior or functioning.

SUGGESTED READINGS

Cooper, S. (1995). *The clinical use and interpretation of the Weschler Intelligence Scale for Children–Third Edition*. Springfield, Illinois: Charles C. Thomas.

Edelman, S. (1996). A review of the Wechsler Intelligence Scale for Children–Third Edition (WISC-III). *Measurement and Evaluation in Counseling and Development, 28*, 219–224.

Jones, D. R., & James, S. (1993). Best uses of the WISC-III. In H. Booney Vance (Ed.). *Best practices in assessment for school and clinical settings* (pp. 231–269). Vermont: Clinical Psychology Publishing Company, Inc.

Journal of Psychoeducational Assessment, Monograph Series. 1993. *Advances in Psychoeducational Assessment, Wechsler Intelligence Scale for Children: Third Edition*. Author.

Kaufman, A. (1994). *Intelligent testing with the WISC-III*. New York: John Wiley & Sons, Inc.

Sattler, J. (1992). *Assessment of children: WISC-III and WPPSI-R*. San Diego: Jerome M. Sattler.

Sattler, J. (1988). *Assessment of children* (3rd edition). San Diego, California: Jerome M. Sattler.

Truch, S. (1993). *The WISC-III companion: A guide to interpretation and educational intervention*. Austin, Texas: PRO-ED.

Wechsler, D. (1991). *Weschler Intelligence Scale for Children: Third Edition manual*. San Antonio, TX: The Psychological Corporation.

APPENDIX
WISC-III SCORING TABLE WITH JOHN DOE'S SCORE ENTERED

Name __John Doe__   Sex __Male__

School _____   Grade _____

Examiner _____   Handedness _____

WISC-III®
Wechsler Intelligence Scale for Children®–Third Edition

Subtests	Raw Scores	Scaled Scores					
Picture Completion	23		12		12		
Information	16	10		10			
Coding	34		6			6	W
Similarities	22	13		13			S
Picture Arrangement	28		9		9		
Arithmetic	16	8				8	
Block Design	52		14		14		S
Vocabulary	32	11		11			
Object Assembly	31		11		11		
Comprehension	23	11		11			
(Symbol Search)	19		(7)			7	W
(Digit Span)	11	(7)			7		W
(Mazes)			( )				
Sum of Scaled Scores		53	52	45	46	15	13
		Verbal	Perfor.	VC	PO	FD	PS

Full Scale Score **105**   OPTIONAL

	Year	Month	Day
Date Tested	96	07	18
Date of Birth	85	05	04
Age	11	2	12

	Score	IQ/Index	%ile	95% Confidence Interval
Verbal	53	104	61	98 – 110
Performance	52	103	58	95 – 111
Full Scale	105	104	61	98 – 109
VC	45	107	68	100 – 113
PO	46	110	75	101 – 117
FD	15	87	19	79 – 98
PS	13	83	13	76 – 95

Subtest Scores

Verbal						Performance						
Inf	Sim	Ari	Voc	Com	DS	PC	Cd	PA	BD	OA	SS	Mz
10	13	8	11	11	7	12	6	9	14	11	7	

IQ Scores			Index Scores (Optional)			
VIQ	PIQ	FSIQ	VCI	POI	FDI	PSI
104	103	104	107	110	87	83

THE PSYCHOLOGICAL CORPORATION®
HARCOURT BRACE JOVANOVICH, INC.

09–980004

12

Cognitive Assessment System (CAS)

Jack A. Naglieri

INTRODUCTION

The purpose of this chapter is to discuss the use and interpretation of the Cognitive Assessment System. In writing this chapter I will encourage practitioners to take a technological step from traditional IQ tests to a modern approach to ability and its measurement. I view the CAS as a new technology that reflects advances made in psychology during the past 50 years and a tool that propels the field into the twenty-first century. The CAS is based on a strong theory and at the same time incorporates what has been learned in applied psychology and especially psychometrics. Most importantly, research presented in this chapter will show that the CAS is highly related to achievement, yields PASS profiles that are diagnostically important, and is relevant to intervention.

This chapter is designed to give professionals a way to obtain some knowledge of the CAS in a brief and easy-to-read format. Interested readers should consult other sources, such as Naglieri and Das or Naglieri, listed in Suggested Readings. The chapter includes an introduction, discussion of the tests' technical qualities, administration, scoring, and interpretation, and a case study. The goal is to describe both the CAS and the Planning, Attention, Simultaneous, and Successive (PASS) theory upon which the test is built. Emphasis will be given to the importance of the PASS theory and application of the theory using the CAS.

Background

Traditional IQ tests were initially formulated by the seminal work of Binet and Wechsler and others who played a critical role during the initial years of making intelligence tests. Although the tests have been effective, their most serious shortcoming is that they do not reflect what has been learned about specific human abilities in the past 60 years. During this time there has been a significant movement toward measuring specific abilities and a new breed of tests to

Jack A. Naglieri • George Mason University, Fairfax, Virginia 22030-4444.

Understanding Psychological Assessment, edited by Dorfman and Hersen. Kluwer Academic/Plenum Publishers, New York, 2001.

measure specific constructs has emerged. This includes the CAS, Differential Ability Scales (DAS), Kaufman Adolescent and Adult Intelligence Test (KAIT), K-ABC, and the Woodcock-Johnson Test of Cognitive Abilities–Revised. Their authors have each made efforts to modernize the old IQ tests that have dominated the field during this century. The CAS is the most recent of these efforts to encourage an evolutionary step from the general ability approach represented by traditional IQ to a theory-based multidimensional view based on the PASS theory of cognitive processing.

TEST CONSTRUCTION AND DEVELOPMENT

PASS Theory

The Planning, Attention, Simultaneous, and Successive (PASS) theory is based on the neuropsychological research of A. R. Luria. His work is considered very influential in American psychology. His view of the basic cognitive processes associated with different brain areas forms the basis of the PASS theory and CAS. Luria described the basic building blocks of intelligence as PASS cognitive processes, which provide us with the ability to act.

The PASS theory is very different from the approach used in traditional IQ tests that use the general ability concept. In this new approach the Planning, Attention, Simultaneous, and Successive cognitive processes are considered the basic building blocks of human ability. These four processes are described by Naglieri as follows:

> *Planning* processes provide cognitive control, utilization of processes and knowledge, intentionality and self-regulation to achieve a desired goal; *attentional* processes provide focused, selective cognitive activity over time; and simultaneous and successive processes are the two forms of operating on information.

Planning

Planning is described as "a mental process by which the individual determines, selects, applies, and evaluates solutions to problems." This provides the person with a way to solve problems that demands the use of strategies and may involve attentional, simultaneous, and successive processes as well as knowledge. All planning subtests on the CAS require the child to develop a plan of action, evaluate the value of the method, monitor its effectiveness, revise or reject an old plan as the task demands change, and control the impulse to act without careful consideration. Planning demands the development and use of strategies to solve problems, whether they are on the CAS or are classroom activities. The processes will be involved whenever the person has to make decisions about how something can be done, what methods can be applied, whether they are working, and what can be done to make the task more efficient.

Planning is well-illustrated by the Planned Codes test on the CAS (see Figure 12.1). This test requires the child to write a code (e.g., OO or XO) that corresponds to a letter (e.g., A or B). Because of the way the page is formatted, children often develop strategies to complete the test and therefore do so in an efficient and timely manner. For example, many children complete the page by doing all the As first, then the Bs, and so on. This strategy is also associated with high scores on the subtest, but those who do not use strategies earn lower scores. The subtest is sensitive to planning because the score the child earns reflects how the demands of the task were met.

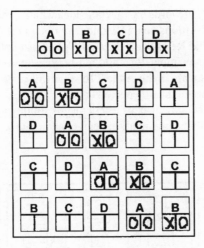

Figure 12.1. Example of a planning test.

Attention

Attention is described as "a mental process by which the individual selectively focuses on particular stimuli while inhibiting responses to competing stimuli presented over time." CAS subtests that measure attention demand focused, selective, sustained, and effortful cognitive activity. The child must direct concentration toward a particular aspect of a stimulus and inhibit responses to distracting stimuli. All CAS attention subtests are designed demand attention and require sustained focus of effort.

The CAS Number Detection subtest is a good test to illustrate attentional processes. The test is illustrated in Figure 12.2. The child is instructed to underline all the numbers 1, 2, 4, and 5 when they are printed in a particular font. Each number has two dimensions, the number and the font and the child is instructed to focus on these aspects. For example, the child may find the number 1, but unless it is printed in the correct font, it is not a target (a number that should be underlined). This environment places strong demands on attention.

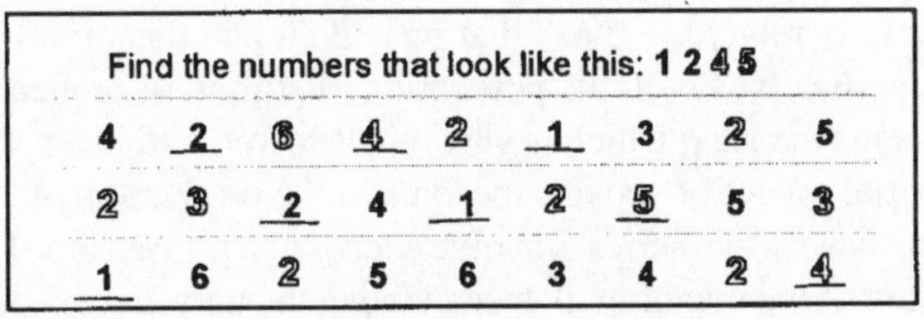

Figure 12.2. Example of an attention test.

Simultaneous

Simultaneous processing is described as "a mental process by which the individual integrates separate stimuli into a single whole or group. The essential aspect of this type of processing is that all the separate elements of the task must be interrelated into a conceptual whole. Simultaneous processing has a spatial aspect. The spatial aspect includes perception of stimuli as a whole. This is also found in tasks that involve grammatical statements because they demand the integration of words into a whole idea which in turn involves comprehension of word relationships, prepositions, and inflections to obtain meaning.

The CAS Verbal Spatial Relations subtest is a good example of a task that involves simultaneous processing. For example, the child must choose one of the six options that shows "the arrow pointing to the square in the circle." To solve this problem, the person must understand the relationships between the objects (an arrow, circle, and square) to determine which option matches the written statement. This test demands simultaneous processing because the child must see the relationships among all the parts and organize the parts into a whole. (See Figure 12.3).

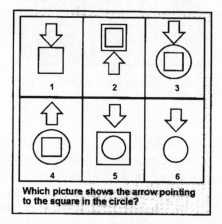

Figure 12.3. Example of a simultaneous processing test.

Successive

Successive processing is "a mental process by which the individual integrates stimuli into a specific serial order that forms a chain-like progression." This process is involved when a person must arrange things in a specific order. The most important aspect of this process is that each element is only related to those that precede it and the stimuli are not interrelated. Successive processing involves both the perception of stimuli in sequence and the formation of sounds or movements in order, which is why it is involved with the syntax of language. For example, the sequential aspect of spoken speech and the production of "separate sounds and motor impulses into consecutive series" involve successive processing. This process provides for the comprehension of the meaning of speech when the narrative involves information that must be related in a certain successive series. The CAS subtests are sensitive to successive processing because they require the reproduction of the serial aspects of the stimuli or demand understanding of statements based on syntactic relationships. For example, the CAS subtest Word Series demands that the child repeat words in the same order as spoken by the examiner. A more complex successive subtest is Sentence Questions, which requires the child answer a question about a statement said by the examiner. For example, the examiner says: "The blue greened the white with a red. Who used the red?" and the child should say "the blue." This demands comprehension of the statement based on analysis of the sequence of the words, making it an excellent measure of successive processing.

Cognitive Assessment System

The CAS was built on the PASS theory to provide an individually administered instrument for assessing ability for children aged 5–17 years. The PASS theory was used to guide construction of the CAS on the assumption that a new test should : (a) be based on a theory of ability; (b) redefine intelligence as basic cognitive processes; (c) inform the user about specific abilities that are related to academic and job successes and difficulties; (d) have relevance to differential diagnosis; (e) provide guidance to the selection and/or development of effective programming for intervention; (f) be firmly based on a sizable research base and have been proposed, tested, modified, and shown to have several kinds of validity; (g) follow closely from the theory of cognition on which it is based: (h) evaluate an individual using items that are as free from acquired knowledge as possible. The CAS was developed with these goals in mind. Most importantly, however, the test is organized according to the PASS theory and is comprised of four scales, each of which is designed to assess the corresponding process. In addition, there is a total score, called a Full Scale, which is obtained from the sum of all the subtests. Each of these is more fully described below:

Cognitive Assessment System Description

Full Scale. The Full Scale (FS) score is an overall measure of cognitive functioning with a mean set at 100 and a standard deviation set at 15. The score yields a measure of the child's level of cognitive functioning based on the four PASS scales.

PASS Scales. The PASS scales (each with a mean of 100 and a standard deviation of 15) are comprised of the sum of the scaled scores of subjects included in each respective scale. These scales represent a child's cognitive functioning in specific areas and are used to examine the possibility of specific strengths and weaknesses in cognitive processing. The PASS scales, not the PASS subtests, are the focus of CAS interpretation.

Subtests. The subtests (set at a mean of 10 and a standard deviation of 3) are measures of the specific PASS process corresponding to the scale on which they are found. They are not considered to represent their own set of specific abilities, but rather are measures of one of the four types of processes. They do vary in content (some are verbal, some not; some involve memory, others not, etc.), but the most important point is that each is an effective measure of a specific PASS process.

The PASS scales and Full Scale scores can be obtained using two combination of subtests, the Basic Battery and the Standard Battery. The Basic Battery includes eight of the subtests (two per PASS Scale) and the Standard Battery includes all twelve of the subtests shown in Table 12.1 (an asterisk indicates which subtests are included in the Basic Battery).

Standardization

The CAS was standardized for children aged 5–17 years using a stratified random sampling plan which resulted in a sample that closely matches the U.S. population. Children from both regular education and special education settings were included. During the standardization and validity study data collection program, a total of 3,072 children were administered the CAS. Of that sample 2,200 children made up the normative sample and an additional 872 children participated in reliability and validity studies. A subsample of 1,600 from the 2,200

Table 12.1. Organization of the CAS Scales and Subtests

Full Scale	Scales	Subscales
	Planning	
	*	Matching Numbers
	*	Planned Codes
		Planned Connections
	Simultaneous	
	*	Nonverbal Matrices
	*	Verbal-Spatial Relations
		Figure Memory
	Attention	
	*	Expressive Attention
	*	Number Detection
		Receptive Attention
	Successive	
	*	Word Series, and
	*	Sentence Repetition
		Speech Rate (children 5–7 years) or Sentence Questions, (children 8–17 years)

standardization group was also administered a series of achievement tests. The CAS standardization sample was stratified on the basis of: age (5 years 0 months through 17 years 11 months); gender; race (black, white, Asian, Native American, other); Hispanic origin (Hispanic, Non-Hispanic); region (Midwest, Northeast, South, West); community setting (urban/suburban, rural); classroom placement (full-time regular classroom, part-time special education resource, full-time self-contained special education); educational classification (learning disability, speech/language impairment, social-emotional disability, mental retardation, giftedness, and non-special education); and parental educational attainment level (less than high school degree, high school graduate or equivalent, some college or technical school, four or more years of college). The methods used to collect the data were designed to yield high quality data on a sample that closely represents the U.S. population. For details on the representativeness of the sample, see the *CAS Interpretive Handbook*.

Reliability

Naglieri and Das provide information about the reliability of the CAS subtests and scales which shows that they have high reliability and meet or exceed minimum values suggested by Bracken. The Full Scale reliability coefficients range from .95 to .97 and the average reliabilities for the Standard Battery PASS scales are .88 (Planning and Attention scales) and .93 (Simultaneous and Successive scales).

Validity

Naglieri and Das provide considerable information about the validity of the CAS in their Interpretive Manual, including a summary of some of the most important validity findings for the CAS. They show that the CAS offers many advantages and make three points related to validity. First, that different PASS profiles are found for children with attention deficit hyperactivity disorders and reading disabilities and that these groups do not show different profiles on the WISC-III or Woodcock Johnson Revised Cognitive Battery. Second, that the CAS has been shown to have intervention implications (see sections later in this chapter for more information on this topic). Finally, that the CAS is more strongly related to achievement than similar tests. Two topics will be presented here—PASS profiles and correlations with achievement. The relevance to intervention will be referred to at the end of this chapter.

PASS Profiles

Naglieri provides a discussion of cognitive profiles for children with attention deficit and learning disabilities for the WISC-III, WJ-R Cognitive, and CAS taken from the test manuals and a recent publication by Woodcock. In the WISC-III Manual, Wechsler provides three studies involving children with learning disabilities (N = 65), reading disabilities (N = 34), and attention deficit hyperactivity disorder (N = 68). The profiles of WISC-III Index scores for the LD, RD, and ADHD children were essentially the same. Similarly, in a study reported by Woodcock in 1998, children with learning disabilities (N= 62) and attention deficit disorders (N = 67) have similar profiles for the seven GfGc clusters. Therefore, the seven factor GfGc, like the four WISC-III Index level scores, does not yield distinctive profiles of scores for the LD and ADHD samples used. In contrast are the results for the CAS. In the studies reported by Naglieri and Das, children with attention deficit (n = 66) and reading disorders (n=24) earned PASS scores that show a different pattern. The ADHD children were poor in planning and somewhat lower in attention while the RD sample was poor in Successive processing. Thus, the profiles for the CAS, shown in Figure 12.4, were different from those obtained for the Wechsler and from Woodcock.

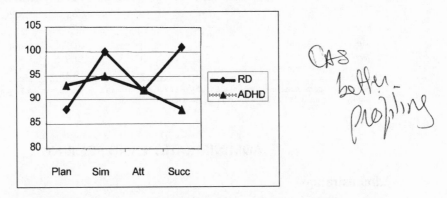

CAS
better
profiling

Figure 12.4. PASS profiles for children with attention deficit hyperactivity disorder and reading disabilities.

Relationships to Achievement

The Full Scale of the CAS correlates more highly with achievement than do any intelligence tests. This finding is especially important because one of the most important dimensions of validity for a test of cognitive ability is the relationship to achievement. Naglieri summarizes several studies involving large numbers of children and several important tests and found the following:

- The median correlation between the WISC-III and WIAT is .59. (n = 1,284 children aged 5–19 years from all regions of the country, different racial and ethnic groups, and each parental educational level).
- The median correlation between the Differential Ability scales and achievement in Basic Number Skills, Spelling, and Word Reading is .60 (n = 2,400 children included in the standardization sample).
- The median correlation between the K-ABC Mental Processing Composite (MPC) and the K-ABC Achievement, Woodcock Reading Mastery Test, and KeyMath Diagnostic Math Test is .63 for several large samples of children across the ages for which the test is used.
- The median correlation between the Woodcock-Johnson Revised Cognitive and Woodcock-Johnson Revised Achievement Test Batteries was .63 (n = 888 children aged 6, 9, and 13 years).
- The median correlation between the CAS Full Scale and the WJ-R Test of Achievement was .70 (for a representative sample of 1,600 children who closely match the U.S. population).

These results showed that the CAS Full Scale score was the most powerful predictor of achievement, accounting for considerably more variance in achievement than any of the measures included (see Table 12.2). This finding, in conjunction with separate profiles for ADHD and reading disabled children and the intervention implications of PASS performance, provide strong support for the validity of the CAS.

Table 12.2. Relationships Between Achievement and Several Different Measures of Ability[a]

	WISC-III	DAS	WJ-R	K-ABC	CAS
	FSIQ	GCA	Cog	MPC	FS
N	1,284	2,400	888	2,636	1,600
Median Correlation	.59	.60	.63	.63	.70
% of Variance	35%	36%	39%	40%	49%
Increase over WISC-III	–	3%	12%	14%	41%

[a]All data are the median correlations of the ability test total score with all achievement variables reported in the respective ability test manual. WISC-III WIAT data are from the WIAT manual.

ADMINISTRATION AND SCORING

Administration

The CAS must be administered and scored as prescribed in the test's administration and scoring manual. It is, of course, the obligation of the user to ensure that administration is consistent with applicable professional standards and that an appropriate environment is maintained. For example, development and maintenance of rapport, as well as following directions precisely, is important. In this chapter only a few important points will be discussed.

Seating Arrangement. Administration is facilitated if the examiner is within reach of the child and can closely observe the child's actions. This is particularly important for the Planning subtests where recording how the child completes the tasks (see section below on strategy assessment). Examiners likely to find sitting across from the child or across the corner of a table most appropriate for this instrument.

Administration Directions. Instructions to the child include both verbal statements and nonverbal actions by the examiner. Examiners must carefully follow the instructions for gestures (indicated in parenthetical statements following or preceding the text) corresponding to the oral directions. The combination of oral and nonverbal communication is designed to ensure that the children understand the task.

Subtest Order. It is important to administer the CAS subtests in the prescribed order to retain the integrity of the test and reduce the influence of extraneous variables on the child's performance. For example, the Planning tests are administered first because they give the child flexibility to solve the subtest in any manner. In contrast, the Attention subtests must be completed in the prescribed order (e.g., left to right, top to bottom). By administering the Planning subtests before the Attention subtests, the amount of constraint increases over time. If the Attention subtests were administered before the Planning ones, some children could be inhibited by the more rigid instruction.

Strategy Assessment. All the CAS Planning subtests include a phase called "strategy assessment" wherein the examiner observes if the child used strategies to complete the items. Strategy Assessment was developed to gather information about how the child completed the items. In addition, it is used to help describe the standard scores that were obtained (see section on interpretation). This information allows the examiner to describe the standard score in relation to the percentage of children who used that strategy in the standardization sample. This can help explain a particularly high or low Planning score and be integrated into the entire evaluation.

Strategy Assessment is conducted for each Planning subtest in two ways. Observed Strategies are those seen by the examiner through careful observation as the child completes the items. Reported Strategies are obtained following completion of the item(s). The examiner obtains this information by saying, "Tell me how you did these," or "How did you find what you were looking for?" or some similar statement. The child can communicate the strategies by either verbal or nonverbal (gesturing) means. These are recorded in the "Observed" and "Reported" sections of the Strategy Assessment Checklist included in the Record Form.

Provide Help Guidelines. Several methods have been used to ensure that the child understands what is being requested. Those include samples and demonstration items as well as opportunities for the examiner to clarify the requirements of the task. However, if the child does not seem ready or appears in any way confused or uncertain, the examiner is instructed to "provide a brief explanation if necessary." This instruction gives the examiner the freedom to explain what the child must do in whatever terms are considered necessary so as to ensure that the child understands the task. This can be done in any form including gestures and verbal communication in any language. The intent is to give the examiner full rein to clarify the demands of the subtest and to allow the examiner to be certain that the child understands what to do. This instruction, however, is not intended to teach the child how to do the test.

Bilingual or Hearing-Impaired Children. Instructions for administration were designed so that a child with an adequate working knowledge of English and can benefit from the samples and demonstrations provided. In those cases where additional help is needed, examiners may augment the English instructions when the statement "provide additional help when needed" is given. Examiners who know a child's native language or can use sign language, may do so when instructed to provide assistance. In these cases, the examiner must decide whether to use the alternative method of communication.

Age Partition. Children aged 5–7 and 8–17 years are given different instructions and in some cases sets of items to allow tailoring of specific items to particular age groups. For example, two of the Attention subtests have different types of stimuli so that the content of the test will be more appropriate to each age groups. Specialized content was selected to ensure that 5–7-year-olds would easily understand the items and that older children would not view subtests as too infantile. For example, the Expressive Attention subtest contains pictures of animals for 5–7-year-olds but is composed of words for the 8–17-year-olds. Similarly, Speech Rate is administered to ages 5–7 years and Sentence Questions to ages 8–17 years so that the most appropriate task is given for the specific ages. In addition, children aged 8–17 typically begin with more advanced items on some of the subtests.

Discontinue Rule. Administration of some subtests is discontinued after four consecutive item failures. This applies to all Simultaneous subtests and all but one of the Successive subtests (Speech Rate).

Time Limits. The time limits for various items vary as shown in the Administration Directions Manual and the Record Form. These limits are provided in total seconds (e.g., 150") as well as minutes and seconds (e.g., 2:30) to accommodate professionals who use digital or analog stop watches. The point at which to begin timing is indicted within the directions found in the administration and scoring manual. Following these instructions carefully will ensure accurate evaluation of the time children take to complete the items. Where time limits are not provided (e.g., Nonverbal Matrices) examiners should exercise good judgment when encouraging the child to attempt the next item.

Rates of Presentation. Six subtests require stimuli be presented at a specific rate or for an exact period of time. Word Series requires administration at the rate of one word per second, and Sentence Repetition and Sentence Questions are presented at the rate of two words per second. Figure Memory involves stimuli that are presented for exactly five seconds. There is also a 30-second exposure time limit for each item in the Verbal-Spatial Relations subtest. These time limits must be followed exactly.

Spoiled Subtests. If one of the three regularly administered subtests in the Standard Battery is spoiled, examiners should use the remaining two subtests and compute the PASS scale using the Basic Battery norms. Because the Full Scale requires either eight or twelve subtests, the calculation of the Full Scale would have to be computed on the basis of the Basic Battery, not the Standard Battery. Alternatively, examiners may prorate the sum of three subtests in the PASS scale. A prorating table is provided in *Essentials of CAS Assessment* by Naglieri (1999).

Scoring

The CAS is scored using procedures that are typical in the field of intellectual assessment. The following steps are used and are described in this section.

1. Subtest raw scores are obtained.
2. Raw scores are converted to subtest scaled scores.
3. PASS Scale and CAS Full Scale standard scores are obtained from the sum of the respective subtest scaled scores.

Subtest Raw Scores to Scaled Scores

The CAS subtest raw scores are calculated using one or more of the following dimensions: (a) the number correct; (b) time to complete; and (c) number of false detections. These measurements are used either in isolation or in combination, depending upon the goals of the subtest. Some subtest raw scores are based on number correct and others on total time, while some are the combination of number correct and total time, or number correct, total time, and number of false detections. Each of the types of raw score methods is more fully described below:

Number Correct. Nonverbal Matrices, Verbal-Spatial Relations, Figure Memory, Word Series, Sentence Repetition, and Sentence Questions subtests are scored using the number of items correct. This is obtained by summing the number of correct items and assigning credit for those items not administered below any starting point.

Time in Seconds. The raw score for Planned Connections and Speech Rate is the sum of the time in seconds to complete all items. Simply add the time scores for the items administered to compute the raw score.

Time and Number Correct. The raw score for the Matching Numbers, Planned Codes, and Expressive Attention subtests is based on the combination of time and number correct. The number correct and time are combined into a ratio score using a Ratio Score Conversion Table included in the record form. This table has the heading "Accuracy Score" at the top and the left-most column contains time scores for three-second intervals. To combine the number correct and time into a ratio score, enter the row that contains the item time in seconds, then find the column for the Accuracy Score earned by the child. The number at the juncture of the row and column is the ratio score for that item. For example, if a child earned a total time score of 43 seconds with an accuracy score of 38, then the ratio score is 54. The ratio scores for each item are summed, as indicated on the Record Form, to obtain a raw score for the subtest.

Time, Number Correct, and Number of False Detections. The raw scores for Number Detection and Receptive Attention are obtained using ratio scores. In these subtests, however, the Accuracy Score is the number of correct responses minus the number of false detections (the number of times the child underlined a stimulus that is not a target).

Converting Raw Scores to Subtest Scaled Scores

The CAS subtest scaled scores (mean of 10 and SD of 3) are obtained using age-based tables included in the administration and scoring manual. The norms tables are divided according to the child's chronological age in years, months, and days.

PASS Scale Standard Scores from the Sum of Subtest Scaled Scores

Each PASS scale (mean of 100 and SD of 15) is derived from the sum of the appropriate subtest scaled scores. The Standard Battery is calculated from the sum of all three subtest scaled scores within each PASS scale (the Basic Battery, from the sum of the first two subtests within each PASS Scale). The Full Scale (mean of 100 and SD of 15) is obtained from the sum of the subtest scaled scores from either the Standard or Basic Batteries. All these scores are obtained from the appropriate norms table, which also includes percentile ranks and confidence intervals (90% and 95%).

INTERPRETIVE GUIDELINES

This section presents a set of methods that can be used as a guide to interpret the CAS. These interpretative steps should be applied within the context of all available information about the child so that a comprehensive view of the child is achieved and a thorough plan for treatment, if appropriate, can be developed, implemented and evaluated. This section includes the essential steps for interpreting results and will be followed by an illustration of how the CAS results can be used to identify a cognitive problem and an intervention.

Steps for Interpreting CAS Results

Interpretation steps of CAS scores vary according to the specific purposes of the assessment. They include an examination of the PASS Scales and subtests, comparison of CAS results with tests of achievement and comparisons of CAS scores obtained over time. These topics are covered in the following sections.

1. Examine the child's performance on the Full Scale and PASS Scale standard scores in relation to peers.
2. Compare the four PASS standard scores for meaningful discrepancies.
3. Compare subtest scores within each PASS Scale for meaningful discrepancies, if appropriate.
4. Compare the child's Full Scale and PASS standard scores with achievement scores.

Step 1— The CAS Full Scale and PASS Scale Standard Scores

Evaluate the child's overall levels of performance by describing the PASS and Full Scale standard scores using the descriptive categories, confidence intervals, and percentile ranks. All this information should be recorded on the front of the CAS Record Form as shown in Figure 12.5.

It is important to remember that the Full Scale score is intended to be an overall measure of processing based on the combination of the four PASS areas. It will be a good overall description of a child's cognitive processing when the four PASS Scale scores are similar. However, when there is significant variability among the PASS Scale standard scores, the Full Scale will not show important relative strengths and weaknesses (as discussed in the section that follows). When this happens, the Full Scale score should be described as a midpoint between extreme scores and de-emphasized.

Step 2—Compare the Four PASS Standard Scores

One of the main goals of the CAS is to determine differences in PASS scores for an individual child so that cognitive strengths or weaknesses are found. This is accomplished by examining the statistical significance of the variation in PASS scores. Also, it is accomplished using an intraindividual or ipsative method. This approach allows the professional to determine when the variation in PASS scores is meaningful. When variation is not significant, any differences are assumed to reflect measurement error. Meaningful, or reliable, variation can be interpreted within the context of the theory, related to strategy use, and evaluated in relation to achievement tests.

When a PASS score is significantly above the child's mean score then a cognitive processing strength is indictated. When a PASS score is significantly lower than the child's mean score, a weakness is detected. Note that the strengths and weaknesses are determined relative to the child's own average level of performance which this tells us about relative strengths or weaknesses. This approach has been used in intelligence testing for some time. The steps needed to determine if a child's PASS profile is significant are numerated below and illustrated using PASS scores presented in Table 12.3. The values needed at different levels of significance and for the Standard and Basic Batteries are shown in Table 12.4.

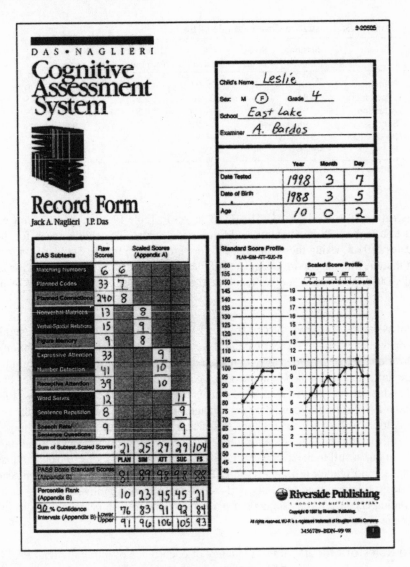

Figure 12.5. Complete CAS Record Form.

1. Calculate the average of the four PASS standard scores.
2. Subtract the mean from each of the PASS standard scores to obtain the intraindividual difference scores.
3. Compare the intraindividual difference scores (ignore the sign) to the values in Table 12.4 or the more detailed tables in the *CAS Administration and Scoring Manual*. When the difference score is equal to or greater than the tabled values, the score differs significantly from the child's average PASS Scale standard score.
4. Label any significant score that is above the mean as a strength and any below the mean as a weakness.
5. Any variation from the mean that is not significant should be considered chance fluctuation.

Table 12.3. Illustrative Case Example of Leslie[a]

	Standard Score	90% %tile	CI range	Difference from mean	Difference Needed	
Planning	81	10	76–91	–10.5	9.7	Sig
Simultaneous	89	23	83–96	–2.5	8.6	NS
Attention	98	45	91–106	6.5	9.9	NS
Successive	98	45	92–105	6.5	8.6	NS
PASS Mean	91.5					
Full Scale	88	21	84–93			

[a]Differences needed are at the .05 level

Illustration of the Method. The PASS scores in Table 12.3 range from a low of 81 in Planning to a high of 98 in Attention and Successive Scales. The child's mean for the four PASS scales is 91.5. Using the values needed for significance for the Standard Battery, it is apparent that the Planning score is significantly lower than the child's mean. This means that the child's Planning score is a significant weakness relative to the overall level of performance.

Relative and Cognitive Strengths and Weaknesses. When there is a significant strength or weakness in the PASS Scale profile, the level of performance in relation to the standardization sample should also be considered. If a child has a significant intraindividual difference score that also falls below a score of 90 (in the Low Average range or lower), then it should be labeled a *cognitive weakness*. This is true for the case of Leslie whose Planning scale standard score is significantly lower than her mean PASS scores *and* below the Average category. Alternatively, when a child has a significant weakness that falls in the average range (90–110), this should be viewed as a *relative weakness* because it is low in relation to the child's mean but is still in the average range of normative expectations. In such an instance, the finding is important for different reasons. For example, it could explain uneven academic performance for a child who typically performs very well. A cognitive weakness is a more serious finding because it represents poor performance relative to peers, as well as in comparison to the child's own level.

Base Rates of Occurrence. Frequency of occurrence of intraindividual PASS scale differences can also be examined. This is determined through use of actuarial tables in Appendix D of the *CAS Administration and Scoring Manual*. These tables provide the frequencies of

Table 12.4. Intraindividual Differences Needed for Significance Between each PASS Score and the Child's Mean PASS score for All Ages[a]

	Standard Battery		Basic Battery	
	.10	.05	.10	.05
Planning	9.7	10.8	10.9	12.1
Simultaneous	8.6	9.6	10.0	11.2
Attention	9.9	11.1	11.5	12.8
Successive	8.6	9.5	9.7	10.8

[a]Data from Naglieri and Das (1997b), Tables D.1 and D.3. See those tables for the differences needed by age.

occurrence of all possible intraindividual difference scores in the standardization sample and can help determine how typical the PASS profile is. For example, using data provided in the illustration for Leslie, the difference of 10.5 found for the Planning Scale occurred in about 25% of the CAS standardization sample. The importance of this finding is therefore augmented by the fact that a weakness of this size is uncommon among those included in the normative group.

Step 3—Compare Subtest Scores within Each Scale for Meaningful Discrepancies

Variation in CAS subtests is examined with the same method used for studying the PASS profile. The subtest scaled scores are compared to the child's mean subtest score and the significance of the differences is evaluated. In addition, the frequency of occurrence of subtest differences is compared to that found for the normal standardization sample. These variations should also be interpreted within the context of the theory and strategy used and other relevant factors. It is important to note, however, that the approach described so far in this chapter is based on the assumption that the four theoretically derived PASS scales will provide the most important interpretive information. When the professional chooses to go further and examine the variation of the CAS subtests, the prescribed method should be followed. Although this level of analysis gives a more specific examination of the child's performance, it has the disadvantage of involving scores with lower reliability than the PASS scales. Subtest level analysis is only considered when there is specific reason to do so. For example, the significance of the difference between the child's subtest scaled scores can be important if a weakness in Planning is the result of poor performance on a single subtest or reflects consistently low scores. This may reflect the child's failure to use a strategy on one of the Planning subtests in contrast to the other two subtests.

Step 4—Compare the Full Scale and PASS Standard Scores with Achievement Scores

The scores a child obtains on the CAS can be compared to those obtained from achievement scores to help determine if achievement is below expectations. This can also assist when interventions are being planned, as well as when eligibility for special education services is being considered. There are two methods for comparing the CAS to achievement—a simple and a predicted difference method. Both of these approaches fit within a theoretical framework designed to discover if the child has a PASS cognitive weakness and an associated academic weakness. First, the simple different method for comparing CAS with achievement will be presented, then a theoretical system for interpretation of these differences will be discussed.

Ability Achievement Discrepancy

The CAS scores can be compared to achievement tests using the Simple-Difference method and the values provided in Table 12.5. This table includes the values needed for significance at the .05 level for both the Standard and Basic Batteries. These values are used in the following manner. First, compare the difference between the two scores to the tabled values (ignore the sign). Any difference that is equal to or greater than the tabled value is significant. For example, Leslie (see Table 12.6) earned a CAS Full Scale standard score of 88 on the Standard

Table 12.5. Differences between CAS and Achievement Scores Required for Significance Using the Simple-Difference Method (p = .05)

	STANDARD BATTERY					BASIC BATTERY				
	Plan	Sim	Att	Succ	FS	Plan	Sim	Att	Succ	FS
DAB - 2										
Listening	12	11	12	11	9	13	12	14	12	13
Speaking	12	10	12	10	9	13	11	13	11	12
Reading	11	9	11	9	8	12	11	13	11	12
Writing	11	8	11	8	7	12	10	12	10	11
Mathematics	13	11	13	11	10	14	12	14	12	13
Spoken Language	12	10	12	10	8	13	11	13	11	12
Written Language	11	8	11	8	7	12	10	12	10	11
TOTAL	11	9	11	9	7	12	10	12	10	11
K-TEA										
Reading Decoding	12	11	12	10	9	13	12	14	11	12
Reading Comprehension	13	12	13	11	10	14	13	14	12	13
Reading Composite	11	10	12	10	8	12	11	13	11	12
Math Applications	13	12	13	12	10	14	13	15	13	14
Math Computation	13	12	13	12	10	14	13	15	13	13
Math Composite	12	11	12	10	9	13	12	14	11	12
Spelling	12	11	13	11	9	13	12	14	12	13
Battery Composite	11	9	11	9	7	12	11	13	10	11
PIAT-R										
General Information	11	10	12	10	8	12	11	13	11	12
Reading Recognition	11	9	11	9	7	12	11	13	10	11
Reading Comprehension	11	10	12	10	8	13	11	13	11	12
Total Reading	12	11	13	11	9	13	12	14	12	13
Mathematics	11	10	11	9	8	12	11	13	11	12
Spelling	11	10	11	9	8	12	11	13	11	12
TOTAL TEST	15	14	15	14	13	16	15	17	15	16
WIAT										
Basic Reading	13	11	13	11	10	14	12	14	12	13
Mathematics Reasoning	14	12	14	12	11	15	13	15	13	14
Spelling	14	12	14	12	11	15	13	15	13	14
Reading Comprehension	14	13	14	13	12	15	14	16	14	15
Numerical Operations	15	14	15	14	13	16	15	16	15	16
Listening comprehension	16	14	16	14	13	17	15	17	15	16
Oral Expression	13	12	13	12	11	14	13	15	13	14
Written Expression	16	15	16	15	14	17	16	17	16	17
READING	12	10	12	10	9	13	11	13	11	12
MATHEMATICS	13	11	13	11	10	14	12	14	12	13
LANGUAGE	14	12	14	12	11	15	13	15	13	14
WRITING	14	12	14	12	11	15	13	15	13	14
SCREENER	12	10	12	10	8	13	11	13	11	12
TOTAL	11	9	11	9	8	12	11	13	11	12
WJ-R										
Broad Reading	12	10	12	10	9	13	11	14	11	13
Basic Reading	12	10	12	10	8	13	11	13	11	12
Reading Comprehension	12	10	12	10	9	13	11	14	11	13
Broad Math	13	11	13	11	9	14	12	14	12	13
Basic Math	13	11	13	11	10	14	12	14	12	13
Math Reasoning	14	12	14	12	11	15	13	15	13	14
Writing Skills	12	10	12	10	9	13	12	14	11	13
Skills Cluster	12	10	12	10	8	13	11	13	11	12
Letter Word Identification	13	11	13	11	9	14	12	14	11	13

Table 12.5. Continued

	STANDARD BATTERY					BASIC BATTERY				
	Plan	Sim	Att	Succ	FS	Plan	Sim	Att	Succ	FS
Passage Comprehension	14	13	14	13	12	15	14	15	13	15
Calculation	13	12	13	12	11	14	13	15	12	14
Applied Problems	14	12	14	12	11	15	13	15	13	14
Dictation	14	12	14	12	11	15	13	15	13	14
Word Attack	14	12	14	12	11	14	13	15	13	14
Reading Vocabulary	13	11	13	11	10	14	12	14	12	13
Quantitative Concepts	15	14	15	14	13	16	15	17	15	16
Proofing	14	12	14	12	11	15	13	15	13	14
WRAT-3 BLUE										
Reading	13	12	14	12	11	14	13	15	13	14
Spelling	14	13	14	13	11	15	14	15	13	14
Arithmetic	15	14	15	14	13	16	15	17	15	15
WRAT-3 TAN										
Reading	14	12	14	12	11	14	13	15	13	14
Spelling	14	13	14	13	11	15	14	15	13	14
Arithmetic	15	14	16	14	13	16	15	17	15	16

Battery and a K-TEA Computation score of 72. The 16 point difference between the two cores is significant (a 10 point difference is needed).

CAS and the Ability/Achievement Discrepancy/Consistency: A New Method

The significance of the difference between PASS and achievement can be used to determine if an ability achievement discrepancy is present. This is done in much the same way as has been done with traditional IQ tests. This often contributes to the decision that the child may be eligible for special services because the discrepancy has provided information that the child's actual level of achievement is not consistent with the level predicted by the IQ score. This method, however, only tells if there is an unexplained difference between ability and academic performance and yields little information about why the discrepancy is found. Assuming that the academic weakness is not due to poor instruction, sensory limitations, emotional problems, and so forth, the discrepancy model identifies a child as disabled when no

Table 12.6. CAS Achievement Comparisons Using the Simple Difference Method for the Case of Leslie

	PASS Scores	Difference Scores	Differences Needed	
Planning	81	9	13	NS
Simultaneous	89	17	12	Sig
Attention	98	26	13	Sig
Successive	98	26	12	Sig
Full Scale	88	16	10	Sig
K-TEA Achievement Scores				
Math Applications	91			
Math Computation	72			

intellectual problem has been detected. That is, because the IQ scores are high (no problems found) and achievement is low (academic problems were found) a discrepancy results.

The CAS often indicates whether there is a cognitive explanation for an academic problem as well as an ability/achievement discrepancy. When a child's Full Scale or separate PASS Scale standard scores are significantly higher than achievement, then a traditional discrepancy is found. In addition, the CAS can help determine when there is a weakness in a specific area of achievement (e.g., Reading-Decoding) that is related to a specific weakness in a PASS area (e.g., Successive Processing). Thus, it is possible to find a *consistency* between two scores (Successive Processing and Reading-Decoding) as well as a *discrepancy* between other CAS scales and achievement. The consistency between Successive Processing and Reading-Decoding is indicated by a nonsignificant difference between these scores. This finding allows the practitioner to suggest that successive processing and reading-decoding were related, which has intervention implications (discussed later in this chapter).

To apply this method, compare each of the PASS and Full Scale scores to achievement. In the example of Leslie, her Math Calculation score is significantly lower than her Full, Simultaneous, Attention and Successive scales. Her Planning score, however, is not significantly different from her achievement in Math. Lack of a significant difference between Planning and Math Calculation provides an explanation for the academic problem. Considering the strong relationships found between Math Calculation and Planning processing, this connection is warranted.

The consistency/discrepancy relationship is illustrated in Figure 12.6. This shows the triangular relationship among the variables. At the base of the triangle are the two weaknesses, one in achievement (K-TEA Math Calculation) and one in cognitive processing (Planning). At the top of the triangle are the child's high scores. When this relationship is found, the practitioner has detected a cognitive weakness and associated academic weakness that warrant intervention. Should an academic weakness be found but not an associated PASS processing difficulty, it would be appropriate to consider variables in the environment that may be responsible for academic failure, such as quantity and quality of instruction, motivation of the child, and so on. In such an instance, direct instruction in the academic area should be considered.

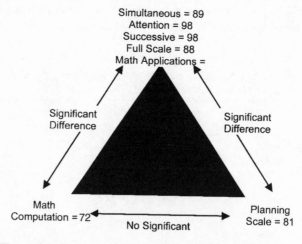

Figure 12.6. Illustration of the discrepancy and consistency approach.

Communication of CAS Results

A good understanding of the PASS theory and the nature of the four types of processes is needed by the practitioner to adequately use the CAS and communicate the results in oral and written form. Readers of this chapter might want to refer to other sources such as Naglieri, Naglieri and Das, or Das, Naglieri and Kirby for more information on PASS or its foundation. In the next section, I will provide a case example to illustrate how the information about the processes can be communicated.

CASE EXAMPLE

This example reports on a young girl named Leslie who attends a school for children with learning disabilities. This child, whose name has been changed, is one of the subjects who participated in a math intervention study reported by Naglieri and Gottling. Results of the classroom intervention will be provided in this example. Her actual CAS scores have already been reported in Table 12.3. This text describes her performance on the CAS without additional test results that might normally be included in a full report. Thus, this example is not intended to provide a complete case study. My aim is to show how the PASS and Full Scale results might be described, then used to identify an appropriate instructional approach.

Test Results and Interpretation

Leslie earned a Cognitive Assessment System (CAS) Full Scale standard score of 88, which falls within the Low Average classification and is ranked at the 21st percentile. This means that her overall score is equal to or greater than 21% of the scores obtained by the children her age who were included in the standardization group. There is a 90% probability that Leslie's true Full Scale score falls within the range of 84–93. There was, however, significant variation among the four separate PASS scales that comprise the CAS, which means that the Full Scale will be higher or lower than the separate scales included in the test. For example, her scores ranged from an 81 in Planning to a 98 in the Attention and Successive scales. Because the Full Scale score is not always representative of the separate scores from which it is made, it should be cautiously interpreted. The range of scores does indicate, however, that there is important variation within Leslie's PASS scales that warrants consideration, especially the Planning Scale which is significantly lower than the mean of the four PASS scales. This indicates that an important cognitive weakness has been found.

Leslie earned a significantly low score on the CAS Planning scale. This cognitive weakness reflects the difficulty she had using efficient and effective strategies for problem solving, self-monitoring, and revising her plans of action. She had difficulty making decisions about how to complete many of the questions and failed to monitor the quality of her work. For example, when required to record a specific code that corresponded to one of four different letters, she did so in a way that showed no apparent plan or method. This is in contrast to about 90% of children her age who made an effective plan to solve these questions.

Leslie's poor performance in Planning is particularly important because it is a weakness both in relation to her average PASS score and relative to her peers. The cognitive weakness in Planning suggests that Leslie will have difficulty with tasks that demand development of strategies to solve problems, making decisions about how to do things, general control of behavior, self-monitoring and self-correction. These activities are especially important, for example, in academic areas such as mathematics computation.

Leslie's poor performance on the K-TEA Mathematics Computation (76, 5th percentile) is consistent with her Planning score of 81 (there is no significant difference between these scores). These two low scores are both significantly lower than her Simultaneous, Attention, and Successive scores which provides evidence of an ability–achievement discrepancy. The her low scores in Mathematics Computation and Planning Processing are likely related and this has implications for intervention (see later section of this report).

Leslie's Attention was assessed by subtests that required her to focus on specific features of test questions and resist reacting to distracting parts of the tests. She was able to focus concentration well enough to earn a score of 98 on the CAS Attention Scale, which ranks at the 45th percentile and falls within the Average classification (90% range is 91–106). Attention was measured by subtests that required her to respond only to specific stimuli (for example, the number 1 when it appeared in an outline typeface) and not to respond to distracting stimuli (when the number 1 appeared in a regular typeface). Leslie's Attention score indicates that she demonstrated typical performance in both identifying targets and avoiding responses to distracting stimuli.

Leslie earned a score of 89 on the Simultaneous Processing Scale (90% confidence interval = 83–96). This score ranks her at the 23rd percentile and falls at the juncture of Average and Low Average classifications. These tests required that she relate parts into a group or whole, understand relationships among words and diagrams, and work with spatial relationships. Leslie's score on the Simultaneous Processing Scale illustrates that she can integrate information into groups at a level that is just below average.

Leslie also earned an Average score of 98 on the Successive Processing Scale which is ranked at the 45th percentile (90% confidence interval = 92–105). Her Successive Processing was assessed by tests that required her to work with information in a specific linear order. For example, repeating words in order as spoken by the examiner or comprehending information that is based on word order.

In conclusion, Leslie earned CAS scores that ranged from 81 to 98 and showed evidence of a cognitive weakness in Planning. This cognitive weakness in Planning is accompanied by a comparable score on the K-TEA Math Computation subtest because both measures demand careful control of thinking and acting, selection of appropriate strategies to complete the math or nonacademic problems, and checking her work (self-monitoring). These results indicate that interventions that address both the mathematical and Planning Processing demands of these tasks should be considered.

Intervention Design

In order to improve Leslie's use of planning processes when doing math computation, the intervention described by Naglieri and Gottling was applied. Consultation between the school psychologist and the teacher resulted in an intervention plan to assist Leslie within the context of an instruction given to the entire class. The teacher taught in half-hour sessions following the format of 10 minutes of math worksheet activity, 10 minutes of discussion, and 10 minutes of math worksheets (see Figure 12.7). The math worksheets included problems covered in the class during the previous weeks. During the 10-minute discussion period, the teacher facilitated an interaction that encouraged all the children to reflect on how they completed the work and how they would go about completing the pages in the future. The teacher did not attempt to reinforce or otherwise encourage the children to complete the math in any special way. Instead, the children were encouraged to think about how they did the work, what methods were effective, why some methods work better than others, and so on. The goal was to teach

DEFINITION of a Group Facilitation "Session"
   Step 1: 10 minutes of math (first data point)
   Step 2: 10 minutes of discussion
   Step 3: 10 minutes of math (second data point)

BASELINE (3 sessions):
   Baseline Step 1: Begin by giving math pages and 10 minutes for completion. The teacher simply says "Here is a math worksheet for you to do. Please try to get as many of the problems correct as you can. You will have 10 minutes." Slight variations on this instruction are permitted, but do not give any additional information.

   Baseline Step 2: During Baseline the discussion is unrelated to the math worksheets. Teachers may facilitate any discussion except those related to the task.

   Baseline Step 3: The teacher gives another math worksheet and says "Here is another math worksheet for you to do. Please try to get as many of the problems correct as you can. You will have 10 minutes." Slight variations on this instruction are permitted, but do not give any additional information.

INTERVENTION (7–10 sessions)
   Intervention Step 1: The teacher gives each child a worksheet and says "Here is another math worksheet for you to do. Please try to get as many of the problems correct as you can. You will have 10 minutes." Slight variations on this instruction are permitted, but do not give any additional information

   Intervention Step 2: The Discussion step requires that the teacher facilitate a discussion which probes the children regarding how they completed the worksheet and how they will go about completing the pages in the future. Teachers do not attempt to reinforce the children. For example, if a child says "I used xyz strategy" the teacher should not say "Good, and be sure to do that next time." Instead, the teacher may probe, saying "and did that work for you?" or some statement designed to encourage the child to consider the effectiveness of the strategy. The general goals are to encourage the children to:
Describe how they did the worksheet
Encourage the children to verbalize ideas (this facilitates planning)
Explain why some methods work better
Encourage the children to be self-reflective
Encourage the children to think about what they will do the next time they get the worksheet

   Suggested probes:
      How did you do the page?
      What do you notice about how this page was completed?
      What is a good way to do these pages?
      Why did you do it that way?
      Did it work as you expected? What did this teach you?
      How are you going to complete the page next time so you get as many correct as possible?
      What do you want to do next time?
      What are some reasons why people makes mistakes on problems like these?
      Do think you will do anything differently next time?

   Intervention Step 3: The teacher gives each child a worksheet and says "Here is another math worksheet for you to do. Please try to get as many of the problems correct as you can. You will have 10 minutes." Slight variations on this instruction are pennitted, but do not give any additional information.

   What teachers should not do:
   Watch me, this is how to do it.
   Math instruction.
   That's right, good, now your getting it!
   Remember to use your favorite strategy.
   Do no direct instruction.

Figure 12.7. Planning facilitation method.

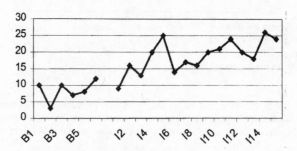

Figure 12.8. Number of math calculation problems correct during baseline and invention for Leslie.

the children to be self-reflective and self-evaluative when they think about what they are doing (see intervention method described in Figure 12.7).

Response to Intervention

Leslie reported that she used several strategies for completing math pages. First, she found it difficult to concentrate because she was sitting next to someone who was disruptive. Her solution was to move to a more quiet part of the room. Second, she noticed that she often did not keep the columns of numbers straight, so she drew light lines to make columns. Third, Leslie realized that she used did the mathematics problems quickly and with little checking, which caused errors. Finally, she realized it was better to get the problems done correctly rather than just get as many finished as she could in the time allotted. These new plans were applied to the math pages she completed during the intervention phase.

Results of intervention with Leslie are shown in Figure 12.8. The graph shows the number of problems Leslie got correct per page over the course of the 10-minute baseline sessions and intervention sessions. These results show that, by improving Leslie's use of planning processes, her performance in math calculation improved considerably over her initial level.

SUMMARY

The purpose of this chapter was to provide a brief summary of the CAS. This included the PASS theory, structure of the test, reliability, validity, interpretation, and intervention. Only the highlights of these topics could be presented due to space limitations. Nevertheless the information described here gives the reader some idea about how CAS and the PASS scales can be used to determine if a child has significant cognitive variation that may have relevance to diagnosis and instruction. This brings the test user to the point of examining different educational treatment methods that could be applied to assist the child. In combination with other information about the child, the CAS can greatly augment the effectiveness of the practitioner.

SUGGESTED READINGS

Bracken (1987). Limitations of preschool instruments and standards for minimal levels of technical adequacy. *Journal of Psychoeducational Assessment, 5,* 313–326.
Brody, N. (1992). *Intelligence.* San Diego: Academic Press.

Cohen, R. J., Swerdlik, M. E., & Smith, D. K. (1992). *Psychological testing and assessment (second edition)*. Mountain View, CA: Mayfield.

Das, J. P., Naglieri, J. A., & Kirby, J. R. (1994). *Assessment of cognitive processes*. Needham Heights, MA: Allyn & Bacon.

Elliott, C. D. (1990). *Differential Ability Scales (DAS) Introductory and technical handbook*. San Antonio, TX: Psychological Corporation.

Gindis, B. (1996). [Review of the book Assessment of cognitive processing: the PASS theory of intelligence]. *School Psychology International, 17*, 305–308.

Kaufman, A. S., & Kaufman, N. L. (1983). *Kaufman Assessment Battery for Children*. Circle Pines, MN: American Guidance Service.

Kaufman, A. S., & Kaufman, N. L. (1993). *Kaufman Adolescent & Adult Intelligence Test*. Circle Pines, MN: American Guidance Service, Inc.

Kaufman, A. S. (1994). *Intelligent testing with the wisc-iii*. New York: John Wiley & Sons.

Kirby, J. R., & Williams, N. H. (1991). *Learning problems: A cognitive approach*. Toronto: Kagan and Woo.

Luria. A. R., & Tsvetkova, L. S. (A. Mikheyev & S. Mikheyev, Transl.)(1990). *The neuropsychological analysis of problem solving*. Orlando, FL: Paul M. Deutsch Press.

Luria, A. R. (1966). *Human brain and psychological processes*. New York: Harper & Row.

Luria, A. R. (1973). *The working brain: An introduction to neuropsychology*. New York: Basic Books.

Luria, A. R. (1980). *Higher cortical functions in man (second edition, Revised and Expanded)*. New York: Basic Books.

Luria, A. R. (1982). *Language and Cognition*. New York: Wiley.

McGrew, K. S., Werder, J. K., & Woodcock, R. W. (1991). Woodcock-Johnson technical manual. Itasca, IL: Riverside Publishing Company.

McGrew, K. S., Keith, T. Z., Flanagan, D. P., & Vanderwood, M. (1997). Beyond g: The impact of Gf-Gc specific cognitive abilities research on the future use and interpretation of intelligence tests in the schools. *School Psychology Review, 26*, 189–210.

Naglieri, J. A. (1993). Pairwise and ipsative WISC-III IQ and index score Comparisons. *Psychological Assessment, 5*, 133–116.

Naglieri, J. A. (1997). Intelligence knowns and unknowns: Hits and misses. *American Psychologist, 25*, 75–76.

Naglieri, J. A., (1999). *Essentials of CAS assessment*. New York: Wiley & Sons.

Naglieri, J. A., & Das, J. P. (1997a). *Cognitive Assessment System*. Itasca, IL: Riverside Publishing Company.

Naglieri, J. A., & Das, J. P. (1997b). *Cognitive Assessment System interpretive handbook*. Itasca, IL: Riverside Publishing Company.

Naglieri, J. A. & Gottling, S. H. (1995). A cognitive education approach to math instruction for the learning disabled: An individual study. *Psychological Reports, 76*, 1343–1354.

Naglieri, J. A. & Gottling, S. H. (1997). Mathematics instruction and PASS cognitive processes: An intervention study. *Journal of Learning Disabilities, 30*, 513–520.

Sattler, J. M. (1988). *Assessment of Children*. San Diego: Author.

Solso, R. L., & Hoffman, C. A. (1991). Influence of Soviet scholars. *American Psychologist, 46*, 251–253.

Wechsler, D. (1991). *Manual for the Wechsler Intelligence Scale for Children-Third Edition*. San Antonio, TX: Psychological Corporation.

Wechsler, D. (1992). *Manual for the Wechsler Intelligence Achievement Test*. San Antonio, TX: Psychological Corporation.

Woodcock, R. W., & Johnson, M. B. (1989). *Woodcock-Johnson—Revised Tests of Cognitive Abilities*. Itasca, IL: Riverside Publishing.

Woodcock, R. W. (1998). *WJ-R and Bateria-R in neuropsychological assessment: Research report Number 1*. Itasca, IL: Riverside Publishing.

Yoakum, C. S., & Yerkes, R. M. (1920). *Army mental tests*. New York: Henry Holt and Company.

13

Wide Range Achievement Test 3 (WRAT3)

Alisa J. Snelbaker, Gary S. Wilkinson,
Gary J. Robertson, and Joseph J. Glutting

INTRODUCTION

The Wide Range Achievement Test 3 (WRAT3) is the most recent edition in a series of instruments which measure codes necessary to learn the basic skills of reading, spelling, and arithmetic. These codes—reading decoding, written encoding, and math computation—are fundamental building blocks of academic achievement, and the assessment of these skills is a vital component of psychological evaluations conducted in clinical and school settings. The WRAT3 and its predecessors, the Wide Range Achievement Test (WRAT) and the Wide Range Achievement Test-Revised (WRAT-R), have been among the most widely used instruments of psychological measurement for over forty years. As but one example, the WRAT tests have been used extensively in the investigation of learning disabilities and neurological impairments in children and adults.

The fundamental nature of skills measured and the extensive age range over which performance can be assessed, contribute to the WRAT3's utility and popularity. The format of the WRAT3 is particularly useful for longitudinal measurement of an individual's basic academic skills over time. The WRAT3 offers two parallel forms (BLUE and TAN), which provide an excellent methodology for pre- and posttesting academic skills that, in turn, can be used to measure intervention effectiveness. Each form spans the ages of 5 to 74 years and allows the comparison of academic skills over substantial periods of time without using multiple instruments.

Alisa J. Snelbaker, Gary S. Wilkinson, Gary J. Robertson, and Joseph J. Glutting • School of Education, University of Delaware, Newark, Delaware 19711.

Understanding Psychological Assessment, edited by Dorfman and Hersen. Kluwer Academic/Plenum Publishers, New York, 2001.

TEST CONSTRUCTION AND DEVELOPMENT

Item Selection

The WRAT3 has direct lines to its heritage; the concepts of the test, like the basic skills necessary for reading, spelling, and math computation, have changed very little since the WRAT's inception nearly 60 years ago. Items selected for this instrument are samples of the domains of all words in the English language for reading and spelling and the arithmetic computation skills taught in kindergarten through high school for arithmetic. Many items from previous editions are incorporated in the WRAT3. Additionally, several new items were selected for each of the two forms (BLUE and TAN) to mirror like items on the alternate form, or to include more difficult items for the scales.

Each form of the WRAT3 was constructed to have an adequate range of item difficulty without significant item overlap or duplication. In other words, the WRAT3 was designed to measure the full range of the domain (i.e., reading decoding, spelling from dictation, or math computation) and do so using the least number of items necessary to assess the skill in question. The previous logit scores from Rasch analyses of the WRAT-R served as the guide for item selection on the new forms and verification of this item selection was done in separate studies early in the WRAT3's development.

A Rasch analysis was performed in conjunction with the standardization project for each of the WRAT3's three tests (i.e. Reading/Word Decoding, Spelling/Written Encoding, and Arithmetic) on both Blue and Tan forms and on the COMBINED form. Specifically, Rasch analysis measures both item separation and person separation. Item separation indicates how well the test items define the variable being measured. Person separation indicates how well the items differentiate between individual performances and is related to the traditional (i.e., classical, true-score) conception of reliability. Item separation indices for each of the nine tests were measured to be 1.00, the highest score possible, and person separation indices ranged from .98 to .99. These results confirmed that each test on all three forms (BLUE, TAN, COMBINED) is well constructed in terms of spread of item difficulty and the ability to measure individuals on the respective items.

Standardization

The WRAT3 was nationally standardized in 1992 and 1993 on a sample of 4,433 individuals. The sample was stratified according to 1990 U.S. census data on the variables of age, regional residence, gender, ethnicity, and socioeconomic group. Randomization was introduced into the selection of subjects once the controlled factors were addressed. Individuals currently, or previously, served in special education were included in the sample so far as randomization would allow. Subjects were excluded only if they were unable to physically respond to test items.

The instrument's age range (i.e., 5 through 74 years) was evaluated by using smaller intervals for the younger age groups to obtain more measurements during peak growth periods of the academic skills. Ages 5 through 8 were each divided into six-month increments and ages 9 through 16 were grouped by full years. Beginning with age 17, ages were collapsed together into groups: 17–19, 20–24, 25–34, 35–44, and so on, thereafter in 9-year groupings, up to age 74.

The United States was divided into four regions, with a minimum of four states in each region, for the purposes of the norm sample. These regions, East, North Central, South, and

West, conform to those used by the 1990 U.S. census data. The total sample percentage ratio of males to females is 50.7% to 49.3%. This is representative to the overall U.S. population where males outnumber females in each age interval up to the 20-through 24-year age interval.

The WRAT3 sample was controlled for an appropriate inclusion of individuals based upon ethnicity: 71.7% of the individuals in the sample were white, 13.6% were black, 10.7% were Hispanic, and 3.9% of the sample was comprised of individuals of "other" ethnicity. For the purposes of this standardization, persons of Hispanic origin were considered separately regardless of whether they might further be classified as one of the other ethnicities. Only individuals who were able to speak and use English effectively were included in this sample.

The sample was also controlled for socioeconomic level of the parent for child participants, or the individual for adult participants. Occupational categories used by the 1990 U.S. Census Report (i.e., managerial and professional; technical, sales, and administrative support; precision production, craft, and repair; operators, fabricators, and laborers; and service, farming, and fishing occupations) were employed and the highest occupational level of the custodial parent, stepparent, or guardian was used in this process. If an individual was unemployed at the time of standardization, the participant was ranked according to the highest previous job held. The obtained percentages of the standardization sample were found to be representative of the U.S. population for all occupational categories.

Individuals participating in the standardization effort were given each test form at the same sitting. Presentations were counterbalanced (i.e., BLUE-TAN or TAN-BLUE) to guard against ordering effects. Administration of the Spelling and Arithmetic tests were given in small groups of appropriate size depending on the age of the subjects. Examination conditions (e.g., environment and rapport with examiners) were optimized, and examiners were trained thoroughly in the administration of the WRAT3 and had at least one year's experience with relevant age ranges.

Reliability

The WRAT3's reliabilities are quite good and remain so across four types of indices: coefficient alpha, alternate form, person separation, and test-retest. Coefficient alpha is a measure of internal consistency and is considered to be a conservative estimate of reliability. The median test coefficients alpha range from .85 to .95 over the nine WRAT3 tests. For the three COMBINED tests, the range is from .92 to .95. Additionally, Rasch person separation indices are equivalent to the Kuder-Richardson 20 coefficients that are often used in the estimation of internal consistency. As noted earlier, the range of person separation indices on the nine WRAT3 tests is from .98 to .99.

Providing further evidence, correlations among the WRAT3's forms (BLUE and TAN) substantiate the test's reliability. Total sample ($N = 4,433$) alternate-form correlations among raw scores for Reading, Spelling, and Arithmetic are .98, .98, and .98. Similarly, test-retest stability coefficients (corrected for attenuation) range from .91 to .98 on the nine tests of the WRAT3 given to a sample of 142 individuals (ages 6 through 16) from the standardization group.

Standard Errors of Measurement

Standard errors of measurement (SEM) and "confidence bands" derived from SEMs are the reliability issues most likely to affect everyday practice. For the WRAT3, coefficient alpha data were used to calculate the SEMs for standard scores, providing a conservative estimate of the fallibility of the scores. COMBINED scores have the lowest mean SEMs, 3.4, 3.6, and 4.4 for Reading, Spelling, and Arithmetic scores, respectively. BLUE and TAN Reading and Spelling scores have mean SEMs ranging from 4.5 to 4.9, and BLUE and TAN Arithmetic scores were found to have mean SEMs of 5.7 and 5.9, respectively. For younger children, SEMs for certain test scores may be slightly higher; the WRAT3 provides a separate SEM and related confidence band for each age group.

Validity

Support for the content and construct validity of the WRAT3 comes from a substantial amount of convergent evidence. Content validity refers to whether items on a test are representative of the domain that the test purports to measure. As noted earlier, the WRAT3 intends to measure the basic academic skills of word recognition, spelling from dictation, and arithmetic computation. To adequately sample these domains, test items should be representative of the entire range of difficulty within each domain. Rasch item-separation statistics, previously discussed in detail, measure the degree to which this is achieved. For each test on the WRAT3, the highest item separation score possible (1.00) was found, giving strong evidence of sufficient breadth and completeness of coverage of items.

Much further evidence is available to support the hypothesis that the WRAT3 is measuring the constructs of the basic academic codes of reading, spelling, and math computation. In particular, investigations have addressed developmental changes in raw scores by age, correlations with IQ, other achievement tests, and score differences between the standardization sample and children with exceptionalities (i.e., learning disabilities, educable mental handicaps, gifted). The skills measured by the WRAT3 are developmental in nature. As one would expect, each of the nine tests shows a steady increase in mean raw scores across the norm age groups until the 45- to 54-year-old age group; from there the scores begin to fall. Using the data from the standardization sample ($N = 4,433$), there is a significant correlation between each WRAT3 test raw score and the age in months of the test-taker, supporting the hypothesis that there is a developmental component to the measurement of academic codes.

Academic skills are positively associated with general cognitive ability and, more specifically, with measures of verbal ability. For 100 children, ranging in age from 6 to 16, WRAT3 COMBINED test standard scores were compared with the Verbal (VIQ), Performance (PIQ), and Full Scale (FSIQ) IQ scores from the Wechsler Intelligence Scale for Children–Third Edition. The COMBINED Reading, Spelling, and Arithmetic scores correlated at the .66, .66, and .57 level, respectively, with the WISC-III FSIQ score. All WRAT3 test scores correlated more highly with the VIQ score than the PIQ score. One study found the same pattern of moderate positive correlations between WRAT3 test scores and WISC-III VIQ, PIQ, and FSIQ scores for children who were referred for special education services ($N = 60$, ages 6 through 15). Similar correlations were found for a sample of 40 adults (age 16 through 63) using the Wechsler Adult Intelligence Scale–Revised, with the exception that the COMBINED Arithmetic score was correlated more highly with the PIQ score than the VIQ score.

Similarly, scores obtained from the WRAT3 show moderate to high correlations with other standardized tests of academic achievement. For groups of children in the standardization sample, information was gathered from the results of three standardized group achievement tests: the Comprehensive Test of Basic Skills–Fourth Edition, the California Achievement Test–Form E, and the Stanford Achievement Test. Table 13.1 shows Pearson correlations based on standard scores for each of the corresponding subtests. Additionally, independent research

Table 13.1. Pearson Correlations of the WRAT3, CTBs-4, CAT-Form E, and SAT scores

	WRAT3-COMBINED Form		
	Reading	Arithmetic	Spelling
CTBS-4[a]			
Total Reading	.69		
Total Math		.79	
Spelling			.84
CAT-Form E[b]			
Total Reading	.72		
Total Math		.41	
Spelling			.77
SAT[c]			
Total Reading	.87		
Total Math		.81	
Spelling			.76

[a] $N = 49$; Age Range = 8-16 years ($M = 11.4$ years; $SD = 3.2$ years)
[b] $N = 46$; Age Range = 8-16 years ($M = 11.1$ years; $SD = 2.1$ years)
[c] $N = 31$; Age Range = 9-15 years ($M = 12.7$ years; $SD = 1.6$ years)

compared a group of university students's performances on the WRAT3 and two recently developed academic screening instruments: the Kaufman Functional Academic Skills Test and the Woodcock-McGrew-Werder Mini-Battery of Achievement. Table 13.2 shows the correlations, based on standard scores for each of the corresponding subtests.

The WRAT3 has also shown the ability to correctly discriminate between groups of children with exceptionalities. Children receiving special education, ranging in age from 8 to 12, (22 students placed in gifted programs, 24 children identified with learning disabilities, and 24 children identified with educable mental handicaps) were compared with an equal number of matched controls without disability from the standardization sample. For each individual group, performance on the WRAT3 BLUE form correctly predicted group membership for 85% of the children receiving gifted programming, 72% of children with learning disabilities, 83% of children with educable mental handicaps, and 56% of controls without disability.

Table 13.2. Pearson Correlations of the WRAT3, MBA, and K-FAST Scores[a]

	WRAT3-TAN Form		
	Reading	Arithmetic	Spelling
MBA			
Reading	.48		
Math		.52	
Writing			.24
K-FAST			
Reading	.31		
Math		.54	

$N = 62$; age range = 19–45 years ($M = 22.7$ years; $SD = 4.0$ years)

ADMINISTRATION AND SCORING

A unique feature of the WRAT3 is that it provides two parallel forms (BLUE and TAN), which may be used apart from, or in conjunction with each other. Each form may be used across the entire age range of the test (i.e., ages 5 through 74). To our knowledge, no individually administered achievement test, other than the WRAT3, provides parallel forms. When the BLUE and TAN forms are used together, this is called to be the COMBINED form. Each of the individual forms contains three tests: Reading, Spelling, and Arithmetic. The individual forms take an average of 15 to 30 minutes to complete, depending on the skill level and working speed of the individual being tested.

Administration of the WRAT3 is simple, and its materials are compact and well organized. The content, administration, and scoring for each test will be discussed below according to the order in which they appear on the BLUE and TAN forms in the context of single-form administration. COMBINED form administration and scoring will be discussed separately.

Spelling Test

The Spelling test was developed to measure written encoding, or the ability to write letters and words from dictation. The test may be taken individually or in groups. It consists of two sections Name/Letter Writing and Word Spelling. Name/Letter Writing requires test-takers to write their names and a series of single letters. Word Spelling asks each individual to spell words that are presented first in isolation, then in a sentence, and again in isolation (e.g., go—Children go to school.—go).

Children age seven and under begin with the first item in Name/Letter Writing; individuals age 8 and over begin with Word Spelling and are asked to complete Name/Letter Writing only if they do not spell at least five words correctly. For all ages, testing should be discontinued when 10 consecutive errors have be made.

Reversals, omissions, substitutions, and additions of letters are to be scored as errors. In the Name/Letter Writing Section, an individual can receive up to two points for successfully writing at least two letters of his or her name and one point for each correctly formed letter, for a maximum of 15 points. In the Word Spelling section, each successfully spelled word earns one point, for a maximum of 40 points. The total raw score for the Spelling test is the sum of each section, with a maximum score of 55 points. Test-takers who are not required to complete the Name/Letter Writing should receive full credit for the section (i.e., 15 points) in calculation of their Spelling test raw score.

Arithmetic Test

The Arithmetic test measures the basic skills of counting, reading number symbols, solving orally presented word problems, and performing written computations. It consists of two sections: Oral Arithmetic and Written Arithmetic. Oral Arithmetic requires the test taker to count series of objects and identify numerals which are printed on the BLUE and TAN forms. Each form contains orally presented questions such as, "Which is more, 9 or 6?" and "How many are 3 and 4 apples?" Written Arithmetic consists of two pages of arithmetic computation questions printed on the BLUE and TAN forms. Items range in difficulty from single-digit addition problems to algebra problems containing variables. Administration time for this section should not exceed 15 minutes; testing may be discontinued early if the individual indicates that he or she has completed all items of which they are capable.

Children age seven and under begin with the first item in Oral Arithmetic (15 items); individuals age 8 and over begin with the first item in Written Arithmetic (40 items) and are asked to complete Oral Arithmetic only if they do not answer at least five computation problems correctly. Each item in the Arithmetic test is worth one point for a maximum total score of 55 points. Test-takers who are not required to complete the Oral Arithmetic section should receive full credit for the section (i.e., 15 points) in calculation of their Arithmetic test raw score.

Reading Test

The Reading test is designed to measure recognition and naming of letters and decoding of words in isolation. It consists of two sections: Letter Reading and Word Reading. Letter Reading (15 items) requires the test taker to identify a series of single letters presented on a separate, plastic Reading Card. Word Reading (42 items) asks individuals to decode words that are presented in isolation on the Reading Card. Test takers must not read the letters and words from the BLUE or TAN form because they contain pronunciation keys. Children age seven or under begin with the first item in Letter Reading; individuals age 8 and over begin with the first item in Word Reading and are asked to complete Letter Reading only if they do not decode at least five items correctly. For all ages, testing should be discontinued when 10 consecutive errors have been made.

Pronunciation of words must be accurate; however, consistent dialect or articulation difficulties may be considered in scoring. Each item in the Reading test is worth one point for a maximum total score of 57 points. Test-takers who are not required to complete the Letter Reading section should receive full credit for the section (i.e., 15 points) in calculation of their Arithmetic test raw score.

COMBINED Form

The COMBINED form consists of administering both forms of the WRAT3 in a single examination. This more extensive evaluation provides a more in-depth assessment of academic skills and allows greater opportunity for performance observation.

The first sections of the Spelling, Arithmetic, and Reading tests (i.e., Name/Letter Writing, Oral Arithmetic, and Letter Reading) are identical on both the BLUE and TAN forms. Therefore, when administering the COMBINED form, each of these sections is only administered once. The second sections of each test (Word Spelling, Written Arithmetic, and Word Reading) contain different items on each form. Thus, a COMBINED form Spelling test would consist of either BLUE *or* TAN Name/Letter Writing (15 items), BLUE Word Spelling (40 items), and TAN Word Spelling (40 items) for a total of 95 items. The same pattern is followed for the Arithmetic and Reading tests, resulting in a COMBINED maximum score of 95 and 99 points, respectively.

INTERPRETIVE GUIDELINES

Norm-Referenced Scoring

The WRAT3 offers five types of derived scores to be used for interpretion of individual performance. Raw scores may be converted into standard scores, absolute scores, grade-equivalents, percentile ranks, and normal curve equivalents. Standard scores (M = 100, SD = 15) are the recommended mode of comparison within and between individuals. The WRAT3 provides standard scores ranging from 45 to 155 for all three forms across 32 age groups interpolated from the 23 age groups used in the norm sample.

The RASCH item analysis performed in conjunction with the standardization of the WRAT3 provided the opportunity to form an interval or absolute scale of the difficulty of each item on each test of the instrument. Absolute scores (M = 500, Spelling SD = 36, Mathematics SD = 34, Reading SD = 37) derived from this scale give a measurement of each academic domain across the whole continuum of that domain regardless of age or grade. Therefore, the WRAT3 absolute scale provides a ruler for the measurement of basic skills which can be used to compare individuals or groups. Interpretation of absolute scores and standard scores will be discussed later, in greater detail.

A grade equivalent indicates the school grade for which a given raw score is average or typical. The WRAT3 provides grade equivalents ranging from preschool through twelfth grade. For the COMBINED form, each grade level is broken down into months of school within the level. For the BLUE and TAN forms, monthly intervals within the grade level are not provided. Grade equivalents have limited utility; they are ordinal and should be used cautiously when interpreting test results.

Percentile ranks, ranging from 1 to 99 (median = 50), indicate the percentage of the standardization sample at a given age who scored at or below a given raw score. Normal curve equivalents are derived from percentile ranks into an interval scale and have the same range and median score. They are most commonly used to evaluate the progress of groups of children.

Interpretation of Individual Performance

The WRAT3 provides qualitative ratings for obtained standard scores and a Profile/Analysis form to aid in interpretation of individual performance and communication of findings to others (e.g., parents, teachers). The ratings of standard scores are identical in name and corresponding score range to those used on the WISC-III, providing continuity of interpretation across instruments which enhances the ease of comparison of IQ-achievement differences.

The Profile/Analysis form aids in the presentation and communication of standard and absolute scores by providing a graphic depiction of an individual's performance: (a) in comparison to same-age peers (i.e., standard scores) and (b) across the whole continuum of each academic domain regardless of age or grade (i.e., absolute scores). A graph of a normal curve with corresponding standard scores and percentiles allows the clinician to plot test-takers' performances on each test on the WRAT3 and on verbal, nonverbal, and full-scale measures of cognitive ability. This facilitates comparison between measured levels of cognitive functioning and academic achievement. An item map, which includes corresponding absolute scores, and grade- and age-levels for successful performance of the items, provides an additional method of interpretation and communication, focusing on individuals' skills in each academic domain.

CASE EXAMPLES

These case examples illustrate how the WRAT3 can be used to assess, quantitatively and qualitatively, basic skills in academic achievement, and how the test's results can be used to assist in the diagnosis of children with exceptionalities (i.e., learning disabilities, mild mental retardation).

Case #1

Sarah is an 8-year-3-month-old girl in the second grade who was referred for intellectual and academic assessment by her teacher to assist in planning an appropriate educational program. Specific areas of concern included: slow but satisfactory progress in reading and language arts and significantly below-grade-level performance in mathematics. Her teacher noted that Sarah has not yet committed to memory addition and subtraction facts of numbers to ten.

As part of the comprehensive evaluation, Sarah was administered the WISC-III and the WRAT3. Table 13.3 contains the results from these measures. The following are excerpts of the Cognitive, Academic, and Conclusion sections of a psychological report based on the findings from these tests.

Cognitive Functioning

Sarah was administered the WISC-III. She achieved a Full Scale IQ (FSIQ) classified in the low average range. Her obtained a Verbal IQ (VIQ) and Performance IQ (PIQ) were measured to be in the average and low average ranges, respectively. The difference between Sarah's VIQ and PIQ is not significant, suggesting evenly developed verbal and visual-perceptual skills. Analysis of her pattern of individual factor and subtest scores was unremarkable. Therefore, Sarah's overall FSIQ score was considered to be the best predictor of her scholastic aptitude.

Academic Functioning

Sarah completed the BLUE form of the WRAT3, and the results indicate that her reading and spelling skills were in the low average range (9th and 14th percentiles, respectively), commensurate with her estimated cognitive ability. The words she correctly read and spelled are representative of skills taught in a first-grade curriculum. When asked to decode individual words, Sarah recognized a few words on sight (e.g., in, cat, book). For those she did not, she attempted to sound out the words phonetically. She pronounced the long vowels in "size" and "lame" as short vowels and successfully read only the first syllable of multisyllable

Table 13.3. WISC-III and WRAT3 scores for case #1

Scales	Scores
Wechsler Intelligence Scale for Children-III (WISC-III) Standard Score	
Verbal Scale IQ (VIQ)	90 (95% Confidence Interval 84-97)
Performance Scale IQ (PIQ)	82 (95% Confidence Interval 76-92)
Full Scale IQ (FSIQ)	85 (95% Confidence Interval 80-91)

	Wide Range Achievement Test 3 (WRAT3) BLUE Form			
	Standard Score	Percentile	Grade Equivalent	Absolute Score
Reading	80	9	1	473
Spelling	84	14	1	477
Arithmetic	65	1	K	457

words (e.g., animal, finger). When asked to spell individual words, she omitted the final "e" in "make" and did not correctly spell some vowel and consonant clusters (e.g., oo, ght).

Sarah's arithmetic skills appear to be less developed than her reading and spelling skills. In formal testing, her performance was measured to be in the deficient range (1st percentile), significantly below her obtained cognitive ability. Sarah's demonstrated arithmetic computation skills are representative of those taught in a kindergarten curriculum. She read the number "41" as "14." Additionally, she added on all subtraction problems and would not attempt any problems with sums greater than ten because, she did "not have enough fingers."

Conclusion

Results of this assessment suggest that Sarah functions in the low average range of general intellectual ability. Using the univariate regression method of comparing IQ and achievement obtained scores (using 5% prevalence rate), her reading and spelling skills were found to be commensurate with her measured cognitive ability. Conversely, Sarah's arithmetic skills were found to be significantly ($p \leq .05$) below the expected range of functioning, given her obtained cognitive ability.

Therefore, based on the most widely employed definition of a learning disability (an unexpected and/or severe discrepancy between expected versus observed level of achievement), the results of the present evaluation indicate that Sarah is eligible for special education services as a student with a learning disability in the area of arithmetic computation.

Case #2

Amy is a 9-year-4-month-old girl in the fourth grade who is presently identified as a student with mild mental retardation. She receives special education services in a self-contained classroom. She was referred for intellectual and academic assessment as part of a triennial reevaluation to assist in determining if her current classification and special education programming are appropriate.

As part of the comprehensive evaluation, Amy was administered the WISC-III and the WRAT3, and her mother completed the *Vineland Adaptive Behavior Scales-Interview Edition, Survey Form.* Table 13.4 contains the results from these measures. The following are excerpts of the Cognitive, Adaptive, Academic, and Conclusion sections of a psychological report based on the findings from these instruments.

Cognitive Functioning

Amy was administered the WISC-III. She achieved a Full Scale IQ (FSIQ) classified in the deficient range. Her obtained Verbal IQ (VIQ) and Performance IQ (PIQ) were measured to be in the deficient range. The difference between Amy's VIQ and PIQ is not significant, suggesting evenly developed but significantly delayed verbal and visual-perceptual skills. Analysis of her pattern of individual factor and subtest scores was unremarkable. Therefore, Amy's overall, FSIQ score was considered to be the best predictor of her scholastic aptitude.

Adaptive Functioning

To assess Amy's personal and community independence and aspects of her social performance and adjustment, her mother provided information for the VABS. Her obtained Adaptive

Table 13.4. WISC-III, VABS, and WRAT3 Scores for Case #2

Scales	Scores
Wechsler Intelligence Scale for Children-III (WISC-III) Standard Score	
Verbal Scale IQ (VIQ)	63 (95% Confidence Interval 59-71)
Performance Scale IQ (PIQ)	68 (95% Confidence Interval 63-79)
Full Scale IQ (FSIQ)	62 (95% Confidence Interval 58-69)
Vineland Adaptive Behavior Scales-Interview Edition, Survey Form (VABS) Standard Score	
Communication Domain	58
Daily Living Scales Domain	59
Socialization Domain	68
Adaptive Behavior Composite	60

Wide Range Achievement Test 3 (WRAT3) BLUE Form

	Standard Score	Percentile	Grade Equivalent	Absolute Score
Reading	51	<1	K	446
Spelling	61	<1	K	456
Arithmetic	50	<1	K	455

Behavior Composite score was measured to be in the deficient range. Amy's skills in the domains of communication, daily living skills, and socialization were estimated to be in the deficient range. The differences between her obtained scores across all domains are not significant, suggesting that Amy demonstrates evenly developed but significantly delayed skills in all adaptive functioning areas assessed.

Academic Functioning

Amy completed the BLUE form of the WRAT3, and the results of testing indicate that her academic skills are significantly delayed in all areas assessed. Her reading, spelling, and mathematics skills were measured to be in the deficient range (less than 1st percentile), commensurate with her estimated cognitive ability.

In formal testing, Amy's reading and spelling skills show a similar pattern and are representative of those taught in a kindergarten curriculum. She correctly identified letters presented in isolation. While reading individual words, she pronounced the first phoneme and did not attempt to decode the rest of the word. Similarly, Amy correctly wrote most letters dictated to her; she reversed the lowercase letter "d" and wrote an uppercase "T" when asked to write an "I." When asked to spell single words, she correctly wrote the first letter and, occasionally, the last letter (all consonants), but omitted the middle vowel (e.g., ct for cat).

Amy's computation skills are also representative of those taught in a kindergarten curriculum. She counted objects up to 15 and recognized all numbers presented to her. Amy did not successfully answer any verbally or visually presented addition or subtraction problems except "1 + 1 = 2."

Conclusion

Results of this assessment suggest that Amy functions in the deficient range of general intellectual ability. Significant developmental delays were found in the adaptive skill areas of communication, daily living, and socialization. Similarly, Amy's academic skills were measured to be in the deficient range, commensurate with her estimated cognitive and adaptive abilities, and indicate that Amy is experiencing significant difficulties in reading, spelling, and mathematics.

Therefore, the results of the present evaluation indicate that Amy remains eligible for special education services as student with mild mental retardation based upon significant delays in cognitive functioning and adaptive and academic skills.

FUTURE DIRECTIONS: THE WRAT-EXPANDED

Work began in 1994 on a new battery of achievement measures designed to extend the scope and format of the WRAT3. The Wide Range Achievement Test–Expanded Edition (WRAT-Expanded) provides increased content coverage for Grades K through Adult (i.e., ages 5 through 24) in the areas of reading comprehension, mathematics, listening comprehension, oral expression, and written language. Group- and individually-administered test formats, standardized with an overlapping norm sample, allow for increased flexibility of use and greater comparability of results, which allow for a number of technical benefits. These three features—expanded content, availability of group- and individually-administered formats, and enhanced technical quality—are discussed more fully below.

Expanded Coverage

The five broad achievement content domains assessed by the WRAT-Expanded are: Reading, Mathematics, Oral Language, Written Language, and Nonverbal Reasoning.

Reading

Reading skills are assessed using three tests: Prereading, Beginning Reading, and Reading Comprehension. The Prereading section includes alphabetic recognition, matching letter combinations and words, and knowledge of beginning, ending, and vowel sounds. A special Beginning Reading section tests comprehension of words and sentences, as well as recognition of dictated words. At grades 2 and above, Reading Comprehension is measured using passages with questions that test both literal and inferential reading skills. Passages sample textbook, recreational, and functional reading (i.e., reading required in daily living) content.

Mathematics

The Mathematics test assesses conceptual understanding and reasoning, with an emphasis on problem-solving. Computation has intentionally been minimized. Content domains include numeration and number sense, operations, measurement, geometry, data analysis and interpretation, probability and discrete mathematics, and patterns and algebra. Beginning mathematics skills receive special emphasis, with a greater concentration of material than is typically found in individually administered achievement batteries.

Oral Language

Oral language skills are assessed by two tests: Listening Comprehension and Oral Expression. Listening Comprehension measures receptive language skills and includes items that assess vocabulary, grammar, and comprehension of complex linguistic structures. Oral Expression tests expressive language skills, through items measuring vocabulary, grammar, and sociolinguistics. These oral language tests, in particular, provide valuable information needed in understanding the nature of reading difficulties, as well as other language disabilities.

Written Language

Areas assessed in Written Language include mechanics (i.e., punctuation, capitalization, spelling, and grammar), written vocabulary, word and ideational fluency, sentence transformations, and sentence and paragraph construction. All items in this domain require constructed responses. This section, when used together with the Reading Comprehension, Listening Comprehension, and Oral Expression tests, provides a comprehensive assessment of language skills.

Nonverbal Reasoning

The Nonverbal Reasoning test measures the ability to reason with symbolic and figural content without the use of language. Items are all of the classification type in which the individual must identify the object which does not follow the rule linking the other elements (i.e., odd one out). This test provides important information in assessing the achievement of students whose oral and written language skills are very limited.

Group and Individual Test Formats

The tests outlined in the previous section are available either in a group-administered format (Form G), an individually-administered format (Form I), or are available in both formats. This unique feature of the WRAT-Expanded offers a greater flexibility in test-administration methods. Table 13.5 shows the various tests available in the Form G and Form I batteries.

Group Form (Form G)

The Group Form is available in five levels designed for use in Grades 2 through 12. Each of the levels requires approximately 22 hours and is designed to be administered to small groups by classroom teachers. As shown in Table 13.5, each level contains four subtests: Reading Comprehension, Mathematics, Written Language, and Nonverbal Reasoning. The

Table 13.5. Tests Available on the WRAT-Expanded Form G and Form I

Test	Form G (Group) (Grades 2 and above)	Form I (Individual) (Grades K and above)
Prereading Skill		X
Beginning Reading		X
Reading Comprehension	X	X
Mathematics	X	X
Listening Comprehension	X	
Oral Expression	X	
Written Language	X	
Nonverbal Reasoning	X	

Group Form is not available below second grade because younger students especially those who are experiencing difficulty with beginning reading and mathematics, often have difficulty in responding to items presented in group test formats.

The Reading, Mathematics, and Nonverbal Reasoning tests use multiple-choice items and can be scored easily and quickly. The Written Language test requires the student to construct a response for each item. Scoring is aided by the use of a checklist containing objective criteria which greatly reduces the burdensome task of scoring usually found in constructed-response writing tests.

Form G was standardized during the 1997–1998 school year on a carefully selected, nationally stratified sample of U.S. school districts. Norms available for the interpretation of results include: age- and grade-based standard scores, percentile ranks, stanines, normal curve equivalents, and age and grade equivalents.

Individual Form (Form I)

The Individual Form is designed for use from ages 5 through 24. As shown in Table 13.5, Form I contains tests assessing Pre-reading Skill, Beginning Reading, Reading Comprehension, Mathematics, Listening Comprehension, and Oral Expression. Although, the Written Language Test is designed to be group-administered, it can be administered individually, if desired. As stated earlier, special effort was made to include content more suitable for assessing beginning reading and math skills than is typically found in individually administered achievement measures. Tests in Form I are housed in a specially designed "flipbook" to facilitate the testing process. Each test contains items covering a wide range of difficulty, and basal and ceiling rules tailor assessment to individual skill levels.

Form I was standardized nationally on a carefully selected sample of children, adolescents, and adults during the 1997–1998 school year. Norms available for the interpretation of results include age- and grade-based standard scores, percentile ranks, stanines, normal curve equivalents, and age and grade equivalents.

The soon-to-be-available Wide Range Intelligence Test (WRIT) was standardized concurrently with Form I. Thus, results from the WRAT-Expanded and the WRIT can be compared. In addition, the WRAT3 was renormed in the same program, thereby resulting in a multifaceted battery of achievement and ability measures that can be used separately and in combination, as a particular assessment need warrants.

Enhanced Technical Quality

The common standardization sample for the WRAT-Expanded, the WRIT, and the renorming of the WRAT3 greatly enhances the technical quality of all the tests and permits increased comparability of performance across measures. State-of-the-art technical methodology, such as latent trait item calibration, test equating, and application of item response theory, ensures the highest quality of psychometric properties for the instruments. Several examples of the benefits from this increased ability to compare an individual's performance across conormed measures will be discussed below.

Joint Use of Form G and Form I

Forms G and I of the WRAT-Expanded may be used in a number of ways. Form G may be used as the first stage in screening a class to determine students in need of in-depth assessment with Form I. The fact that results from Forms G and I are comparable greatly facilitates the use of the forms in this way and overcomes a major obstacle faced when group-administered tests are used to screen for follow-up assessment with individually administered tests. The WRAT-Expanded Forms G and I are the only tests available with such group-individual test linkage.

A second possible joint use of the forms is to consider the tests available on Forms G and I as a single battery of tests, some of which may be administered individually and some of which may be administered in a group. It then becomes possible to accomplish different types of assessment outcomes by choosing a particular test configuration, depending on one's assessment needs. For example, a student may be given Form G followed only by Form I Reading, assuming Reading was the only result on Form G needing in-depth follow-up. Another student may be given Form G Reading, Written Language, and Nonverbal Reasoning if those were the only tests needed. These tests may then be followed up by Form I Listening Comprehension and Oral Expression to gain greater insight into the relationship of the written language measures to the oral language measures. Additionally, performance on all of the language-based measures could be compared to Nonverbal Reasoning performance. In another application, a student having difficulties with mathematics could be given Form G Mathematics, followed by Form I Mathematics if results on Form G warranted in-depth follow-up. Thus, the availability of Form G means that the amount of individual testing can be reduced, thereby decreasing the amount of time that trained staff must spend in assessment activities. The capability of accomplishing some assessment in small groups achieves a savings in both staff time and cost of testing.

Separate Use of Form G and Form I

Forms G and I on the WRAT-Expanded can both be used independently of one another to meet traditional assessment needs. Form G can be used within the same context as any group achievement measure to survey reading, mathematics, and language domains. The added feature of the Nonverbal Reasoning test offers a special advantage for assessing students whose language and reading skills are severely limited. The availability of both grade- and age-based standard scores facilitates the use of Form G to check results from other previously administered group tests where such information is usually not provided in similar form.

Form I can be used in situations where any comprehensive individually administered achievement battery is needed. The battery includes the areas important for identifying learning disabilities. Moreover, the availability of the major curricular areas required for learning disability assessment in a single instrument normed on the same sample greatly facilitates the use of the WRAT-Expanded in this context. This is not possible with most other individually administered achievement batteries where two or three different tests might be needed to cover all areas necessary to identify a learning disability.

Use of Forms G and I with the WRIT and WRAT3

As stated earlier, the common norming sample for the WRAT-Expanded, the WRIT, and the WRAT3 results in a number of gains for the test-user. Comparability of results on the WRAT-Expanded and WRIT greatly facilitates the use of an appropriate discrepancy model for identifying significant differences between measured cognitive ability and achievement in the diagnosis of learning disabilities. Users of the WRAT3 can select tests from the WRAT-Expanded, as desired, to round out their assessment battery, and vice versa. For example, the Reading Comprehension Test on the WRAT-Expanded Form I can be added to a WRAT3 evaluation. Similarly, users of the WRAT-Expanded Form I may wish to administer the WRAT3 Arithmetic test to assess mathematical computation skills. Various other test permutations are possible, depending upon the user's specific needs.

SUMMARY

The WRAT series of assessment measures are among the most widely used instruments of psychological measurement. Their distinguished history of assessing the codes necessary to learn the basic skills of reading, spelling, and arithmetic, and their promising future of extended scope and format can be attributed to their advanced technical quality and ease of use. The WRAT3 is unique in its offering of two equated forms (BLUE and TAN) which greatly increases the flexibility of its use and its application in pre- and posttesting situations. Additionally, it sets itself apart by providing an absolute scale, derived from Rasch item analysis, which provides a ruler for the measurement of the basic skills, regardless of age or grade. This scale can be used to compare individuals or groups, providing an additional method of performance interpretation not found in other measures of achievement.

This use of state-of-the-art psychometric methodology has set the stage for the next wave of instruments, the WRAT-Expanded, the renormed WRAT3, and the WRIT. The future of the WRAT3 lies in a multifaceted battery of achievement and ability measures which were co-normed to allow greater comparability of results and flexibility of use. The WRAT-Expanded contains greater breadth of academic curriculum and is the only achievement test available with both group- and individually-administered formats (Forms G and I). When used together, the WRAT3 and the WRAT-Expanded create the most comprehensive co-normed achievement test battery available. When used in conjunction with the WRIT, the battery becomes the most technically sound method available for making achievement-ability comparisons for the identification of learning disabilities. Thus, the tradition set forty years ago with the WRAT will be carried into the next century with a group of co-normed instruments covering the full extent of academic curricula and cognitive ability assessment.

SUGGESTED READINGS

CTB Macmillian/McGraw-Hill. (1988). *California Achievement Tests, Form E.* Monterey, CA: Author.

CTB Macmillian/McGraw-Hill. (1989). *Comprehensive tests of basic skills-fourth edition.* Monterey, CA: Author.

Gardener, E. F., Madden, R., Rudman, H. C., Karlsen, B., Merwin, J. C., Callis, R., & Collins, C. S. (1987). *Stanford Achievement Test, Seventh Edition Plus.* San Antonio, TX: The Psychological Corporation.

Jastek, J., & Jastek. S. (1965, 1976, & 1978). *Wide Range Achievement Test.* Wilmington, DE: Jastek Associates, Inc.

Jastek, J., & Wilkinson, G. S. (1984). *Wide Range Achievement Test-Revised.* Wilmington, DE: Jastek Associates, Inc.

Kaufman, A. S., & Kaufman, N. L. (1994). *The Functional Academic Skills Test.* Circle Pines, MN: American Guidance Service, Inc.

Sparrow, S. S., Balla, D. A., & Cicchetti, D. V. (1984). *Vineland Adaptive Behavior Scales, interview edition, survey form.* Circle Pines, MN: American Guidance Services, Inc.

Wechsler, D. (1981). *Wechsler Adult Intelligence Scale-Revised.* New York: Psychological Corporation.

Wechsler, D. (1991). *Wechsler Intelligence Scale for Children-Third Edition: manual.* San Antonio, TX: Psychological Corporation.

Wilkinson, G. S. (1993). *Wide Range Achievement Test 3.* Wilmington, DE: Wide Range, Inc.

Woodcock, R. W., McGrew, K. S., & Werder, J. K. (1994). *Woodcock-McGrew-Werder Mini-Battery of Achievement.* Chicago: Riverside.

14

Human Figure Drawings and the Draw-A-Person: Screening Procedure for Emotional Disturbance

Achilles N. Bardos and Shawn Powell

INTRODUCTION

Human figure drawings (HFD) have been used for almost a century as ways to gather information about an individual's cognitive as well as personality functioning. In 1926, Goodenough submitted one of the first scoring systems which could be used to determine mental abilities through drawings. From this early work, the use of HFD as measures of mental ability, or developmental level, has involved reviewing the content of drawings to obtain an estimate of a person's mental abilities. When used for this purpose, an individual's drawings are reviewed for specific content items such as represented body parts and clothes.

The second way projective drawings have been used is as a measure of personality functioning. As personality assessment techniques, drawings allow individuals to describe themselves by projecting their emotional characteristics through their picture drawings. The premise of projective drawings is that, when people are asked to draw human figures, their drawing reflects something about themselves. Acquiring personality information from the content of projective drawings has been a subject in the literature for many years. Incorporation of projective drawings in individual assessments has been supported through the development of two systematic approaches: House-Tree-Person Drawings and the Machover's Draw-A-Person Test.

While, Machover's approach to the interpretation of human figure drawings prompted other works on this subject, Machover's approach to the interpretation of projective figure drawings remains the most widely cited in the literature. As Machover's approach has served

Achilles N. Bardos and Shawn Powell • Division of Professional Psychology, University of Northern Colorado, Greeley, Colorado 80639.

Understanding Psychological Assessment, edited by Dorfman and Hersen. Kluwer Academic/Plenum Publishers, New York, 2001.

as a foundation for later works for incorporating projective drawings into personality assessments, it deserves some explanation.

Machover contended that individual aspects of a person's drawing can assist in gaining an understanding of the individual who produced the drawing. She developed general guidelines for human figure drawings, that could be applied to a person's drawings in order to obtain insight into that individual's personality. These guidelines (e.g., placement on the page, body part content, size, line quality, erasures) were used to identify specific aspects of an individual's drawings and were interpreted as signs of personality functioning. For clarification, it should be noted that Machover's guidelines, or signs, were qualitative in nature and were not derived from a normative database. It was assumed these signs would indicate the presence of specific personality functions. These signs were developed through comparison to existing personality constructs in a theoretical context which has become known as the body-image hypothesis. For example, a large drawing was assumed to serve as a sign which indicated the presence of an exaggerated self-concept, while a small drawing was assumed to serve as a sign which indicated a low opinion of oneself.

While Machover's approach has become a seminal work in human figure drawings, Koppitz advanced the use of human figure drawings by developing a quantitative scoring system for interpreting such projective drawings. Machover's approach involved looking at a specific aspect of a person's drawings and then making conclusions about the individual's personality on the basis of the signs that were present or absent in the drawing. Koppitz encouraged the application of a set of emotional indicators and then the making of interpretations about personality functioning on the basis of the number of emotional indicators present in the drawing. In this way, Koppitz discouraged the interpretation of single specific signs of emotionality and emphasized the importance of viewing the whole drawing in terms of personality functioning.

From the beginning of human figure drawings to current times the widespread use of projective drawings in the assessment of children and adolescents as measures of personality is well documented. In a 1992 national survey of practicing school psychologists, it was reported that projective drawings were used most frequently to gather information about the social-emotional functioning of students referred for assessments.

CRITICISMS OF HFD

Although projective drawings have a long history and are widely used in psychological assessments, there have been numerous criticisms made as to their use. Early critics of using projective drawings as a measure of personality believed that the concept of people projecting their personality into their drawings lacked empirical evidence. Recently Motta, Little, & Tobin (1993) argued that, in addition to lacking empirical support, HFD scoring systems designed for projective drawings are not truly exposed to experimental designs. Several authors have pointed out the inadequacies of using projective drawings in psychological assessments, claiming they do not adequately distinguish between populations who have emotional difficulties and those who do not.

As the majority of reviews written about projective drawings indicate, they lack empirical research and have poor psychometrics. The use of projective drawing techniques in psychological assessment has been cited as unethical on the grounds that they are not valid instruments. On the other hand, Anne Anastasi wrote that the Draw-A-Person test (DAP) can serve best, not as a psychometric instrument, but as part of a clinical interview, in which the drawings are interpreted in the context of other information about the individual.

If we accept the criticisms of the review studies that highlight the inadequacies of human figure drawings, it is puzzling how this technique has not only survived over one hundred years but continues to be ranked in the top ten list of frequently used instruments in psychological evaluations. Many of the arguments brought by researchers over the years are reasonable based on the literature. However, at issue here is the definition of a test's validity. Validity of a test refers to the quality of inferences that are made by a test score or procedure. To test the quality of inferences, we typically select an external criterion and relate the test score to this criterion. If we entertain popularity with practitioners as the external criterion, there must be something with the HFD responsible for its continued use. Of course, popularity alone should not be seen as the sole validity criterion, but the procedure is just not popular with laymen's but has been demonstrated and supported by individuals with advanced degrees in the field of psychology. After all, it is hard to dismiss the practices of thousands of psychologists who interact with children and adolescents on a daily basis. If indeed there is absolutely no merit in the technique, it should have disappeared from the practices of today's psychologists.

Probably the most recent debate about the usefulness of the HFD in evaluations occurred in 1993 in an issue of the *School Psychology Quarterly* entitled "The use and abuse of Human Figure Drawings" with responses from a number of individuals, including the senior author of this article. The reader is referred to this source for a review of the various positions. Our main objection to the 1993 review is that various scoring procedures, old and new, were grouped under one category, human figure drawings, and the evaluation did not treat every instrument or scoring procedure independently. This is similar to saying that intelligence tests are not sensitive in the diagnosis of learning disabilities, supporting the argument with research that includes all intelligence tests published since the early 1900's and offering the conclusion that psychologists should not be using intelligence tests because the old ones do not seem to be effective. A conclusion of this nature ignores some of the recent advances proposed by new, theoretically sound instruments of cognitive ability. More importantly it is a frightening message to those researchers and practitioners who believe that our tools, integral components of our evaluations, can be improved and subsequently alter the way we conduct psychological evaluations and understand our clients.

TEST CONSTRUCTION AND DEVELOPMENT

In light of the criticisms of the use of projective drawings, a need for a normative derived human figure drawing technique arose. In responding to this need, the Draw-A-Person: Screening Procedure for Emotional Disturbance (DAP: SPED) was developed to be used as a screening tool for children and adolescents manifesting emotional or behavioral disorders. The first goal of the DAP: SPED was to supply an objective scoring system for human figure drawings that was easy to score and standardized on a current, nationally based normative group. Another goal was for the scoring system to be reliable and to be able to adequately differentiate between normal and clinical populations. Finally, as a screening measure the DAP: SPED can be administered individually or in group settings by a variety of mental health professionals properly trained in the administration and interpretation of psychological tests. It requires approximately 15 minutes to administer, and 3 to 5 minutes per client to score. In the next few paragraphs, we will present some specifics regarding these goals. We begin with the development of the DAP: SPED.

Development: Philosophy and Methodology

Following the work of Koppitz, the DAP: SPED was developed as a screening device to determine the possible presence of emotional disturbances by looking at entire pictures individuals produce. It extended Koppitz's work, since its administration and scoring involves three projective drawings: a drawing of a man, a drawing of a woman and a drawing of self. In this way, an actuarial system is applied to an individual's projective drawings to assist in determining if additional emotional or behavioral assessments are warranted. The DAP: SPED's scoring system provides an objective indication of the presence of items laden with indications of emotionality.

We began our work by reviewing the literature, identifying a total of 93 signs that have been reported or hypothesized to have a link to emotional disturbance or psychopathology. Using the normative sample of over 2,260 children aged 6–17, we examined the frequency of occurrence of all 93 items across 6,780 drawings. Only items/signs that appeared less than 16% of the time (one standard deviation) in the normative sample were selected for the final scoring system. The remaining items, which occurred frequently in the standardization sample, were judged as items drawn by many children and therefore were not included as signs of possible emotional difficulties. By applying this philosophy and these criteria, we were able to describe how children, free of formally identified emotional difficulties, draw. We examined gender differences and found that males had an overall higher number of signs in their drawings than females. Therefore, separate norms were developed for each gender. In addition, three age groups were identified: 6–8, 9–12 and 13–17 years. The final DAP: SPED scoring system includes 55 items. These 55 items include 47 content items (e.g., legs together, transparency, eyes omitted), and 8 measurement items (e.g., tall figure, top placement, right placement). All items are presented in the case study below.

Standardized Sample

The DAP: SPED was normed on a total sample population of 2,260 children and adolescents ranging in age from 6 to 17 selected to reflect the 1980 census. Therefore, this sample was systematically drawn with specific attention given to area of the country and community size, including students from each age group across the range of 6 to 17-years old, taking into consideration ethnicity, parent's occupation, and household income. This sampling procedure resulted in a normative sample that closely resembled the census data.

Psychometric Properties

Many opponents of using projective drawings in psychological assessments base their criticisms on limited psychometric data for such techniques. When the DAP: SPED was developed, specific attention was given to its psychometric properties. The first of these properties to be considered is reliability. Reliability refers to a test's ability to provide accurate and consistent results and the reliability of projective techniques has historically been low, often in the mid .20's.

Two types of errors, systematic error, which can be controlled, and random error, which can not be controlled, can effect a test's reliability. In development of the DAP: SPED, caution was exercised to reduce the types of systematic errors which can influence test results. This caution is evident in the specific instructions that were written for the administration and scoring of the DAP: SPED. In addition, a drawing of the child's self was included which, along with the drawings of a man and a woman, forms the basis for the calculation of a total score. This increased the reliability of the evaluation procedure by enlarging the sample of the behavior domain measured by the test. The result of these efforts to minimize the instrument's systematic error is evident in the reported reliability estimates for the instrument. Three types of reliability are reported. The first is the DAP: SPED's internal consistency. This indicates the extent to which individual test items relate and thus contribute to the test's overall total score and is reported in the form of coefficients alpha. The reported internal consistency coefficients alpha for the three age groups were as follows: Age 6–9 = .76; Age 9–12 = .77; Age 13–17 = .71. These internal consistency coefficients represent adequate coefficients for an instrument intended to serve as a screening tool of emotional difficulties.

A second type of reliability is test-retest reliability which indicates the stability of an instrument over time. The DAP: SPED was administered twice to a sample of 67 students with a one week interval between administrations. The first administration resulted in a group mean T-score of 54.6, and the second administration yielded a group mean T-score of 52.9. These two test scores did not vary significantly ($t = 1.8$, $p > .05$). Additionally, a Pearson correlation of these two administrations resulted in a stability correlation of .67. These results indicate DAP: SPED scores have adequate stability over time.

The third type of reliability is interrater and intrarater reliability. Historically, one weakness of projective assessment techniques has been the poor interrater reliability of such measures. Interrater reliability indicates the extent to which two independent raters, or observers, report similar findings after scoring the same test or observing the same behavior. The interrater reliability of the DAP: SPED was obtained by having two raters score the same 54 protocols. A correlation of .84 was found between these two raters. Intrarater reliability indicates the extent to which a single rater remains consistent over time. In obtaining intrarater reliability, a single rater scored the same 54 protocols after one-month interval. A correlation of .83 was obtained between the two rating sessions. In summary, the present evidence regarding the DAP: SPED's reliability is satisfactory based on multiple evidence presented. These reliability estimates are substantially higher than the ones reported for projective tests in general. The DAP: SPED is a reliable instrument for use as a screening procedure for emotional disturbance.

Once the reliability of any psychological instrument has been demonstrated, the second psychometric property that has to be established is validity. Validity refers to the quality of inferences that can be made by a test's obtained scores. As the DAP: SPED was designed to serve as a screening device to determine if additional personality evaluations are required, studies have been conducted to demonstrate the test's discriminant power using regular education and clinical groups of students. Such studies were conducted and reported in the technical manual as well as by other independent researchers. These studies included samples of children identified with emotional disturbance in both residential and public schools settings, students with learning disabilities, drawings of students who were sexually abused, students with hearing impairments, and Native Americans. In most studies, in addition to the DAP: SPED, additional personality evaluation tools were administered, such as measures of self-concept, behavior rating scales, and self-report inventories. A brief review of some of these validity studies is presented in Appendix A. Readers are also invited to visit the senior author's home page http://web.edtech.unco.edu/abardos. In summary, these studies demonstrate that the DAP: SPED can differentiate between normal and clinical populations and provide substantial support for the use of the DAP: SPED as a screening instrument for emotional difficulties.

ADMINISTRATION AND SCORING

Administration

Administration of the DAP: SPED is quite simple. Students are asked to produce three drawings in the following sequence: first of a man, then of a woman, and last of self. The examiner reads a set of instructions printed on the record form for each drawing. Each drawing is allowed a maximum of five minutes, so the entire procedure can be completed in a maximum of 15 minutes. This can be accomplished in individual or group settings and the instructions in either setting are identical.

Scoring

After the three drawings are complete, scoring can be accomplished fairly quickly, usually in three to five minutes. To score the instrument, evaluators refer to the DAP: SPED examiner's manual to determine the presence or absence of 55 items (47 content items, and 8 measurement items). Three sets of scoring templates, based on three age groups (6–8, 9–12, and 13–17) are provided to assist in scoring the measurement items. The examiner's manual contains detailed descriptions regarding the scoring of the measurement and content items. Additionally, the examiner's manual contains five practice cases and five competency cases which can be used to learn the scoring system with detailed descriptions of the specific items scored and not scored in each case. These practice and competency cases were used in the training of the raters hired to score all 6,780 drawings of the 2,260 children included in the standardization sample. After one learns how to administer and score the DAP: SPED, these examples can be of assistance as comparison examples.

After the three drawings are scored, the raw scores for each drawing are combined to yield a total DAP: SPED raw score. Through the use of an age- and gender-based norm table in the examiner's manual, raw scores are transposed into T-scores. In addition to T-scores, the manual provides percentile rankings and confidence intervals.

As the DAP: SPED is intended to be used as a screening device to indicate the need for further emotional or behavioral evaluation, three predetermined cut scores are given. If an individual's T-score is less than 55, no further evaluation is indicated. If the individual's T-score is 55 to 65, then further evaluation is indicated. Finally, if an individual's T-score is greater than 65, further evaluation is strongly indicated. A case that demonstrates the scoring system follows.

CASE EXAMPLE

Figures 14.1, 14.2, and 14.3 present the drawings of a 14-year-old child. Due to space limitations, only one of the drawings, the picture of self, will be evaluated, but a completed cover page of a typical record form will also be presented. A score of 1 indicates that a particular sign is present in the drawing.

The DAP: SPED Scoring System

The first nine items of the scoring procedure relate to measurements of the drawing and require the use of templates (provided in the test kit). The examiner applies the transparent

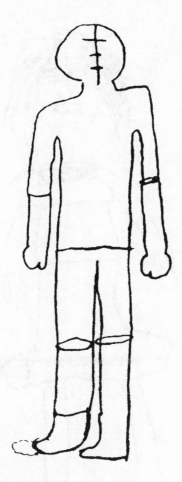

Figure 14.1. Case study: Sample drawing of a man.

templates over each of the drawings (see Figures 14.4–14.8 for illustrations) to determine the score. Templates used must be for appropriate ages.

1. Tall Figure is scored if the distance between the uppermost and the lowermost points of the figure is greater than the height of Line 1. For this and the following measurements, articles of clothing, such as hats or shoes are included in the measurement, although other objects (e.g., handbag, briefcase, backpack, and baseball bat) are not included and the template must be aligned squarely with the page (not rotated).

Score: 1

2. Short Figure is scored if the distance between the uppermost point of the figure and the lowermost point of the figure is less than Line 2.

Score: 0

3. Big Figure is scored if the figure exceeds both the vertical *and* horizontal dimensions of Box 3.

Score: 1

4. Little Figure is scored if the figure fits completely within Box 4.

Score: 0

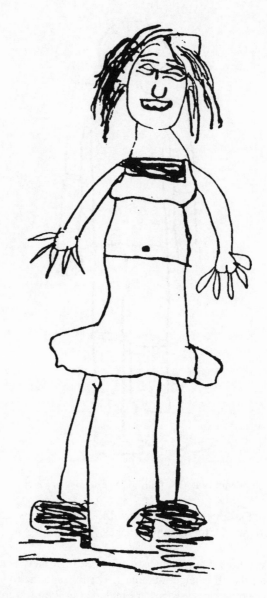

Figure 14.2. Case study: Sample drawing of a woman.

5. Top Placement is scored when any part of the figure is in Box 5 and the figure is entirely above Line 5.

Score: 0

6. Bottom Placement is scored when any part of the figure is in Box 6 and the figure is entirely below Line 6.

Score: 0

7. Left Placement is scored when any part of the figure is in Box 7 and the figure is entirely to the left of Line 7.

Score: 0

8. Right Placement is scored when any part of the figure is in Box 8 and the figure is entirely to the right of Line 8.

Score: 0

9. Slanting Figure is scored if the vertical axis of the figure (i.e., the line from midpoint of head width to midpoint of stance width) deviates by 15 degrees or more from a perpendicular to the bottom edge of the page (use the Item 9 template).

Score: 1

10. Legs Together is scored if the legs are drawn together with no visible space between legs or if only one leg is visible in profile.

Score: 0

11. Baseline Drawn is scored if a ground line (e.g., grass) is drawn.

Score: 1

12. Lettering/Numbering is scored if letters, words, phrases, or numbers appear anywhere on the page *other than* on the figure (on the figure to include worn accessories).

Score: 0

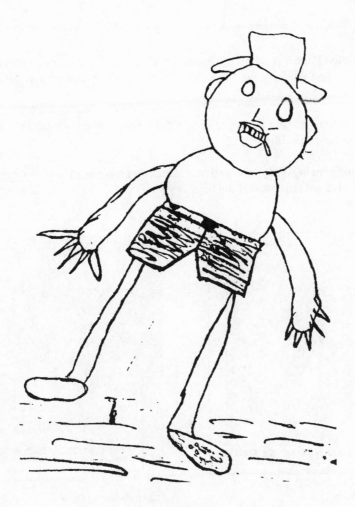

Figure 14.3. Case study: Sample drawing of self.

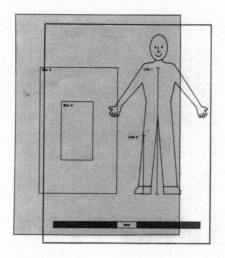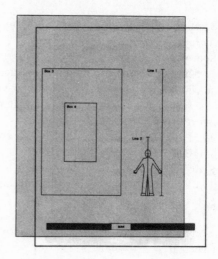

Score Tall Figure   Score Short Figure

Figure 14.4. Examples of using the templates to score Items 1 and 2. The shading represents the template.

13. Rotated Page is scored if the figure is drawn with the longest dimension of the page on the top (i.e., the folded edge of the Record Form is at the bottom or top instead of on the side).
Score: 0
14. Left/Right-Facing Figure is scored if the entire figure or head only is in the left-facing or right-facing profile.
Score: 0
15. Figure Facing Away is scored if the entire figure, or head only, is facing away from the viewer so that only the back of the head is visible.
Score: 0

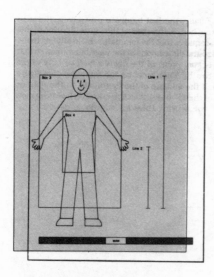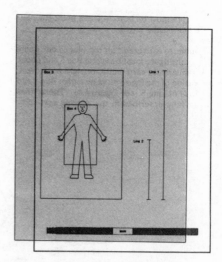

Score Big Figure   Do Not Score Big Figure

Figure 14.5. Examples of using the templates to score Item 3. The shading represents the template.

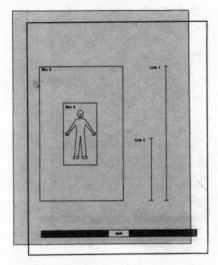 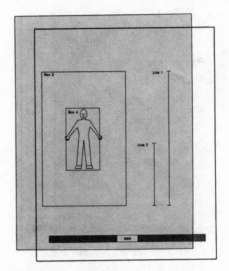

Score Little Figure   Do Not Score Little Figure

Figure 14.6. Examples of using the templates to score Item 4. The shading represents the template.

16. Failed Integration is scored if any of the following are present but not attached:

- head is attached to neck or top of torso
- two arms (one if in profile) are attached to the top half of the torso (above the halfway mark in the vertical measurement of the torso or bottom of a dress). The torso extends from the top of the trunk, where it meets the head or neck, to the bottom, where it meets the legs or crotch.
- two legs (one if in profile) are attached at the bottom of the torso (below the halfway mark in the vertical measurement of the torso or bottom of a dress).

Score: 0

17. Transparencies is scored if any body part shows through clothing or another body part.

Score: 0

18. Restart is scored if one or more human figures are obviously abandoned (erased, scratched out, or merely left incomplete) and a more complete figure appears on the page.

Score: 0

19. Head Omitted is scored if the figure's head is absent. Any attempted representation of a head cannot be scored as an omission.

Score: 0

20. Hair Omitted is scored if the figure has no hair on its head. Any attempted representation of hair on head, including beard, etc., cannot be scored as an omission.

Score: 1

21. Eyes Omitted is scored if the figure's eyes are absent. Any attempted representation of eyes (including only one eye) cannot be scored as an omission.

Score: 0

22. Nose Omitted is scored if the figure's nose is absent. Any attempted representation of a nose cannot be scored as an omission.

Score: 0

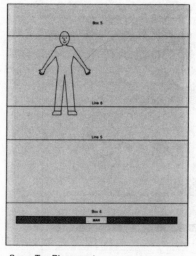

Score Top Placement

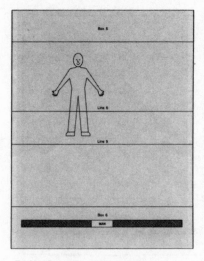

Do Not Score Top Placement

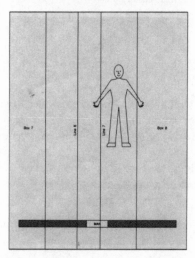

Score Right Placement

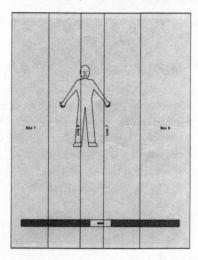

Do Not Score Right Placement

Figure 14.7. Examples of using the templates to score Items 5 through 8. The shading represents the template.

23. Mouth Omitted is scored if the figure's mouth is absent. Any attempted representation of a mouth cannot be scored as an omission.

Score: 0

24. Torso Omitted is scored if the figure's torso is absent. Any attempted representation of a torso cannot be scored as an omission.

Score: 0

25. Arms Omitted is scored if the figure has no arms. Any attempted representation of arms (including only one arm) cannot be scored as an omission.

Score: 0

26. Fingers Omitted is scored if the figure has no fingers. Any attempted representation of fingers cannot be scored as an omission.

Score: 0

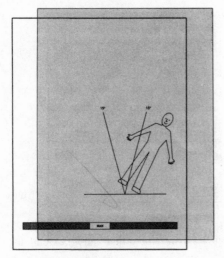
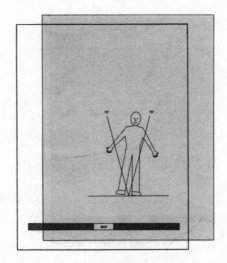

Score Slanting Figure   Do Not Score Slanting Figure

Figure 14.8. Examples of using the templates to score Item 9. The shading represents the template.

27. Legs Omitted is scored if the figure has no legs. Any attempted representation of legs (including only one leg) cannot be scored as an omission.

Score: 0

28. Feet Omitted is scored if the figure has no feet. Any attempted representation of feet (including only one foot) cannot be scored as an omission.

Score: 0

29. Crotch Erasure is scored if erasure is apparent in the area of the figure's crotch (below the waistline or belt and above the knee area of the leg).

Score: 0

30. Crotch Shading is scored if pencil strokes are present on the figure's crotch area (below the waistline or belt and above the knee area of the leg) which fill in an area by coloring or darkening (including stripes or checks on clothing).

Score: 1

31. Hand Shading is scored if pencil strokes are present on the figure's hand(s) which fill in an area by coloring or darkening.

Score: 0

32. Feet Shading is scored if pencil strokes are present on the figure's feet (foot) which fill in an area by coloring or darkening. (Shoelaces are not scored as shading.)

Score: 1

33. Outside Shading is scored if pencil strokes are present outside of the figure which fill in an area by coloring or darkening.

Score: 1

34. Vacant Eyes is scored if both the figure's eyes (one if in profile) are empty (i.e. open circles).

Score: 1

35. Closed Eyes is scored if both the figure's eyes are closed.

Score: 0

36. Crossed Eyes is scored if both the figure's eyes are crossed.
Score: 0
37. Gazing Left/Right is scored if both the figure's eyes (one if in profile) are gazing toward the rater's left or right.
Score: 0
38. Frowning Mouth is scored if the figure's mouth is frowning.
Score: 0
39. Slash Mouth is scored if the figure's mouth is a straight line or slash.
Score: 0
40. Teeth is scored if teeth are present in the figure's mouth.
Score: 1
41. Object in Mouth is scored if an object (cigar, pipe, etc.) is present in the figure's mouth.
Score: 1
42. Reaching Arms is scored if both the figure's arms (including hands) extend above the top of the figure's head.
Score: 0
43. Pressed to Torso is scored if both the figure's arms are down at the side of figure with no visible space between the torso of the figure and the arms.
Score: 0
44. Inconsistent Position is scored if each of the figure's arms is in a different position (i.e., reaching, outstretched, hanging, or pressed to torso, as defined below).

- a reaching arm extends above the figure's head
- an outstretched arm is approximately horizontal
- a hanging arm points downward
- an arm is pressed to torso if there is no space between it and the torso

Score: 0
45. Hands Cut Off is scored if there are no hands or fingers at the ends of the arms. (Hands hidden behind back of figure or in pockets not scored.)
Score: 0
46. Hidden Hands is scored if the hands are hidden behind the back of the figure or in pockets.
Score: 0
47. Fists is scored if the hands are made into fists.
Score: 0
48. Talons is scored if one or more fingers are clearly pointed (like a claw) or knife-like.
Score: 1
49. Aggressive Symbols is scored for the presence of one or more aggressive symbols, gestures, or written statements (e.g., guns, knives, clubs, written profanity, or other symbols of aggression).
Score: 0
50. Object Attached is scored for the presence of one or more objects attached to, or being held by, the figure (e.g., handbag, briefcase, backpack, baseball bat, but excluding aggressive symbols and articles such as eyeglasses and jewelry).
Score: 0
51. Background Filled In is scored for the presence of anything drawn in addition to

the human figure which is not attached to or being held by the figure (e.g., animal, automobile, building, tree, sun, moon, clouds, raindrops).

Score: 1

52. Monster is scored if the figure is drawn as a nonhuman or monster.

Score: 0

53. Multiple Figures is scored for the presence of more than one complete person (or monster) on the page.

Score: 0

54. Nude Figure is scored if a fully or partially unclothed figure is drawn. This item includes any representation of genitalia, for example, but bare feet, short pants, or short sleeve shirt are *not* scored.

Score: 1

55. Uniformed Figure is scored for a figure drawn as a soldier, cowboy/cowgirl, policeman, etc. Sports figures or cheerleaders are *not* scored.

Score: 0

DAP: SPED: Interpretation

Figure 14.9 shows the completed front cover page of a DAP: SPED record form 0. The raw score of 28 in this case was translated to a T-score of 78. Next, the examiner completes the range of scores based on the confidence intervals. In this case, the scores ranged from 69 to 87. The examiner should use the cut-off criteria presented in the front of the record form to describe the child's score as "like normal" or "typical of children" or "atypical" (with possibilities of emotional problems) in comparison to children of the same age. In our case, the DAP: SPED score strongly suggests that this child should be referred for an evaluation. An example of how DAP: SPED findings can be integrated in a psychological report is presented next.

> Theresa's emotional status was assessed using several different kinds of measures. She earned a T-score of 78 (90% confidence range is 69 to 87) on the Draw-A-Person: Screening Procedure for Emotional Disturbance. This score falls at the 99th percentile, meaning that she had more signs of emotional problems in her drawings than about 99% of the children the same age in the general population. Similarly, she earned very high scores on the.... (The examiner must present additional data and relate the DAP: SPED scores to other measures of emotional status. Consistency across projective and behavioral rating scale method scales is not necessarily expected. An indication of a problem in either type of evaluation system is cause for concern and further examination of the case).

DAP not use alone

In the lower part of the record form (see Figure 14.9) the examiner may choose to evaluate the drawings from a different perspective using the Naglieri Draw-A-Person: Quantitative Scoring System (DAP: QSS) which examines the exact three drawings from a cognitive ability perspective by applying 14 criteria to each. The total DAP: QSS score is organized with a mean of 100 and a standard deviation of 15.

SUMMARY

Psychologists have used human figure drawings for over a century. Despite the criticisms, the technique has survived the test of time and remains popular with those who work

DAP:SPED

RECORD FORM

Jack A. Naglieri, Timothy J. McNeish,
and Achilles N. Bardos

Identifying Information

Name _____

Address _____

_____

Home Telephone _____

Grade/Teacher _____

School _____

Examiner _____

Gender _____

	Year	Month	Day
Date of Testing	_____	_____	_____
Date of Birth	_____	_____	_____
Age (yr. only)	_____	_____	_____

Summary of Scores

Drawing	Raw Score
Man (M)	*14*
Woman (W)	*7*
Self (S)	*7*
Total DAP:SPED RAW SCORE (M + W + S)	*28*

DAP:SPED *T* score _*78*_   Percentile Rank _*99*_

Confidence interval at _*90*_ % level of confidence = ± _*9*_

Standard score range = _*69*_ to _*87*_

Examinee status (check one): Further evaluation is

not indicated (<55)   _____

indicated (55–65)   _____

strongly indicated (>65)   *X*

Examiner comments:

Other Information:

Draw A Person: A Quantitative Scoring System

Man _____ Woman _____ Self _____ DAP:QSS Total score = _____

© 1991 by PRO-ED, Inc.
3 4 5 6 7 8   97 96 95 94 93

Additional copies of this form (#5122) are available from PRO-ED, Inc.
8700 Shoal Creek Boulevard, Austin, Texas 78757 USA 512/451-3246

Figure 14.9. Case study: The front page of the DAP: SPED record form.

with children and adolescents. There are many scoring systems available for the evaluation of children's drawings and each one must be evaluated independently. In this chapter, we presented a recently developed scoring procedure, the DAP: SPED which is intended to serve as a screening procedure to determine if further evaluation for the presence of emotional disturbance is warranted. The DAP: SPED's major goal was the determination and description of how normal children draw so that atypical drawings can be identified and serve as additional evidence in the assessment process. This was accomplished with a sound standardization sample and the DAP: SPED provides an objective basis from which to make recommendations for further evaluation. Many of the criticisms regarding HFD were addressed through the construction of this instrument to ensure it had adequate psychometric properties. Some authors have suggested, that projective drawings can be used in personality assessments, in that they allow an evaluator to start the assessment process in a fairly nonthreatening manner and can serve as a guide for professionals in deciding if projective drawings are useful for their purposes. In determining if human figure drawings and this instrument in particular represent an advancement in the use of drawings in psychological evaluations, users should ultimately make this decision based on the instrument's psychometric properties. We have presented such evidence for the intended purpose of the DAP: SPED, that is, as a screening procedure for emotional difficulties.

For mental health professionals who want to determine if a child or adolescent should be referred for comprehensive evaluation, or who might want to screen large groups of children, the DAP: SPED can assist in this decision. For psychologists conducting personality assessments, the DAP: SPED can be incorporated into their evaluations in order to provide an objective measure of the individual's need for a complete evaluation. In these times of increasing case loads and pressure to identify children and adolescents with emotional or behavioral disorders, this instrument provides useful information in a short time.

SUGGESTED READINGS

Anastasi, A. (1988). *Psychological testing* (6th ed.) New York: Macmillan.

Bardos, A. N. (1993). Human figure drawings: Abusing the Abused. *School Psychology Quarterly, 8(3)*, 177–181.

Buck, J. N. (1948). The H-T-P technique: A qualitative and quantitative scoring manual. *Journal of Clinical Psychology, 4,* 317–396.

Burns, R., & Kaufman, S. (1970). *Kinetic Family Drawings (K-F-D): An introduction to understanding children through kinetic drawings.* New York: Brunner/Mazel.

Finch, A. J., & Belter, R. W. (1993). Projective techniques. In T. H. Ollendick and M. Hersen (Eds.) *Handbook of Child and Adolescent Assessment*, (pp. 224–236). Boston: Allyn and Bacon.

Goodenough, F. L. (1926). *Measurement of intelligence in drawings.* New York: Harcourt Brace and World.

Hammer, E. (1958). *The clinical application of projective drawings.* Springfield, IL: Charles C. Thomas.

Koppitz, E. (1968). *Psychological evaluation of children's human figure drawings.* New York: Grune & Stratton

Machover, K. (1949). *Personality projection in the drawing of a human figure.* Springfield, IL: Charles C. Thomas.

Motta, R. W., Little, S. G., & Tobin, M. I. (1993). The use and abuse of human figure drawings. *School Psychology Quarterly, 8(3)*, 162–169.

Naglieri, J. A (1988). *Draw A Person: A quantitative scoring System.* San Antonio, TX. The Psychological Corporation.

Naglieri, J. A., McNeish, T. J., & Bardos, A. N. (1991). *Draw a Person: Screening procedure for emotional disturbance examiner's manual.* Austin. TX: Pro-ed.

Naglieri, J. A., Pfeifer, S. & LeBuffe, P. (1993). *Devereux Behavior Rating Scale- School Form.* San Antonio, TX: The Psychological Corporation.

Neal, V. (1992). Situational stress and children's performance on the Draw A person: Screening Procedure for Emotional Disturbance considering parental stress levels, gender, and socio-economic conditions. Unpublished Doctoral dissertation, Texas Women's University.

Norford, B. C., & Barakat, L. P. (1990). The relationship of human figure drawings to aggressive behaviors in preschool children. *Psychology in the Schools, 27,* 318–325.

Politikos, N. (1997). Performance of Greek children on the Draw A Person: Screening Procedure for Emotional Disturbance. Unpublished Doctoral Dissertation, University of Northern Colorado, Greeley, Colorado, USA.

Prout, H. T. (1983). School psychologists and social- emotional assessment techniques: Patterns in training and use. *School Psychology Review, 12,* 377–383.

Ryser, C. Lassiter, K. & Bardos, A. N. (1991, May). *Emotional indicators in the drawings of learning disabled children.* Paper presented at the annual conference of the Colorado Psychological Association, Denver, Colorado.

Salvia, J., & Ysseldyke, J. E. (1991). *Assessment* (5th edition). Boston: Houghton Mifflin Company.

Stinnett, T. A., Harvey, J. M., & Oehler-Stinnett, J. (1994). Current test usage by practicing school psychologists: A national survey. *Journal of Psychoeducational Assessment, 2,* 327–350.

Swensen, C. H.. (1957). Empirical evaluations of human figure drawings. *Psychological Bulletin, 54,* 431–436.

United States Bureau of the Census. (1983). *1980 census of the population* (Publication No. PC80-1-B1 and PC80-1-C1). Washington, D.C.: U. S. Government Printing Office.

Wilson-Ball, B. M. (1989). *Children's human figure drawings: Symbolic communications of self-esteem level.* Unpublished doctoral dissertation, University of Maine.

APPENDIX A.
VALIDITY STUDIES FOR THE DRAW-A-PERSON: SCREENING PROCEDURE FOR EMOTIONAL DISTURBANCE

VALIDITY STUDIES

DAP:SPED Validity

- McNeish & Naglieri (1993) Journal of Special Education, 27, 115-121
  - 81 Special Ed (SED)
  - 81 Regular Ed
  - Matched Groups
  - All males (75% white)
  - 7-13 years of age
- SED earned significantly higher mean T-score (55.3; SD =10.6) than control group (49.5; SD=8.6)

	>55	< 55
SED	49%	51%
Normal	32%	68%

DAP:SPED Validity

- Naglieri, & Pfeiffer, S. I. (1992). Psychological Assessment, 4, 156-159.
- 54 Subjects in psychiatric day treatment at the Devereux Foundation & 54 matched controls
- DSM-III-R Disruptive Behavior Disorders
- Age range 7-17 years, 78% males; 95% white
- DAP:SPED means significantly different
  - 56.6 (SD 10.3) vs 49.4 (SD =8.7)
  - 78% of controls and 48% of DBD correctly identified
  - SPED improves accuracy of prediction by 25%

Study 1.
Psychiatric Residential Sample

		Age		DAP:SPED		Percentages	
Sample	N	Mean	SD	Mean	SD	Males	White
Clinical	49	15.3	1.1	57.0	6.4	67	33
Normal	218	12.9	2.2	49.1	8.1	81	19

T-test = 7.41, p<.001

Study 1
DAP:SPED and Self Concept

	Mean	SD	Pearson Corr.
DAP: SPED	57.0	6.4	
MSCS			
Social	103.9	17.5	.04
Personal Competence	97.8	15.7	.06
Personal Affection	97.6	15.9	-.26*
Achievement	97.3	15.3	.14
Family	92.2	15.0	-.43**
Physical	100.4	18.6	-.19
Total	95.8	16.8	-.17

Note: * p< .05
      ** p< .01

Study 1.
Psychiatric Residential Sample

	Nonreferred (N=22)		Referred (N=26)	
	Mean	SD	Mean	SD
DAP:SPED	51.8	2.1	61.3	5.1
MSCS				
Social	106.3	19.9	101.9	15.3
P. Comp.	97.8	20.3	97.7	11.1
P. Affec.	103.9	18.5	92.5	11.4
Achieve.	95.7	16.1	98.6	14.7
Family	96.0	16.6	88.9	12.9
Physical	106.7	15.5	95.3	19.6
Total	100.4	17.5	92.0	15.4

Study 1
Efficiency of Classification with ED Adolescents

Emotional Classification	Normal	ED
DAP: SPED Decision		
Do not Refer	160	22
Refer for Further Evaluation	56	27

Sensitivity:	.55	55% of children scoring 55 or above will be correctly identified
Specificity:	.74	Accurate screening predictions were made for 74% of the children
Efficiency of outcome "refer"	.33	There is a 33% chance that a child referred will have emotional difficulties
Efficiency of "do not refer"	.85	85% chance that a child referred will be judged as being normal

Study 2.
ED children in a public school

		Mean	SD
WISC-R	VIQ =	96.3	11.1
	PIQ =	95.3	16.8
	FSIQ =	94.9	12.4

(n=58)

Study 2.

Sample	N	Age Mean	SD	DAP:SPED Mean	SD	Males	White
ED	58	12.1	1.2	54.8	9.2	86	91
Normal	262	11.3	1.0	49.7	9.0	86	97

t-test = 3.85, p< . 001

Study 2
Results of DAP:SPED Classification

	Group's Emotional Classification	
	Normal	Emotionally Disturbed
DAP:SPED Decision		
Do Not Refer	191	30
Refer for Further Evaluation	71	28

Study 2
Efficiency of Classification

Hit Rates		What this means:
Sensitivity	.48	48% of those scoring 55 or above will be correctly identified
Specificity:	.73	Accurate screening predictions were made for 73% of the children
Efficiency of screening outcome "refer"	.28	There is a 28% chance that a child referred by DAP:SPED will be judged as having emotional difficulties
Efficiency of screening outcome "do not refer"	.86	There is a 86% chance that a child not being referred by DAP:SPED will be judged as normal

15

Children's Apperception Test (C.A.T.)

Jan Faust and Sara Ehrich

INTRODUCTION

The Children's Apperception Test (C.A.T.) is a projective measure for acquiring information about children's personality and psychological processes. The test, in general, includes a series of 10 quasi-ambiguous pictures to which the child is asked to create a story. This assessment technique was developed from psychoanalytic theory and was designed to obtain information about psychological functioning through the specific mechanism of projection.

Projection is both a process by which an individual's personality is expressed and a specific defense mechanism. With respect to the former, theorists have suggested that external reality is filtered, then ordered or synthesized, by an individual through his or her own subjective perceptions, feelings, cognitions, and a wide range of human experiences. Therefore, when a child is presented with an external ambiguous stimulus such as a C.A.T. picture, the story he or she develops is passed through this subjective filter. Some refer to this projection process as an "apperceptive distortion." It is said to occur in every situation in which external events are experienced subjectively as they pass through the individual's unique filter of previous experiences and perceptions. For example, when a subject responds to a card with an illustration of a father figure, he or she will naturally provide information about this card which reflects experiences and perceptions of similar figures (caretakers, authority figures) in his or her own life.

Projection as a defense mechanism is considered a form of coping activated automatically (unconsciously) by the ego to protect the aware (conscious) self from frightening unconscious thoughts, feelings, and beliefs. These cognitions are thought to be generally sexual and aggressive in nature.

Though the concept of projection was around for centuries before Sigmund Freud, his definition of this construct was pivotal in advancing modern psychoanalysis. He was one of the first to elaborate on this concept, describing projection as a defense mechanism used to

Jan Faust and Sara Ehrich • Center for Psychological Studies, Nova Southeastern University, Fort Lauderdale, Florida 33314

Understanding Psychological Assessment, edited by Dorfman and Hersen. Kluwer Academic/Plenum Publishers, New York, 2001.

externalize unsatisfactory wishes, thoughts, and impulses through attribution of one's inner perceptions and experiences to others. Freud further extended his projection concept to include the projection of various nonthreatening (nondefended) sensations, emotions, and ideas onto outer reality.

Projective techniques involve the use of specific tools designed to elicit projected material. Such techniques include presentation of stimuli, such as C.A.T. drawings. The stimuli are developed or selected for their potential psychological meaning to the subject and not as a result of an arbitrary or random objective experiment. That is, the assessor is interested in a subjective response—the idiosyncratic and unique meaning of the perceived stimuli to the individual. This is unlike scientific experimentation wherein one is interested in the average or normative objective response obtained from a group of individuals.

TEST CONSTRUCTION AND DEVELOPMENT

The Thematic Apperception Test (T.A.T.) was the most widely used projective measure for children until the development of the C.A.T. in 1949. The T.A.T. includes a set of 31 ambiguous drawings depicting mostly human figures in various settings, as well as some landscape and abstract drawings. The T.A.T. is widely used in personality and projective assessment of adolescents and adults. Conceptually, the C.A.T. emanated from a theoretical discussion between Dr. Ernest Kris and Dr. Leopold Bellak regarding projection and the shortcomings of the T.A.T. in its use with children. Dr. Kris believed that children may be able to more freely identify with and project more openly onto animals than human figures. He further exemplified that this process had been observed by Sigmund Freud, citing his seminal work with Little Hans in "The Phobia of a Five Year Old."

After discussing the idea for about one year, the authors had a professional illustrator develop illustrations representative of children in such areas as home life, school, and other environments. Originally, 18 cards were produced. The illustrations included human activity in some scenes with animals (e.g., kangaroo riding a bike) while others depicted activity germane to animal behavior (e.g., bears in a cave). These preliminary cards were then dispersed to various child psychologists to whom Dr. Bellak had previously taught the T.A.T. The authors also used these cards in their own work with children. Subsequently, the psychologists returned C.A.T. responses and patient background information, along with their comments and criticisms of the test. As a result of this feedback, the 18 cards were reduced to the 10 that appeared most promising for eliciting material regarding children's primary relationships and drives. As a direct derivative of the T.A.T., the C.A.T. in no way attempts to replace it. On the contrary, the authors recommend using the C.A.T. for children aged 3–10; the T.A.T is to be used for individuals over the age of 10.

Human versus Animal Supplements

In 1965, the authors developed a human version of the C.A.T. (C.A.T.-H.), contrary to the belief that young children would emit more projected material when given to animal, rather than human, figure drawings. Several artists contributed to the creation of the C.A.T.-H. under the tutelage of Leonard Bellak and Sonya S. Bellak. According to the authors, construction of the C.A.T.-H. presented some unexpected difficulties. The use of animals in the C.A.T.-A. (Animal) allowed for pictures free of age, gender, and cultural stimuli, but with the C.A.T.-H. the illustrators had to go to great lengths to avoid gender and cultural specificity (e.g., by clothing figures in shapeless garments). The authors noted that the gender and cultural attributions of the C.A.T.-H. will vary more than the C.A.T.-A. across various cultures and subcultures. However, they expected that the advantages of using the human figures with certain populations would outweigh any negative implications. Further, in recent years, the C.A.T. has been redrawn to include culturally specific features (e.g., a Japanese version). The human form can be used in addition to the animal form if the tester believes the additional cards could provide additional information. It may also be used in lieu of the animal form if the child is not responding to the animal figures, or as a retest if the child needs to be tested consecutively in a short span of time. However, it is the recommendation of many clinicians that the C.A.T.-H. form should only be administered under the above conditions and should not be routinely given in place of the animal form. Many clinicians have discovered that the animal form provides the examiner with material which is richer in pertinent information than the human form. First, this is because the animals allow children to psychologically distance themselves from real characters who are often the source and target of conflicts (e.g., parents). Hence, the child's resistance should be weaker and information more forthcoming with the animal cards than with the human. Second, children often identify with animals in important ways, since animals are less powerful (more helpless and dependent) than humans and are usually smaller and not able to stand upright (they cannot see eye-to-eye). Further similarities between children and animals include a lack of complex language systems. Also, children and animals rely on behavioral methods of communication (e.g., they rely more directly on external cues than on expressive language). In addition, animals do not place their expectations upon children nor do they discipline as do humans.

Although some research has demonstrated potential superiority of the animal form over the human form, there is also some research demonstrating greater utility of the human form over the animal form. One study of 6- to 10-year-old subjects found that the use of animal figures resulted in higher scores on projection and intellectualization than with the human form, thus suggesting that the C.A.T.-H. may be more productive for older or more mature children than the C.A.T.-A. Consequently, it may be that both forms are equivocally beneficial in assessment and that differences lie in specific characteristics of the individual (e.g., age, type of psychological problem, medical problem, history).

The Children's Apperception Test Supplement (C.A.T.-S.) was added by the original developers of the C.A.T. in 1952. It was recommended for use in a play-therapy context, as opposed to that of formal assessment. The C.A.T.-S. is composed of 10 cards that present animals in situations that some, but not all, children may have experienced. The supplement is a suggested technique for children who are very young or who are too severely disturbed to respond to the more formal testing process. As the C.A.T.-S. is a more informal style of testing, it can also be used to explore specific conflicts (body image, injury, mother's pregnancy) that children may be working on in treatment. Use of these cards is at the discretion of the examiner and is for the purpose of supplementing, not replacing, the C.A.T.-A. or C.A.T.-H.

Psychometric Properties

In the 1950's, numerous validation studies were conducted on projective tests. These studies found that projective techniques did not successfully predict group membership (e.g., psychologically impaired groups). As a result, there has been much debate regarding the validity of projective techniques as assessment instruments. However, many professionals believe that projective techniques are used for the purpose of illuminating unique individual characteristics, not the commonalities of group membership. Some have argued that validity and reliability studies are based on group norms, not individual characteristics, and therefore cannot be effectively used to assess the psychometric integrity of projective techniques.

The C.A.T.'s construction was based on a subject pool of 200 children between the ages of 3 and 10. C.A.T. developers published the measure without psychometric data on the premise that projective techniques are used for the purpose of illuminating a child's fundamental dynamics. Thus, as with most projective measures, establishing norms and assessing validity was deemed unnecessary. With greater advances and sophistication of test construction, research design, and statistics, professionals promulgated future research aimed at developing normative and other psychometric information regarding projective tests. Unfortunately, while such information has become more widely available, there remains a dearth of studies establishing psychometric norms, validity, and reliability for the C.A.T.

Reliability

There are difficulties in establishing test-retest reliability on projective measures with children. If the child is retested after a relatively short span of time, he or she may remember the initial responses. However, with retesting after a relatively long span of time, the child may be in a significantly different period of development. Thus, testing results may reveal different unconscious and conscious processes reflecting growth. In this way, retesting children differs greatly from and can be more onerous than retesting adults.

Validity

The construct validity of the C.A.T., or the extent to which each of the cards is educing the card-specific dynamic material, has been explored in several studies. One study, using preschool subjects, discovered that each of the cards successfully elicited the information it was developed to investigate. For example, cards specifically designed to explore themes of orality (Cards 1, 4, and 8) evoked such themes with much greater frequency than others. Similar themes were also noted in Cards 3, 6, and 9.

With respect to concurrent validity, a study conducted on 12 pairs of identical twins compared results of a battery of tests including the C.A.T., Rorschach, and the Bender Gestalt. Each of these tests were then rank ordered by several judges on the basis of "general adjustment." Results of comparison between the C.A.T. and the Rorschach protocols showed a coefficient of .35; C.A.T. and Bender. The coefficient with Bender was .38. As for discriminative validity, studies discriminating groups, such as children with speech problems, cerebral palsy, and emotional disturbances, have yielded significant results.

ADMINISTRATION AND SCORING

It is important during the administration of the C.A.T. that the examiner be aware of various potential problems that may occur both when testing children and when using projective techniques. For an extensive review see Haworth (1966).

First and foremost, establishing good rapport is crucial. The child should be made to feel comfortable and at ease in the testing situation by providing a comfortable environment, including adequate lighting so as to avoid shadows on the cards which could cause potential falsification of responses. Also, comfortable seating, no interruptions, and intermittent breaks are recommended throughout the process. As the child, in most cases, does not chose to participate in the testing procedure, it is important to make her or him feel psychologically as well as physically comfortable, thus reducing the chance that extraneous feelings about the testing process will influence responses to the cards.

Subsequent to establishing good rapport, the test is introduced as a play activity (game), if at all possible. If the child has already been informed of the nature of the test, it should be emphasized that there are no right or wrong answers, and responses will not result in a grade, score, rewards, or disapproval. A positive attitude should be conveyed to the child throughout this process. Children provide more productive and complete C.A.T. answers when the examiner conveys a positive, rather than negative or neutral, attitude. Depending on the age of the child, it may also be helpful to explain the confidentiality of the examination and to whom the results will be presented. It should be emphasized that if the information is disclosed, recipients will be limited (e.g., only to the therapist or parents).

The cards should be presented to the child one at a time. To avoid distraction and possible contamination of responses, cards not being used should be kept face down and out of sight from the testee during the procedure. As each card is presented, the examiner should request that the child tell a story with a beginning, middle, and end as it pertains to the picture. Some professionals, including those following Bellak's method, believe it may be necessary to prompt the child at different points in their story. The examiner may query as to what happened prior to the beginning of the story and after the end. However, others argue that prompting can distract the patient as well as distort provided material. Many take a minimalist position such that any prompting taints pure projected material, whereas others believe that prompting may be necessary but to be utilized sparingly. This moderate approach tends to be the one most frequently adopted by professionals. Depending upon the age of the child, one may need to more frequently query throughout C.A.T. administration. It is extremely important that the cards be presented in their numbered order, as Bellak ordered the cards with a specific theoretical rationale in obtaining projected material. For example, Card 6 may evoke information suppressed in Card 5 (Haworth, 1966).

Each story and every verbalization throughout the testing process should be recorded, including jokes, slips of the tongue, and any other seemingly superficial comments. Gestures and facial expressions can also provide a consequential amount of information regarding unconscious, or even conscious, responses to particular cards, or the testing process in general. Tape recording is highly recommended but should not replace verbatim transcription of stories during the examination.

Some additional testing techniques for the C.A.T. have been supported in the literature and may be utilized depending on the testing situation. For example, in the manual Bellak (1961) suggests revisiting each of the cards upon completion of the formal testing process to probe for sources of names used for persons or places, elaboration of particular points, and clarification regarding outcomes described.

One author recommends using a "dream technique," specifically for cards 5, 6, and 9, as the characters often appear to the testee as being asleep. It was discovered that by instructing children to develop a dream, children provide unconscious material more freely than with the card as originally presented. Material produced by this format, in impulse and imagery can be likened to responses elicited by the Rorschach.

A tester might add a blank card, similar to the T.A.T. Adding a black card, or a half black and half-white card to the examination, may be helpful in educing additional information. The half-black and half-white card has evoked racial issues in some, typically African-American, children.

Scoring and Interpretative Guidelines

There have been a number of systems developed for C.A.T. scoring purposes. In fact, one reference sites as many as 40 different systems, although very little psychometric data exists for these methods. There are two formal C.A.T. scoring methods that are more widely used than others. These include Bellak's Diagnostic System and L. Chandler's Need Threat Analysis System.

One of the most frequently utilized scoring systems is Bellak's Diagnostic System. Bellak has provided a scoring sheet which delineates 10 different categories of scoring which become integrated into a final diagnostic summary. Bellak's system summarizes the responses to the C.A.T. on 10 different dimensions and is based upon psychoanalytic theory. Each story is analyzed separately, but stories are interpreted in relationship to each other. Further, the sequencing of stories is often important in diagnostic meaning. In fact, most professionals believe the test to be invalid unless all 10 of the cards are used.

Bellak's first dimension of the 10 is *The Main Theme* which delineates the core psychological issues and conflicts for the child. In obtaining *the Main Theme* it is helpful to summarize or describe each response, including the plot and its psychological or diagnostic meaning, as well as to interpret free associations the testee may have made to the story. Bellak and others generally break down the Main Theme into 3 categories: descriptive level which is the manifest or obvious/external content; interpretive level; and diagnostic level (latent/unconscious meaning). Examination of all of these levels contributes to understanding of both the manifest and latent, (conscious and unconscious) meaning of these stories. It is important to note that stories may have multiple themes, which may, or may not, be related.

The second dimension of this system is *the Main Hero*. This dimension reflects the testee's representation of himself in the story. The Main Hero is the primary character around whom the story revolves. Usually, this character is the one most similar to the child in sex, age, appearance, vocation, abilities, and interests. However, Bellak cautions that occasionally a child may include more than one hero in a story and may identify with each of them at different times. He also notes that some children depict the hero of their story as the opposite sex. Both of these occurrences are of note and should be indicated on the scoring sheet and explored. The hero frequently represents the strengths and weaknesses (emotional, physical) that the child has, wants to have, or is afraid he may have. Bellak stresses the importance of examining the hero's feelings about his own adequacy and competence, as this is the best measure of ego strength with the C.A.T. This does not apply, however, in the case of obvious wish fulfillment, in which the child projects onto the hero all the qualities he or she wishes to possess in order to feel truly adequate.

The third dimension is the *Main Needs and Drives of the Hero*. These needs and drives may be overtly or covertly expressed, or indicated by information included or omitted from the child's stories. He or she may attribute to the hero characteristics and behaviors with which he or she already possesses in real life. For example, a very depressed boy may portray the character as depressive and apathetic. On the contrary, a child may attribute characteristics to the hero that reflect the unconscious wishes, impulses and drives of that child. For example, the depressive child may depict the hero as happy and enthusiastic. The unconscious motives behind such attributions to the hero can become very complex and must be teased apart carefully. The repetition of themes and corroborating material from other stories illuminate central issues, drives, impulses and wishes for the child.

Bellak notes that a useful way to deduce whether or not the story reflects "acting out" behavior of the child is to examine the amount of detail the child uses regarding these incidences. If the child describes these behaviors in great detail and vividness, they probably reflect his behaviors in daily life. Whereas, if the story is lacking in detail and is vague, the child is probably not "acting out" these wishes, impulses, and drives in daily life.

It is also clinically worthwhile to scrutinize and attempt to interpret objects or circumstances included, or omitted from, the story. If a child includes a gun in a picture where one does not exist, one may infer that he has a need for aggression. In contrast, if there is a pipe in the picture and the child chooses to omit it from his story this may represent a child's wish that it were not there. On a deeper level, this may also represent a child's anxiety concerning issues of orality.

The fourth dimension is the *Conception of the Environment or World*. This dimension reflects the child's perception of self and world as developed through memory traces of various life experiences. The tester can often find a common theme throughout the stories that represents how the child views the world. Often, a few adjectives can sum up this dimension (hostile, friendly, threatening).

The fifth dimension is entitled *Figures Seen as.* . . . This dimension focuses on examining the patient's object, or primary, relationships. In theory, the patient will project salient and significant past experiences with important figures onto the characters in the pictures. For example, if he or she experienced mother as domineering and controlling, stories including authority or female figures may share this common theme.

The sixth dimension examines *Significant Conflicts*. This dimension includes identifying not only conflicts but also defenses used to tolerate the anxiety that results from such conflicts. These conflicts are unconscious in nature and according to psychotherapists are thought to emerge when the Id drives and the Superego are at odds. Further, the extent of the conflict is related to how well the ego negotiates this battle. By examining significant conflicts, some have emphasized the opportunity to analyze early personality formation.

The seventh dimension is *Nature of Anxieties*. This dimension illuminates the source of the child's major anxieties (bodily harm, loss of parent, disapproval) which emanate from the source of conflict. In addition, the nature of the anxiety illuminates the competency with which the individual defends against such anxiety and the methods used in the defense (denial, passivity, aggression).

The eighth dimension, *Main Defenses against Conflicts and Fears,* is an overview of the main defense mechanisms used by the child. Examining the defense mechanisms or coping styles of the child can contribute to further illumination of the drives motivating them, as the drives are often more difficult to observe when masked by defense and other ego mechanisms. The ninth dimension is *Adequacy of Superego as Manifested by "Punishment for Crime."* Examination of the relationship between an offense (e.g., acting out behavior) and its punishment in the story provides the tester information regarding the strictness or leniency of the child's Superego. It is also helpful to note the degree of integration of the Superego and manifestations of such Superego involvement.

The tenth dimension, *Integration of the Ego,* examines the integration of the child's Ego and his or her ability to cope and function in daily life. The ability of the story's hero to resolve problems are of paramount importance in this dimension. Some authors recommend further scrutiny in this dimension including the 12 ego functions: reality testing, judgement, sense of reality, regulation and control of affects and impulses, object relations, thought processes, adaptive regression in the service of the ego, defensive functioning, stimulus barrier, autonomous ego functioning, synthetic functioning, and mastery-competence.

Another popular method of interpretation is the Need Threat Analysis System. The original version of this system was proffered by Murray in 1938 to be used for scoring the T.A.T. He recommended that each story be evaluated or scored by assessing the hero's needs and environmental presses. Subsequently, the tester would rank order them and use frequency of the various needs and presses to assess the testee's most important issues or concerns. He proposed approximately 40 needs and possibly more than 30 presses per story.

A similar system developed by Cox and Sargent (1950) examines each story for needs, threats, feelings, heroes, action and outcomes. It pairs five combinations of needs and threats, including Independence-Domination, Affiliation-Rejection, Security-Insecurity, Achievement-Failure, Aggression- Punishment. The goal of the Needs Threat Analysis System is to elucidate central needs and threats which evoke anxiety and stress in individuals. Each story is then reviewed and assessed for one or more binary. The frequency of each binary is recorded and rank ordered for significance/importance. Professionals believe that if the needs and threats are matched to actual life events, one can determine the meaningfulness of the stress to the individual. According to Chandler, Shermus & Lempert, one can interpret a child's unmet or quasi-met needs and perceived threat of danger harm, and loss (threats) and, in so doing, the origin and strength of a child's perceived stress can be estimated. Research shows that certain needs and threats are more common than others in evaluating C.A.T. protocols.

Finally, a common scoring method is a qualitative approach to interpretation of the C.A.T. frequently utilized in clinical practice. It involves approaching the C.A.T. line-by-line and word-for-word and examining the context as well as the latency to response and the total time of the stories. In addition, similarly to Bellak's system, the examiner accounts for the previous stories in considering the meaning of the current story coded. It is believed that specific words if used frequently enough or utilized in a specific manner or context can hold unconscious meaning. For example, it is believed that if the story contains references to the distant past (medieval times), the author is attempting to place distance between self and conflict as a defense. The frequent use of the term "thinking" refers to anxiety. Pauses throughout the story can refer to editing of potentially frightening unconscious material.

Often the examiner will circle key words which may hold latent meaning, particularly those that occur more than once or in unusual or salient position to other words. Professionals believe that the repetition of such terms is indicative of an important theme.

With respect to psychometrics, the system is considered reliable. The face validity for this approach for the skilled therapist and examiner is so extensive that it is tempting to believe that one can interpret this instrument as one can an X-ray or other physically concrete measurement. Novices will request a supervisor to "blindly" interpret a C.A.T.—similarly to reading tea leaves or a crystal ball. The C.A.T., like any other psychological test, is only meaningful when placed in the context of the person and should never be interpreted without background information.

The following case example demonstrates the use of the three most frequently used scoring systems for the C.A.T: Bellak's System, Chandler's Need Threat Analysis, and Qualitative Analysis. Administration included presentation of 10 cards; however, for demonstration purposes we have provided specific scoring for 5 cards. In the appendix, the reader will find the responses to the remaining 5 cards. It will be important for the reader to consider the content of the nonscored card responses in "evaluation" of the five scored cards. In addition, as stated above, it is crucial that the C.A.T. is not scored "blindly" but rather in the full context of historical information and any other available test data.

CASE EXAMPLE

"Jared," an attractive 5-year-and-3-month-old boy of multiethnic and racial heritages, was referred for evaluation by his private religious school due to his disruptive and aggressive behaviors. In the spring, the school's administration was so concerned about Jared's behavior they informed his parents that he could not return to school in the fall without evaluation and intervention.

With respect to Jared's history, he was the only son of Mr. and Mrs. Weiss and was adopted shortly after birth. The Weiss' told Jared about his adoption when he was 4½ years old (this was three months prior to the onset of symptoms). In addition, his maternal grandparents, to whom Jared was emotionally close, relocated approximately 1500 miles away when he turned 4 years old. The Weiss' stated that in December, when Jared was 4 years and 9 months, he began to exhibit conduct problems such as frequent "out-of-seat" behavior at school and disruption of other students. These were addressed by a sticker chart. The Weiss' said that both parents and teachers noted a significant improvement while Jared was on the charts until the middle of May (5 months later) wherein Jared's behavior deteriorated. In addition to the out-of-seat behaviors, Jared's behavior became much more aggressive and noncompliant. For example, he knocked down a tower built by another child and he kicked chairs and other children. Furthermore, he refused to comply with the "time-out" procedure at school.

Jared's parents reported that at home he is a very affectionate child, but at times has had difficulty controlling his anger. He also asked his parents when he can be "boss." The Weisses reported using a variety of discipline techniques, including explaining, lecturing, spanking by father, and "time-out" procedure.

The Weisses have been married for 10 years; she is an educator, and he is in the health care profession.

Assessment Measures

- Parent Interview: Mr. and Mrs. Weiss
- Child Interview
- School Personnel Interview: Guidance Counselor Two Teachers
- Behavioral Observation
- McCarthy Scales of Children's Abilities
- House–Tree–Person
- Draw-A-Person of the Opposite Sex
- Draw-A-Family
- Children's Apperception Test
- Revised-Behavior Problem Checklist-Parent Completed
- Child Behavior Checklist-Parent Completed

During the assessment sessions, Jared presented as an attractive pleasant boy who had a curious nature. During testing, however, it became evident that he exhibited somewhat of a low frustration tolerance level (giving up easily on tasks) and had some difficulty attending to the tasks presented him. His resistance seemed more oppositional in nature than as an attentional deficit per se. He did attend much more closely when given an external incentive for completing portions of the tests. Although these findings are reasonably valid indicators of his functioning, it is likely, due to Jared's difficulty in complying with tasks presented him, that the intellectual portion of the assessment was an underestimate of his true abilities.

Observation of his parents interacting with him revealed that both parents engaged in frequent criticizing/controlling behaviors, issued many commands, and delivered very little positive reinforcement, even when Jared complied with their commands. They attended much more closely to his disruptive behaviors than to his compliant behavior. It was also evident that the parents had frequent disagreements about disciplining Jared. Mrs. Weiss disapproved of the physical discipline Mr. Weiss occasionally delivered. In addition, Mr. Weiss presented as the meeker of the two parents and often succumbed to his wife's commands and parenting methods even though they conflicted with his own wishes. In session, some open conflict and hostility were evident between the two parents.

The following includes examples of Jared's responses and the scoring of five (numbers 1,2,4,5,9) of the 10 C.A.T. cards. The remaining cards are located in the appendices and should be considered in conjunction with the five example cards to determine the meaningfulness of Jared's material assessment.

Jared's C.A.T.—Card One

Card 1: (There is a table with a large bowl of food and several chicks sitting at the table. There is a vaguely outlined large chicken in the background.) (10" latency) "Once upon a time these birds were eating all kinds of food. Then when they were done, they were thinking about a chicken to have for their mom." (Examiner: "How did they feel?") "A little bad because they didn't have a mom and didn't have money. And a little good because they had a house and had food, because some other people let them have food." (22" total time)

Bellak's Scoring: Card One

1. Main Theme: nurturance: food and maternal love.
2. Main Hero: Children (self-image): dependency on others for survival.
3. Main Needs and Drives of Hero: maternal nurturance. (Figures and objects introduced in the story and the implication of this): Money, other people: The meaning of these for the patient includes: nurturance needs sought apart from mother. (Figures, objects omitted in background): the large figure in the background is indirectly alluded to as "thinking about" having a mother or as "other people" but not as an active figure in story—this implies that the child has a need for Mother but sees her as unaccessible and nonnurturing, withholding, and devoid of warmth.
   4. Conception of Environment; with respect to a patient's immediate environment (i.e., he sees his parents) as nonnurturing but believes that others in the world are capable of meeting his needs.
   5. Conception of Parental Figures: Patient views his parents as nonnurturing conception of Peer and Junior Figures: Patient views his peers or contemporaries as neutral.
   6. Significant Conflicts: Patient has an ambivalent attachment to Mother and Father
   7. Nature of Anxieties: Patient's source of anxiety includes his sense of feeling unloved as can be detected in the deprivation of food in the story.
   8. Main Defenses Against Conflicts and Fears: repression and denial (if Mother cannot help me survive, strangers will do it, and this feels good).
   9. Adequacy of Superego as Manifested by Punishment for Crime: If the crime in this story included a desire to replace the mother then the punishment would be adequate (they felt

"bad"). If in the story, the desire of the "birds" to rid themselves of the mother was via her death, then the superego is not adequate.

10. Integration of Ego, Manifesting Itself In: The patient's ego integration is ambivalent, unrealistic, however, he views the world as capable of meeting his needs to some extent.

Need Threat Analysis: Card One

Need: emotional nurturance, attachment.
Threat: loss of love, loss of mother/nurturance (food for survival).
Class of Need/Threat Combination: security-insecurity and affiliation-rejection.

Qualitative Interpretation: Card One

The latency time prior to the first response does not appear clinically significant due to the age of the child and because this is his first experience responding to the C.A.T. As the cognitive process of "thinking" can mean avoidance and being uncertain/insecure, it can be referred that Jared may be experiencing anxiety. In addition, this anxiety is the result of Jared's not feeling that his mother can meet his basic survival needs of nurturance and love (via food). There is ambivalence about having a mother as can be discerned by his willingness to accept that other people (in the story) can meet needs that generally are fulfilled by a mother and yet he has "bad" feelings because they (the birds in the story) do not have a mother and money.

Jared's C.A.T.—Card Two

Card 2: (One bear pulling one end of a horizontal rope while a second bear and a baby bear pull the other end of the rope.) (5" latency) "Once upon a time there were bears playing tug-of-war and then the momma bear was all alone pulling and then the momma bear fell inside a tug of war water. The momma bear felt good because she wanted to get wet but she felt bad because she fell and the baby bear and daddy felt good because they didn't fall."(17" total time)

Bellak's Scoring: Card Two

1. Main Theme: Mother pitted against baby and daddy bears. (Diagnostic level: conflict between parents, Oedipal conflict.)
2. Main Hero: The main heroes of the story included the baby and the father. As a result, Jared, identifying with a strong child figure, perceives himself (self-image) as strong. There is also evidence that Jared has become victorious over Mother's Oedipal seduction which results in appropriate identification with the father. Both father and child in this story align together and win the tug of war over the mother.
3. Main Needs and Drives of Hero: to identify/ align with Father; to negotiate anxiety associated with Oedipal conflict.
4. Conception of Environment/World: Jared's view of the world is ambivalent. The victory of Jared's main characters after the struggle felt good because he won. He attempted to rationalize the mother's falling down and loss as positive since she felt good to be wet.
5. Conception of Parental Figures: Mother as weaker than Father.
6. Significant Conflicts: Oedpial conflict.
7. Nature of Anxiety: Oedipal in that he aligns with Father to prevent Father's retaliation

against him for enjoying Mother. However, there remains some anxiety regarding Mother's response to his choosing of Father's side. This can be discerned in his "undoing" of Mother's fall; he felt bad because she fell, but good because she got all wet. His concern over Mother's response to her fall and his shared responsibility with Dad for the fall originate with basic fears of retaliation via abandonment (loss of love, physical abandonment, annihilation, etc.).

8. Main Defenses against Conflicts: undoing, denial.

9. Adequacy of Superego as Manifested by Punishment of the Crime: The superego in this case is too lenient as evidenced by the baby's and the father's feeling good because they didn't fall, even though the mother fell.

10. Integration of the Ego Manifesting Itself: The integration of the ego is adequate, since the child is able to control his id impulses through identifying with Father and rejecting his id impulses for Mother.

Need Threat Analysis: Card Two

Need: affiliation with Father, separation from Mother (growing up).
Threat: potential loss of Mother (she falls but is not injured).
Need/Threat Classification: Independence/domination and affiliation/rejection.

Qualitative Analysis: Card Two

Both the initial response and total latency (latency time and response time together) are insignificant. The child is struggling with Oedipal conflict. He is gravitating toward identifying with the father but is experiencing some concomitant anxiety in separating from his mother as he views her as being "alone," and once she falls, he quickly undoes the "pain" he has inflicted upon her by stating that she feels good for being wet. The water, from analytic theory, is believed to represent Mother's womb. Hence his struggle of separating from Mother to identify with father is further highlighted by introducing "tug of war water." If he had "lost" his Oedipal struggle and fell into the tug of war water, he would have returned to mother's womb and he would have been the Oedipal victor, winning Mother over Father. However, he in fact appropriately aligns with Father, giving the womb back to Mother, where it belongs. As with any conflict, there are other people involved, so whether or not a child successfully negotiates a developmental stage is not solely dependent upon the child. Negotiating developmental conflict involves other people, as is apparent in this vignette; the child also experiences the mother's pull or seduction to keep him in her womb. The term "pull" and his concomitant anxiety are evidence of this fact.

Jared's C.A.T.—Card Four

Card 4 (A small kangaroo is on a tricycle with a large Kangaroo next to the trike. This large kangaroo has a baby kangaroo in her pouch; she is wearing a hat and carrying a purse and a basket with a bottle in it.) (6" initial latency) "What is it? A kangaroo? A dog? (22" total latency to response). "Once upon a time the kangaroo was going to the supermarket, and they forgot they needed to go someplace important. This place was broken and they couldn't go to the place anymore, and they all had wanted to go to the special place." (Examiner: "What was this special place?") The big special place was a place to buy beautiful clothes to get married. The big special place was where they were going to buy beautiful marriage clothes and get married. It was broken." (Examiner: "How did they feel?") "Good." (Total time 97")

Bellak's Scoring: Card Four

1. Main Theme: Forgetting something special, something more special even than food. This special event concerns marriage. But this special place was broken. The broken marriage place reflects Jared's Oedipal conflict over wishing to marry his mother. Similarly, it may reflect conflict within his own parent's marriage. Such "real" conflict would serve to heighten his Oedipal victor anxiety (i.e., if Mother's and Father's marriage fails, then Jared's conquest of Mother is a greater possibility).

2. Main Hero: According to some, this card typically represents sibling rivalry. Since Jared is an only child sibling rivalry would be latent. The heroes in this card are referred to as "they" (the kangaroos). It is apparent that the heroes are viewed as ineffective and powerless as they needed to get to an important place that, once remembered, was broken. Hence Jared probably views himself and his family members as ineffective and powerless, especially in matters of marriage (his parents' real marriage and a fantasied Oedipal union) and unity of family.

3. Main Needs and Drives of the Hero: Id drive for Mother but conflict due to struggle with need to identify with Father. Figures, Objects Introduced and Implications of this: "Supermarket" and "broken place" represent Oedipal conflict.

4. Conception of Environment (immediate environment, parents). Unpredictable, not fulfilling, anxiety provoking since important places tied to survival are broken.

5. Conception of Parent Figures: The marriage is broken. There is conflict between the parents and Oedpial conflict. Conception of Peers and Junior Figures: This is not evident in this story.

6. Significant Conflicts: Oedpial.

7. Nature of Anxieties: Fear of retaliation by Father if Oedipal conflict is not successfully negotiated. This conflict is even greater in light of the marital conflict between parents.

8. Main Defenses Against Anxieties and Fears: repression and denial.

9. Adequacy of Superego: adequate.

10. Integration of Ego, manifesting itself in: somewhat unrealistic. Although Jared realizes he may not marry his mother and that the "marriage place is broken," he denies harboring any negative feelings about the demise of a space that is even more important than the basic necessity of survival—food (as represented by the supermarket).

Need Threat Analysis: Card Four

Need: Love, nurturance, attachment.
Threat: "Forgetting" and "broken" both lead to losses.
Need-Threat configuration: security/insecurity; affiliation/rejection

Qualitative Analysis: Card Four

Jared's anxiety is shown initially by his initial query about the composition of the card presented him and the relatively long latency time. The term "forgetting" is a direct reference to repression. From theory, individuals repress what is too anxiety provoking or threatening. From psychodynamic theory, food represents love, nurturance, and survival. The special place was even more special to Jared than basic love and nurturance/sustenance—this special place of marriage is experienced by Jared as greater in importance than basic survival food. Jared views marriage as broken and this is a reference to difficulties both negotiating Oedipal conflict and his own parents' marriage. Further, Jared denies any painful or rageful feelings he has in order to cope with the above conflicts.

Jared's C.A.T.—Card Five

Card 5 (In the foreground is a picture of a crib with two small bears lying inside and a large lumpy bed in the background. There is no one visible in this bed, but the ambiguous lumpy manner by which the bed is made could be suggestive of someone under the covers.) (an immediate response) "Oh! (pause for 18 seconds) Once upon a time there was a little baby cat who was sleeping in a crib and he thought a bad guy was coming to get him and the bad guy was in a costume. Lions, alligators, crocodiles. Dad, Mom, Grandpa, *Me,* and Sister and Brother all got dead, and they were dying. No, me, the brother and sister lived." (Examiner: "How did baby cat feel?") "Good because he lived and two people lived. The end." (52" total time).

Bellak's Scoring: Card Five

1. Main Theme: loss of loved ones, particularly those responsible for caretaking. Fear of annihilation, feeling not protected and that the environment cannot be trusted. Similarly, people are not as they seem (e.g., "A guy" in costume).

2. Main Hero: Baby cat. In this story, Jared used a diminutive weak animal "Baby cat" as the main hero and infused him with power to survive dangerous interactions (e.g., a bad guy in a costume). Jared sees himself as a survivor with power. It is also evident that he is ambivalent between feeling victimized and feeling empowered, as can be detected through his vacillation between being killed and surviving the traumatic event in this story.

3. Main Needs and Drives of the Hero (figures and objects introduced and implications): survival, protection, aggressive drive killing off all caretakers, rage at caretakers, need to have contemporaries (siblings) live.

4. Conception of Environment: immediate environment: unsafe, not trustworthy, threatening, aggressive.

5. Conception of Parent Figures: not able to protect, rage towards parents. Conception of Contemporary Figures: need to be protected, not safe.

6. Significant Conflicts: struggle between superego and Id that is punishing the self (by death) for aggression towards others. In the end, Id wins as others die, but self remains intact.

7. Nature of Anxieties: aggression, feelings of being overpowered and devoured.

8. Main Defenses: undoing, repression, denial, since he feels good that he and two people lived but all caretakers died.

9. Adequacy of Superego: inappropriate, vacillates between too lenient and too harsh.

10. Integration of Ego:
   Hero: inadequate.
   Outcome: unrealistic, unhappy.
   Drive control: insufficient plot, processes inappropriate.

Need Threat Analysis: Card Five

Need: safety, protection, nurturance.
Threat: rage (self and other).
Need Threat Configuration: security/insecurity, independence/domination.

Qualitative Interpretation: Card Five

Jared's initial response is one of exclamation followed by an 18 second latency to response. This initial reaction and reaction time is indicative of anxiety and is an attempt to negotiate threatening material by the ego. Initially Jared sees himself as a "little baby" animal. These terms represent regression. He does not feel his home environment, including he himself, is safe from overwhelming violence. He "undoes" his death but denies feeling badly even though all the caretaking relatives die. Although this reflects inadequate ego integration and superego functioning, it resolves his anxiety, which includes Oedipal conflict (if both Mom and Dad are dead, the conflict is resolved) as well as his rage at his parents both for their role in problems negotiating his Oedipal conflict as well as their own marital problems and parenting styles.

Card 9 Jared's C.A.T.—Card Nine

(A picture with an open door in the foreground which reveals a small rabbit in a juvenile bed. The rabbit is sitting prone and looking toward the door. The room is dimly lit and on the opposite wall from the door is a window, drapes drawn, and partially open.) (4" latency) "One day there was a rabbit. He was feeling good (4" pause) and then suddenly he didn't feel good because his mom was so angry. She was always so angry. Because she was a crocodile and never wanted to be his mother.(Jared pauses for 22" then puts the card down and appears finished.) (Examiner: "What happened when he grew up?") Nothing, he didn't want to grow up. It was magic. He didn't have to grow up. (46" total time)

Bellak's Scoring: Card Nine

1. Main Theme: aggression, under threat, unloved, dominated to stay young.
2. Main Hero: attempts at self-empowerment. He can decide whether he grows up or not, but he feels diminutive (stays a child) and under threat by angry mother crocodile, especially as he matures and grows.
3. Main Needs and Drives of Hero: safety and love. Aggressive drives which are projected via the mother crocodile.
4. Conception of the Environment: not safe, nonnurturing.
5. Parent Figures: aggressive, hostile, sadistic, nonprotective
6. Significant Conflicts: dependence-independence and maturity. The mother represents the superego. In this story, the mother is successful such that her son stays young to avoid the angry hostile crocodile mother. Hence, the dependency conflict overrides Jared's independence need.
7. Nature of Anxiety: Jared fears physical harm and/or punishment, if he separates and becomes independent. He feels overpowered and "helpless," devoured by his mother. He fears and experiences loss of mother's love. (His mother doesn't want to be a mother).
8. Main Defenses Against Conflicts and Fears: repression, denial, magical thinking.
9. Adequacy of Superego: Jared's superego is too severe in its attempt to control his need for independence and Oedipal strivings. He almost loses his life as he negotiates the conflict between needs and desires.
10. Integration of Ego: Jared's ego functioning is inadequate as depicted by the story's hero's ambivalence and use of undoing. Further the environment which Jared presents and projects is threatening and dangerous. The outcome of the story is unrealistic as the adult

caretakers all die, but the children/babies live despite a killer in the house. While Jared's main hero lives, the story is not a happy one; this is a story of survival and not one of triumph.

Need Threat Analysis: Card Nine

Need: love, nurturance (to be able to grow up), protection.

Threat: Rejecting, angry mother who is extremely dangerous (crocodile).

Need-Threat Configurations: affiliation-rejection, security-insecurity, independence-domination.

Qualitative Analysis: Card Nine

Jared's ambivalence and concomitant anxiety is detected in a switch of affect for the primary character at the beginning of the story. The term "suddenly" often refers to an unexpected occurrence or change of events which creates anxiety by its unpredictability. The ambivalence begins to dissipate and the patient's affect becomes definitive. Further, his primary conflict becomes clear and both affect and conflict match. He doesn't feel "good" because he believes the hostility and anger he experiences from his mother is because she does not want him. The manifest content of the story is very close (near) to the latent meaning. The disguised or symbolic rage expressed in all of the other stories is revealed directly in this story. In addition to his struggle with the Oedipal conflict, he is clearly angry at his mother for her overt hostility and rejection which he may interpret as a response to his disengaging from her as part of the successful negotiation of the Oedipal conflict. Further, his anxiety concerning his conflict is evident in his not wanting to face the future with her.

Assessment Results

The McCarthy Scales of Children's Abilities (MSCA) indicate Jared to be functioning in the bright-normal range with a General Cognitive Index (GCI) Score of 115. This yields a mental age of 6 years and 2 months. Jared performed at one standard deviation above the mean for his normative group on tests of verbal and performance functioning. He also performed at one standard deviation above the mean for both his overall GCI and tests that measure visual and verbal memory.

Tests of emotional and personality functioning suggest that Jared feels that his needs for nurturance are not being satisfactorily met. For example, throughout the Children's Apperception Test (C.A.T.), Jared told stories of vulnerable child animals who did not have parents or whose parents and/or grandparents were killed, enraged or ineffective. Furthermore, he views caretakers with much ambivalence in that they are unaccessible, rejecting, angry, and to be feared (e.g., when mother turned into a crocodile), yet they are available at specific times when the child needs assistance, such as in toilet training.

In calculating the frequency of the need-threat binaries for the five C.A.T. stories, Jared's most frequently told stories included affiliation-rejection and security-insecurity themes. These need-threat binaries, revolving around survival, nurturance, and love, are not only consistent with the other C.A.T. analysis but with other assessment results as well.

His need for nurturance and greater support from his environment was also indicated in the interview when he said that he played by himself some and that this was lonely and made him sad. In addition, when asked what he likes doing with his father, he responded "play with him and eat lots of candy," but stated that with his mother "he didn't know (what he likes doing) that she only works." Furthermore, his House-Tree-Person (H-T-P) also indicated a lack of feelings of support from his environment in that the tree was barren, the house was inaccessible, and the people were without much detail.

Another issue for Jared includes a pervasive sense of anger which more than likely contributes to his sometimes noncompliant and oppositional behavior. Aggressive themes with concomitant anxiety were pervasive throughout the C.A.T., with death and destruction evident in many of his stories. This anxiety may be responsible for Jared's feeling that "all the time you're trapped in a rocket ship and feel like you're going to throw-up." This aggression was also evident on the Child Behavior Checklist and the Revised-Behavior Problem Checklist as evident through Jared's difficulties in bothering others, fighting, disobedience, and arguing.

It is likely that the anger, isolation, and lack of feelings of support from his primary caretakers originate from his parents' overintrusiveness, as well as from attempts at negotiating Oedipal conflict. Jared's parents have low tolerance for any deviation from their ideas and have excessively high expectations of their son; this is evident in their difficulty in allowing Jared to be his own person, as they are critical and controlling of his behavior. His questionning of when does he get to be boss reflects this, as does his statement of feeling trapped and nauseous. Further, his sense of not being his own person is indicated in his family drawing in which he placed himself between his parents, drawing himself without a nose and mouth, whereas his parents have both. Part of his separation and maturity is the result of successful negotiation of Oedipal conflict. Jared's primary mechanisms of defense include denial, repression, and undoing.

SUMMARY

The purpose of this chapter was to describe the Children's Apperception Test and its utility in psychological assessment. In addition, specific nuances of administration were described. Finally, the goal of this paper was to present several scoring systems, and to illustrate their use through actual case material. Three different scoring systems which vary in structure, coverage and process, were presented and applied to actual case material.

SUGGESTED READINGS

Bellak, L. (1993). *The T.A.T., C.A.T., and S.A.T. in clinical use* (5th ed.). Boston, M.A.: Allyn and Bacon.

Bellak, L., & Bellak, S. (1949). *Children's Apperception Test.* New York: C.P.S. Co.

Bellak, L. and Bellak, S. (1965). *The C.A.T.-H.-A human modification.* Larchmont, NY: C.P.S. Inc.

Bellak, L., & Bellak, S. (1952). *Children's Apperception Test-Supplement (C.A.T.-S.).* NY: C.P.S. Co.

Cain, A. (1961). A supplementary dream technique with the Children's Apperception Test. *Journal of Clinical Psychology, 17,* 181-184.

Chandler, L. A., Shermis, M. D., & Lempert, M. E. (1989). *The need-threat analysis: A scoring system for the Children's Apperception Test.* Psychology in the Schools, 26, 47–54.

Exner, J. E. (1974). *The Rorschach: A comprehensive system, Vol. 1.* New York: Wiley.

Haworth, M. (1966). *The C.A.T.: Facts about fantasy.* New York: Grune & Stratton.

APPENDIX A
C.A.T. CARDS

Card 3 (12" latency) "Once upon a time there was a little mouse with a big hole. Every-day the lion was his friend. Everyday, when the lion was smoking, the mouse smelled the smoke and came out to play with him and then the lion roared because he thought it was a new mouse and so the mouse said, "it's your friend—it's your mouse friend, and then the lion played with him because it was his friend and he still needed his thing, cane and pipe." (37" total time)

Card 6 (8" latency) "Once upon a time this little bear was happy because he just had one mom he wasn't happy because he didn't have a dad and then a stranger came and took him and mom jumped up to see what happened and it was a stranger and then the momma bear killed him because he was a bad guy stranger. The momma bear felt good and bad. She felt bad because the stranger took the baby bear and she felt good because she killed the bad guy. The baby bear felt good because the momma bear killed the stranger." (23" total time)

Card 7 (3" latency) "Once upon a time there was this tiger and this monkey was always bothering him. The tiger always tried to kill him, but the monkey was too fast and then the tiger jumped up and then a lion and bear and the man came to kill the tiger because the man always wanted to kill the monkey, and they killed the tiger. (Examiner: "How did the monkey feel?") "Good." (17" total latency)

Card 8 (Jared visibly anxious, 3" latency) "What's this picture?" (45" pause prior to starting the story). "Once upon a time this little baby monkey bear stayed up all the night. He almost died, but didn't, and then he changed into a crocodile. And then this monkey crocodile, he wriggled his tail and killed all the mommas, daddies, grandpas and grandmas. How did the monkey crocodile feel? Good because he was all by himself and they didn't bother him be-cause before they didn't let him stay up all the nights." (71" total time)

Card 10 (5" latency) "One day this doggie was playing with his mother, and he needed to make but couldn't. His mommy picked him up to help him out. He felt good. The end." (15" total time)

16

Minnesota Multiphasic Personality Inventory-Adolescent (MMPI-A)

Johnathan David Forbey and Yossef S. Ben-Porath

INTRODUCTION

The Minnesota Multiphasic Personality Inventory–Adolescent (MMPI-A) is the new adolescent-specific version of the original Minnesota Multiphasic Personality Inventory (MMPI). It was developed during the revision and restandardization of the original MMPI, which also yielded the MMPI-A, the revised adult-specific version of the MMPI. The interested reader is referred to the MMPI-2 chapter found in this text for a thorough review and description of the newly revised MMPI form for adults.

The MMPI-A was developed to address concerns about using the MMPI with adolescents. Before describing the MMPI-A, we first provide a review of the history of MMPI use with adolescents. This overview identifies the reasons why separate instruments were eventually developed for use with adolescents and adults.

A BRIEF HISTORY OF THE USE OF THE MMPI WITH ADOLESCENTS

The MMPI was originally intended for use with individuals 16 and older. However, use of MMPI with adolescent populations began at almost the same time the instrument was originally developed. Initial studies demonstrated the test's ability to differentiate between groups of delinquent and nondelinquent adolescent females based on differences in their scores on specific clinical scales, particularly Clinical Scale 4.

In the late 1940s and early 1950s, two researchers, Starke Hathaway and Elio Monachesi, began an MMPI data collection project targeted specifically at adolescents. Their data collection efforts focused on Minnesota ninth graders, and, over the course of several years, these

Johnathan David Forbey and Yossef S. Ben-Porath • Department of Psychology, Kent State University, Kent, Ohio 44242.

Understanding Psychological Assessment, edited by Dorfman and Hersen. Kluwer Academic/Plenum Publishers, New York, 2001.

investigators accumulated the largest adolescent MMPI data set ever collected, consisting of more than 11,000 ninth graders. In addition, close to 4,000 of these adolescents repeated the MMPI during their senior year of high school. Hathaway and Monachesi collected additional data on all of these adolescents, including school records, teacher ratings, scores on intelligence tests, and results from the Strong Vocational Interest Blank. This extratest data-set was collected to compare adolescent MMPI results with external criteria.

Hathaway and Monachesi sought to identify MMPI predictors that could serves as risk indicators for later development of delinquent behaviors. They found that certain MMPI scales (specifically Clinical Scales 4, 8, and 9) seem to serve "excitatory" functions that are related to acting out or delinquent behavior. Their research also indicated that differences exist between adolescent males and females in terms of item endorsement frequencies, and, more importantly, that large differences exist between adolescents and adults in terms of item endorsement patterns. This led to consideration of developing adolescent-specific norms for the instrument.

DEVELOPMENT OF ADOLESCENT NORMS FOR THE ORIGINAL MMPI

The differences noted in item endorsement patterns between adolescents and adults translated into differences in MMPI results for adolescents. When plotted on adult norms, adolescents (both normal and in clinical settings) consistently generated profiles that were much more elevated than their adult counterparts. Several studies found that adolescents typically had higher elevations on MMPI scales F, 4, 6, 7, 8, and 9 when compared to adults. In addition, in clinical settings, adolescents tended to score significantly higher on scales reflective of serious psychopathology (F, 4, 6, and 8) than did their adult counterparts.

Although researchers were aware of the discrepancies in the endorsement frequencies between adults and adolescents, some felt that the development of a separate set of adolescent norms would "erase" or minimize the contrast between adolescents and adults. Nonetheless, several sets of adolescent norms were developed for the MMPI. The first of these was introduced by Marks and Briggs in 1972. These norms were derived from the responses of about 1,800 normal adolescents and were reported separately for males and females. In addition to separating the norms by gender, Marks and Briggs also separated them into four distinct age groups: 17, 16, 15, and 14 or younger. This set of norms was based on a combination of a selected sample of adolescents from the Hathaway and Monachesi adolescent data set collected during the late 1940s and early 1950s and several samples of adolescents collected throughout the United States in the 1960s.

Two other sets of MMPI adolescent norms were introduced after the Marks and Briggs norms were published. Research comparing the three sets of MMPI norms indicated significant differences in profile elevation by norm set. The absence of a clearly agreed upon set of norms for adolescent MMPI interpretation was a major factor leading to the development of the MMPI-A.

Although it had very early beginnings and was pursued throughout the years by numerous investigators, the research on the use of the MMPI with adolescents was far outpaced by research examining the MMPI's use with adults. As a result, most of the interpretive statements made about adolescents came from research conducted with adults (or a combination of adolescents and adults) and from clinical lore, not from MMPI research done specifically with adolescents. This left unanswered questions about the reliability and validity of interpretations made when using the MMPI with adolescents. As a result of these and other concerns outlined in the next section, in 1982, when the MMPI publisher, the University of Minnesota Press, embarked on a project to update the normative base for the instrument, a separate project was initiated to explore the feasibility of developing an adolescent-specific version of the MMPI.

TEST DEVELOPMENT AND CONSTRUCTION

Beginning in the 1960s, concerns were expressed that the MMPI normative sample was outdated and inappropriate given the expanding population base with which the instrument was being used. Concerns were also voiced regarding the content, wording, and relevance of some of the test items for use with contemporary adults and adolescents. These concerns led to the development of a new adult version of the MMPI, the MMPI-2 (for ages 18 and up), and later, to a new adolescent-specific version of the MMPI, the MMPI-A.

The MMPI-A was developed, in part, to address norming concerns that hampered use of the original MMPI with adolescents. In addition, the MMPI-A authors sought to shorten the length of the test and to add and alter items to make them more relevant for adolescents. Finally, the MMPI developers sought to clarify the wording of some of the original items, drop repeated items, and remove items that may be deemed objectionable or offensive.

Development of the MMPI-A began with the an experimental form labeled MMPI-TX. It contained 704 items, including the original 550 MMPI items as well as 58 new items that were borrowed from the MMPI-2. These 58 items were designed to address issues such as treatment compliance, attitudes toward self-change, alcohol and drug use, and suicide potential. In addition to these 58 items, 96 new items were added that were designed to address adolescent specific concerns. These items were designed to assess problems, behaviors, and attitudes in areas such as identity formation, peer-group influence, school and teachers, relationships with parents and families, and sexuality.

Additional forms were used during the development of the MMPI-A to compare MMPI-A results with extratest data. For the normative sample, these included a biographical information form (designed to obtain demographic information and data on family structure, parental occupation, residence, and family history) and a life events form (in order to determine what, if any, stressful life events had occurred during the last six months of the adolescents' lives). For clinical sample adolescents, in addition to the biographical form and the life events form, the Child Behavior Check List, the Devereux Adolescent Behavior Rating Scale, and a record review form (based on a structured review of each adolescent's clinical chart) were also used.

The MMPI-A normative sample is described in full detail in the test manual. Thus, only a brief description is provided here. In total, 805 boys and 815 girls between the ages of 14 and 18 from 8 states were included in the normative sample. Ethnically, approximately 76% of this sample were White, 12% were African American, 3% were Asian American, 3% were American Indian, 2% were Hispanic, 3% reported having another ethnic identity, and about 1% did not report their ethnicity. In terms of parental education, more than half of the sample reported that their parents had at least some college experience, thus providing a somewhat more educated group of participants than that of the population in general. More than two-thirds of the participants were from intact families, about one quarter lived with their mother only, and about 4% lived with their father only.

The MMPI-A clinical sample consisted of 420 boys and 293 girls aged 14–18. The clinical sample came solely from one state (Minnesota), but from several different types of treatment facilities. The majority of these individuals came from inpatient alcohol and drug treatment units; others came from inpatient mental health facilities, day-treatment programs, and a special school program. Ethnically, the breakdown for the clinical sample is similar to that for the normative sample, with the exception of African Americans (approximately 6%) and American Indians (approximately 6%). This discrepancy between the clinical and normative sample resulted from the fact that more American Indians and fewer African Americans live in Minnesota (as compared to other states).

ADMINISTRATION AND SCORING

The MMPI-A can be administered by trained, licensed psychologists, or under their supervision by other individuals (e.g., technicians) who have been properly trained to administer the instrument. There are three methods for administering the MMPI-A: Paper-and-pencil, using a standard test booklet and answer sheet, by computer, or by audiotape. Before administering the MMPI-A, it is necessary to determine the testability of the adolescent. To provide useful information, the test taker must be able and motivated to comprehend and respond relevantly to the test items. An essential requirement is adequate English language reading and comprehension skills. The minimal recommended reading level is sixth grade. In some instances, when an adolescent has attention deficit hyperactivity symptoms, it may be necessary to provide frequent breaks in test administration. Computerized administration of the test is generally faster and more efficient because there is no need for the test taker to move back and forth between a booklet and answer sheet. Paper-and-pencil administration of the MMPI-A typically requires 45 to 75 minutes, whereas computerized administration of the test can be accomplished in 30 to 60 minutes.

MMPI-A profiles can be scored by hand or by computer. Templates are available to facilitate hand scoring, however this tends to be an arduous, error-prone process. In contrast, computertized scoring is efficient and accurate, particularly when scannable answer sheets are used to avoid the need to hand enter an adolescent's item responses.

Whereas MMPI-A administration and scoring are relatively simple, proper test interpretation requires considerable training and expertise. Individuals who interpret the MMPI-A should have training in test theory and familiarity with adolescent personality structure, development, and psychopathology. In addition, individuals who interpret the MMPI-A results should be aware of the ethical issues regarding test interpretation and the communication of test results. They must have graduate-level training in personality assessment and be licensed to practice psychology. Textbooks are available to assist MMPI-A interpreters (see list of suggested readings at the end of this chapter). In the following section, we provide interpretive guidelines for the MMPI-A. These guidelines will familiarize readers with basic aspects of MMPI-A interpretation. However, they do not relieve the interpreter of the responsibility to acquire the levels of training and expertise just mentioned.

Interpretive Guidelines

The MMPI-A has four sets of scales: Validity, Clinical, Content and Supplementary. In this section, we present interpretive guidelines for each set of scales. The scale descriptors are based on research with adolescents. Most come from data published in the MMPI-A manual based on extratest information collected for the normative and clinical samples. Unless otherwise specified, the descriptors apply to both genders, and elevation refers to T-scores of 60 or greater.

Validity Scale Descriptions

There are eight MMPI-A validity scales. These include the Cannot Say (CNS), Lie (L), Infrequency (F), Defensiveness (K), Variable Response Inconsistency (VRIN), and True Response Inconsistency (TRIN) scales plus the F scale which is divided into to subscales, F1 and F2.

The Cannot Say Index (CNS) is a count of the number of items left unanswered, or answered in both directions ("true" and "false") by an adolescent. It is not a scale, per se, and, therefore, does not have a standard score transformation. MMPI-A protocols where CNS is greater than 15, should be interpreted with caution. The location of item omissions plays a role in their interpretation. All of the items needed to score the MMPI-A basic profile (consisting of scales L, F1, K, and the ten clinical scales) appear within the first 350 items in the test booklet. This is so that it may be possible to administer an abbreviated form of the test to adolescents who are incapable of completing the full 478-item test. Thus, if all or most of the item omissions occur after item 350, it is still possible to interpret the basic profile.

The L scale consists of 14 items and was designed to detect naïve attempts by adolescents to put themselves in a favorable light (unsophisticated "faking good"). Adolescents with high scores on the L scale (T≥65) deny relatively minor flaws or weaknesses. Moderate elevations (T-scores between 60 and 64) suggest a cautionary statement be made about the possibility of a defensive response style. One of the original L items was removed from the MMPI-A version of the test because it was deemed to be developmentally inappropriate.

The F scale on the MMPI-A consists of 66 items that no more than 20% of the adolescents in the MMPI-A normative sample endorsed in the keyed direction. The original MMPI F scale was often highly elevated in adolescents. This is because many of its items did not function appropriately as infrequent response indicators. Therefore, in the process of developing the MMPI-A, its authors eliminated the original MMPI F scale and developed the current F scale based on the criterion just mentioned. The MMPI-A scale is divided into two sub-scales, F1 and F2, that consist of the first and second sets of 33 items as they appear in the test booklet. Comparison of T-scores on F1 and F2 allows the test interpreter to detect whether any significant changes in the adolescent's approach to the test occurred between the first and second half of the inventory.

Three non-mutually-exclusive factors may lead to elevations on the F scale. These include an attempt on the part of the test taker to "fake bad," the presence of severe psychological maladjustment, or a random or careless response set. When the F scale is moderately elevated (T-scores between 80 and 89), concerns about a problematic response pattern should be suggested. When the F scale T-score is 90 or above, it is possible that the resulting MMPI-A profile is invalid. The VRIN scale (described below) helps rule in or out the possibility that random responding may account for an elevated score on F. If F is elevated, but VRIN is not, then random responding can be ruled out, leaving the need to differentiate between faking and exaggeration on the one hand and genuine reporting of significant psychological disturbance on the other. In this task, the clinician must rely on extratest data regarding the adolescent's current level of adjustment.

If, for example, an adolescent, who has been functioning well in school and at home and has no history of significant behavioral problems, produces a very high score on F, coupled with a normal limits score on VRIN, then the possibility of faking or exaggeration should be considered. If the same pattern is found in an adolescent with a documented history of severe psychopathology, then it is more likely that the elevation on F reflects severe psychopathology rather than malingering or exaggeration.

A differential pattern of elevation on F1 and F2 reflects a change in the adolescent's test-taking attitude. Typically, when this occurs, F2 will be substantially higher (at least 20 T-score points) than F1. If this is the case, and the T-score on F2 exceeds 90, the clinician should refrain from interpreting the MMPI-A Content scales that contain many items that appear in the second half of the booklet.

The *K* scale of the MMPI-A consists of 30 items that were selected with the original MMPI to identify individuals in psychiatric settings who displayed significant degrees of psychopathology, but produced MMPI profiles within normal limits . Elevated scores on the K scale indicate a defensive response pattern on the MMPI-A. Unlike with the MMPI and MMPI-A, the MMPI-A does not employ a K correction procedure (where a certain percentage of K is added to some of the clinical scales to correct for defensiveness). An MMPI profile should never be invalidated based solely on a high K score. A T-score greater than or equal to 65 on K is, however, suggestive of a defensive test-taking attitude that may result in an underestimate of the test takers problems as reflected in her or his scores on the substantive scales of the instrument.

Variable Response Inconsistency (VRIN) and True Response Inconsistency (TRIN) are two newly developed validity scales designed to complement the traditional validity indicators. Both VRIN and TRIN are made up of specially selected pairs of items. For VRIN, the item pairs have either similar or opposite content. If a person responds inconsistently to these item pairs, a point is earned on VRIN. High VRIN scores suggest that the adolescent responded to the MMPI-A in a careless manner, and, if high enough, indicates that the profile is uninterpretable.

The TRIN scale is made up exclusively of pairs that are opposite in content. If a person responds inconsistently by answering true to both items, one point is added to the TRIN score. If a person responds inconsistently by answering false to both items, one point is subtracted from the TRIN score. Therefore, a high TRIN raw score suggests the tendency on the part of the test taker to answer true to all of the questions; whereas a low TRIN raw score indicates a tendency to respond in the false direction to all questions. T-scores greater than 75 on VRIN or TRIN are suggestive of an invalid and uninterpretable test protocol. The T-Score on TRIN can never be lower than 50. If it is 50, this means that there was no pervasive pattern of inconsistent "true" or "false" responding. If it is greater than 50, it will be followed by a "T" or and "F," indicating the direction of inconsistent responding.

MMPI-A validity scale interpretation is often accomplished by comparing scores on the validity scales. For example, as was just mentioned, interpretation of scores on F depends upon the score on VRIN. Similarly, the response sets of "yea saying" or "nay saying," detected by TRIN, will likely affect scores on L and K, because all but one of the items scored on these scales are keyed false.

The MMPI-A Clinical Scales

The MMPI-A retains the 10 clinical scales that were developed for use with the original MMPI. With the exception of scales 5 and 0 (where many items were removed to reduce the length of the adolescent version of the inventory), the 10 clinical scales are essentially the same as those found on the MMPI and MMPI-A. However, unlike the MMPI-2, the cutoff for clinically significant elevation on the MMPI-A is a T-score of 60. In the following descriptions, the clinical scales are identified primarily by their numeric designators because their descriptive labels no longer reflect accurately the constructs assessed by these scales. The following descriptions identify some of the most salient, adolescent-specific features associated with elevations on these scales. They are based primarily on research done with the normative and clinical samples collected for the MMPI-A development project. For exhaustive lists of correlates associated with these scales, the reader is referred to the MMPI-A texts listed in the suggested readings at the end of this chapter.

Scale 1 (Hypochondriosis, Hs) consists of 32 items that reflect a preoccupation with health and illness. Scores on Scale 1 are related to many different physical complaints as well as to problems in school for both sexes. In addition, girls with high scores on Scale 1 are likely to report more family problems.

Scale 2 (Depression, D) consists of 57 items that tap issues such as dissatisfaction with life, feelings of discouragement, hopelessness, and low morale. The MMPI-A manual reports that high scores on Scale 2 are related to depression and suicidal ideation in both sexes. Girls in the clinical sample with elevations on Scale 2 were likely to engage in acting-out behaviors, to be socially withdrawn, to have few or no friends, to report somatic concerns, and to have low-esteem. Clinical sample boys with elevation on Scale 2 were described as being guilt-prone, fearful, withdrawn, perfectionistic, clinging, and worrying.

Scale 3 (Hysteria, Hy) is made up of 60 items that were selected originally to identify individuals who respond to stress with hysterical reactions. The MMPI-A manual reports that only clinical sample girls demonstrated an association between somatic complaints and scores on this scale. For clinical sample boys with elevations on Scale 3, the most common symptom was having a history of suicidal ideation or gestures.

Scale 4 (Psychopathic Deviate, Pd) consists of 49 items that reflect antisocial behavior. The MMPI-A manual reports that elevations on Scale 4 are related to school, family, and legal problems, as well as to lying, cheating, stealing, temper outbursts, and aggression. In addition, clinical sample males with high scores on Scale 4 were likely to have run away from home or to have been physically abused. Clinical sample females with elevations on Scale 4 were reported likely to be sexually active and may have been sexually abused.

Correlates involving a history of physical or sexual abuse must be interpreted cautiously because of the implications they raise. The association between elevations on MMPI-A scales and a history of abuse are not sufficiently strong to warrant a direct inference that abuse has indeed occurred. Rather, elevations on scales associated with a possible history of abuse should be viewed as risk indicators that require careful follow-up to explore the possibility that an adolescent has been the victim of abuse. This caveat applies to all MMPI-A scales suggestive of a possible history of abuse.

Scale 5 (Masculinity-Femininity, MF) underwent a significant change from the original MMPI. Sixteen items were removed from this scale to reduce the overall length of the test. Deleted items were redundant, objectionable, irrelevant to adolescents, or did not differentiate between the two genders. Correlates for boys and girls differ for this scale. The MMPI-A manual reports that for clinical sample boys, elevations on Scale 5 were reflective of intelligence, good grades in school, and better school adjustment. For girls, elevations on Scale 5 were associated with behavior problems, suspension from school, a history of learning disabilities, and a number of other acting out behaviors. The MMPI-A manual points out that the finding for girls differs from previous research on the relation between high scores Scale 5 and extratest criteria. Thus, the MMPI-A manual suggests caution when interpreting an elevated on clinical Scale 5 for girls.

Scale 6 (Paranoia, Pa) consists of 40 items selected to identify patients who were manifesting paranoid symptomatology. The MMPI-A manual reports that elevations on Scale 6 were associated with aggressive acting out and argumentative behavior for both genders. For boys in the clinical sample, elevations on Scale 6 were associated with hostile, dependent, and withdrawn behaviors. For girls in this sample, elevations on Scale 6 were also associated with an increase in disagreements with parents.

Scale 7 (*Psychasthenia, Pt*) consists of 48 items that cover a wide variety of symptomatology associated generally with anxiety. The MMPI-A manual reports that for girls in the clinical sample, elevations on Scale 7 were related to depression and increased discord with parents; whereas for clinical sample boys, elevations were related to a history of sexual abuse.

Scale 8 (*Schizophrenia, Sc*) consists of 77 items with content that includes bizarre thought processes, peculiar perceptions, social isolation, disturbances in mood and behavior, and difficulties in concentration and impulse control. The MMPI-A manual reports that elevations on Scale 8 for boys in the clinical sample were related to severe problems such as somatic complaints, behavior problems, internalizing-schizoid behavior, psychotic symptoms, low self-esteem, and a possible history of sexual abuse. For girls in the clinical sample, high scores on Scale 8 were associated with a history of sexual abuse and an increase in disagreements with their parents.

Scale 9 (*Hypomania, Ma*) consists of 46 items developed to identify patients manifesting hypomanic symptoms. The MMPI-A manual reports that for girls in the clinical sample high Scale 9 elevations were related to school behavioral problems; whereas for clinical sample boys, the only significant correlation had to do with amphetamine use.

Scale 0 (*Social Introversion, Si*) consists of 62 items that measure social relationship problems. The MMPI-A manual reports that for both sexes high scores on Scale 0 were related to social withdrawal and low self-esteem. In addition, clinical sample girls with elevations on Scale 0 were more likely to have eating problems, depression, suicidal ideation and/or gestures, and a history of having few or no friends.

When interpreting an adolescent's clinical scale profile, use of the Harris-Lingoes subscales with selected MMPI-A scales (2, 3, 4, 6, 8, 9), and the subscales developed for Scale 0 can enhance profile interpretation. These scales may help to clarify which characteristics to emphasize when describing an individual's elevations on a particular scale. It should be noted that a Harris-Lingoes or Scale 0 subscale score should be interpreted only if the "parent" scale is clinically elevated (i.e., has a T-score of 60 or more) and the Harris-Lingoes or Scale 0 subscale itself is elevated to or above 65. Subscales should never be interpreted if the parent scale is not clinically elevated.

The MMPI-A manual provides adolescent norms for the Harris-Lingoes subscales. Such norms were not available prior to development of the adolescent-specific version of the test. A list of the subscales is provided in Appendix A.

A final issue regarding interpretation of the MMPI-A clinical scales pertains to the use of code types. Much of the original MMPI interpretive literature was based on a code-typing approach to profile interpretation. Code types reflect patterns of scores on the clinical scales. Early MMPI investigators and users noted that there were certain recurring combinations of scores on the test's clinical scales that were associated with the presence of certain symptoms, traits, and behavioral tendencies.

Many of the seminal actuarial guides to MMPI interpretation were based on systems of code-type classification. The early systems of Marks and Seeman, and Gilberstadt and Duker, required that profiles be classified based on complex rules that generated relatively homogeneous groups of individuals. Unfortunately, many profiles did not meet the stringent criteria of any of the code types. Consequently, MMPI investigators began to relax the rules for profile classification so that more cases could be classified into a code type. This involved, typically, classifying profiles into code types based on the two highest scales on the profile. This was the approach used by Marks, Seeman, and Haller who developed the most comprehensive and extensive actuarial data base for interpreting adolescents' MMPI code types.

Williams and Butcher attempted to replicate the Marks, Seeman, and Haller findings with a contemporary sample of adolescents. They identified empirical correlates for only a small number of the original code types and urged caution in relying on code types in adolescent MMPI interpretation. The authors of the MMPI-A manual reiterated the need for further research into the utility of using code types in MMPI-A interpretation. They also presented data demonstrating that two-point code types based on the MMPI-A norms are largely congruent with those generated based on the Marks and Briggs original MMPI adolescent norms when code type classification is based on well-defined two-point code types (i.e., at least five T-score points separate the two highest scales in the profile from the remaining scales). Thus, it is possible to apply the findings of Marks, Seeman, and Haller to MMPI-A code-type interpretation.

The MMPI-A Content Scales

Retention of both the four basic validity scales (CNS, L, F, K) and the 10 clinical scales insured continuity between the original MMPI and the MMPI-A. A new feature of the MMPI-A was the development of a new group of scales that were derived from an item-content-based approach to scale construction. The MMPI-A Content scales assess a broad range of problems that adolescents face, and are similar, but not identical, to the content scales developed for the MMPI-2. Four of the MMPI-A content scales were developed exclusively for use with adolescents. Following, is a brief overview of the primary features associated with elevations on the MMPI-A Content scales.

Adolescent-Anxiety (A-anx) consists of 21 items that measure symptoms of anxiety. Adolescents who score in the elevated range of A-anx often report feelings of tension, frequent worrying, sleeping difficulties, problems with concentration, and an inability to stay on task. A-anx also is a good measure of general maladjustment as well as of symptoms relating to depression and somatic complaints.

Adolescent-Obsessiveness (A-obs) consists of 15 items that describe patterns of obsessive rumination. For boys in the clinical sample, this scale was also related to dependent and anxious behavior. For girls, scores on A-obs were related to an increased risk for suicidal ideation, gestures, or both.

Adolescent-Depression (A-dep) consists of 26 items that measure behavior and experiences related to depression. In the clinical sample, high scores on A-dep were related to behaviors and symptoms of dysphoria and depression as well as suicidal ideation and gestures.

Adolescent-Health Concerns (A-hea) consists of 37 items that are related to reports of physical problems by adolescents. These physical complaints may interfere with the adolescents' participation in after-school activities and contribute to significant school absences. In the clinical sample, elevations on this scale were associated with a variety of somatic complaints.

Adolescent-Alienation (A-aln) consists of 20 items that reflect emotional distance from others. This is one of the new content scales that are unique to the MMPI-A. Adolescents who score in the clinical range on this scale believe that they are getting a raw deal from life and that no one cares about or understands them. In addition, adolescents with high scores on this scale are likely to believe that they are not liked by others, do not get along well with others, and that others are not sympathetic toward them.

Adolescent-Bizarre Mentation (A-biz) consists of 19 items that reflect strange thoughts and experiences. These may include auditory, visual, and olfactory hallucinations and persecutory delusional beliefs. In the clinical sample, elevated scores on A-biz were related to bizarre sensory experiences and other symptoms and behaviors that may be indicative of psychosis.

Adolescent-Anger (*A-ang*) consists of 17 items that reflect problems with anger control. Items on this scale reflect an adolescent's tendency to swear, smash things, start fist fights, and to break and destroy things. These items also assess an adolescent's irritability and impatience with others. Adolescents with high scores on this scale tend to have histories of assault and other acting-out behaviors.

Adolescent-Cynicism (*A-cyn*) consists of 22 items that reflect misanthropic attitudes. High scores on this scale indicate an adolescent's feelings that others are out to get her or him and will use unfair means to gain an advantage. Adolescents who produce elevations on this scale tend to be on the lookout for hidden motives when someone does something nice for them.

Adolescent-Conduct Problems (*A-con*) consists of 23 items reflective of a number of acting out problems among adolescents. These may include stealing, shoplifting, lying, breaking or destroying things, being disrespectful, and being oppositional. In addition, items on this scale are also reflective of negative peer group influences. Clinical sample adolescents who scored high on this scale had numerous significant behavioral problems.

Adolescent-Low Self Esteem (*A-lse*) consists of 18 items reflective of having negative opinions about oneself. These may include feeling unattractive, lacking self-confidence, as well as feelings of uselessness of having little ability, and of having many faults. High scores on this scale were related to adolescents having negative views of themselves and doing poorly in school. In addition, for girls in the clinical sample, high scores on A-lse were suggestive of depression.

Adolescent-Low Aspirations (*A-las*) is another of the new content scales developed especially for use with adolescents. A-las consists of 16 items that assess the degree to which an adolescent lacks interest in being successful. Adolescents who score high on this scale report that they do not like to study and read about things and do not expect to be successful. These adolescents also report having difficulty starting things and giving up quickly when things go wrong. For adolescents in the clinical sample, elevated scores on A-las were related to poor academic achievement and limited participation in school activities. Additionally, high scores on this scale were found to be related to behaviors such as running away, truancy, and sexual acting out.

Adolescent-Social Discomfort (*A-sod*) consists of 24 items that indicate a desire not to be around other people. The item content of A-sod reflects an adolescent's shyness and preference to be left alone. Adolescents who score high on this scale dislike having other people around and frequently avoid others. For adolescents in the clinical sample, high scores on A-sod were related to social discomfort and withdrawal. Additionally, for clinical sample girls, high scores on this scale were related to depression and eating problems and were related negatively to aggression and irresponsibility.

Adolescent-Family Problems (*A-fam*) consists of 35 items that reflect considerable problems with parents and other family members. Discord, jealousy, fault finding, lack of love, anger, and limited communication characterize families of adolescents who score high on this scale. In addition, adolescents who produce elevated A-fam scores feel that they cannot count on their families for help and look forward to the day when they can leave home. High scores on this scale were related to disagreements with and between parents reported by participants in the clinical sample. High scores on A-fam were also related to delinquent behaviors and neurotic symptoms.

Adolescent-School Problems (*A-sch*) consists of 20 items that reflect difficulties in school such as poor grades, suspension, truancy, negative attitudes towards teachers, and a general dislike of school. Additionally, these items reflect a lack of participation in school activities and sports and the belief that school is a waste of time. Scores in the elevated range on A-sch were related to both academic and behavior problems for both boys and girls.

Adolescent-Negative Treatment Indicators (A-trt) consists of 26 items reflective of negative attitudes toward mental health professionals, doctors or both and other potential sources of difficulty in treatment. The items reflect an adolescent's belief that other people are not capable of understanding of them or do not care about what happens to them. Adolescents who score high on this scale report being unwilling to take charge and face their problems and difficulties. Items on this scale also reflect an adolescent's belief that he or she has many faults and bad habits that are insurmountable and that he or she cannot plan his or her own future. Items on this scale also reflect an adolescent's anxiety about being asked personal questions and that the adolescent may have many secrets they feel are best kept to themselves. Elevations on this scale are not necessarily indicative of a negative prognosis for treatment and should not be used to conclude that an adolescent is unlikely to benefit from intervention. Rather, they are intended to alert the clinician to the potential for interference with treatment so that early steps can be taken to surmount these difficulties.

A set of subscales for the MMPI-A Content scales has been developed called the *Content Component scales*. As with the Harris-Lingoes, clinical subscales, the content component scales are designed to serve as aids in determining which correlates to emphasize and which not to emphasize in MMPI-A Content Scale interpretation. Content Component scales were derived for 13 of the 15 content scales. As with the Harris-Lingoes subscales, content component scales should only be interpreted when the parent content scale is elevated (i.e., T-score of 60 or greater) and the content component scale is elevated to or above a T-score of 65. Appendix B provides a list of the MMPI-A Content Component scales.

MMPI-A Supplementary Scales

A number of supplementary scales have been developed for the MMPI-A. Three of these were carried over from the original MMPI with little modification, and three new supplementary scales have been developed specifically for use with the MMPI-A.

Anxiety (A) is one of the traditional MMPI supplementary scales that was retained for use with the MMPI-A. It was developed originally for use with the MMPI by Welsh and consists of 35 items. High scores on A are related to distress, anxiety, discomfort, and general emotional upset. Additionally, high scorers tend to be inhibited and overcontrolled, whereas low scorers tend to be energetic, competitive, and socially outgoing.

Repression (R) is another of the traditional MMPI supplementary scales that was developed by Welsh. The R scale on the MMPI-A consists of 33 items. Adolescents with high scores on R tend to be overcontrolled, inhibited, and less spontaneous than other adolescents, whereas low scorers on R tend to be outgoing, energetic, expressive, and informal people with an enthusiasm for life.

MacAndrew Alcoholism Scale–Revised (MAC-R) is the final original supplementary scale that was retained for use with the MMPI-A. The scale consists of 49 items associated empirically with a proclivity toward substance abuse. High scores on the MAC-R are related to illicit substance abuse but are also found in individuals who are socially extraverted, exhibitionistic, and willing to take risks but are not necessarily substance abusers. Adolescents with low scores on the MAC-R tend to be introverted and shy. An elevated score on this scale should not be interpreted a positive indication that an adolescent is abusing substances, but rather as an indication of an increased risk that this might be happening.

Alcohol and/or Drug Problem Acknowledgment (ACK) is one of the new supplementary scales designed for use with the MMPI-A. ACK consists of 13 items and was developed to assess a young person's willingness to acknowledge problematic use of alcohol or illicit drugs. Scale elevations on ACK indicate the extent to which the adolescent has acknowledged problems with alcohol or drug use. The absence of elevation does not indicate that an adolescent does not use substances, only that she or he has not acknowledged such behavior in responding to the test items. In adolescents who are known to be abusing substances, a nonelevated score on this scale indicates denial of substance abuse problems.

Alcohol and/or Drug Problem Proneness (*PRO*) is another of the new supplementary scales developed for use with the MMPI-A. This scale consists of 36 items and was designed to assess the likelihood of alcohol or drug problems in adolescents. The items were identified through empirical analyses that compared the responses of adolescents in a clinical setting who were known to have substance abuse problems with those who did not have difficulties in this area. Adolescents who have elevations on PRO are at risk for having alcohol or drug problems or both. Unlike high scorers on MAC-R who are at risk for similar problems as part of a pattern of risk taking and sensation seeking, adolescents who score high on PRO tend to develop difficulties in this area due to their susceptibility to negative peer group influences.

Immaturity (*IMM*) is another new supplementary scale developed for use with the MMPI-A. It consists of 43 items and is designed to assess psychological maturation during adolescence. IMM scores are negatively correlated with age, and high scores on IMM are related to having school difficulties and problems. IMM elevation has also been associated with disobedience, defiance, and antisocial behaviors for both boys and girls. Conversely, low scores on IMM tend to be found in adolescents described as controlled, stable, patient, cooperative, and predictable.

MMPI-A Critical Items

MMPI-A interpretation focuses on the validity, clinical, content, and supplementary scales reviewed above. Occasionally, it is helpful to examine responses an adolescent provides to particular items on the test, although no specific conclusions are to be drawn from answers to individuals inventory items. This may be particularly helpful when providing feedback to an adolescent regarding their MMPI-A results or when attempting to determine whether a young person has responded to the items in an idiosyncratic manner.

Several critical item sets were developed for the original MMPI. However, none of these was deemed appropriate for adolescents. Therefore, a new set of critical items has been introduced recently for use with the MMPI-A. This new critical item set was developed through a combination of rational and empirical methods. It consists of 82 items separated into 15 groupings based on their content. Although the critical item sets are not a scale in the traditional sense, there are a number of ways that clinicians can use responses to critical items to aid them in MMPI-A interpretation. First, in the case of an invalid, "faked bad" profile, a clinician may examine the critical item list to gain a sense of which type of problems an adolescent may be faking or exaggerating. Conversely, in the case of a "fake good" profile, the clinician might seek to determine whether there are certain problem areas that an adolescent has been reluctant to acknowledge. Another way critical items may be incorporated in the interpretive process is in giving the clinician a sense of the nature and severity of the problems an adolescent has reported. Finally, in cases where the validity scales indicate that the adolescent has accurately reported significant problems, a review of critical items may facilitate the beginning of a therapeutic discussion of the young person's difficulties. Appendix C provides a list of the 15 areas covered by the MMPI-A critical items.

INTERPRETIVE STRATEGY

MMPI-A interpretation is an integrative process in which the clinician gleans information from all of the sources described in this chapter to generate a description of the adolescent's functioning. A typical MMPI-A interpretation covers the following areas.

Profile Validity: An indication of the adolescent's test-taking attitude and its likely impact on the accuracy of the resulting MMPI-A interpretation.

General Level of Adjustment: A global evaluation of the extent to which the adolescent is functioning adaptively (or maladaptively), the overall level of distress or dysfunction that the young person may be experiencing, and how well she or he is coping with these difficulties.

Symptoms and Traits: This, typically, is the heart of the interpretation and includes issues such as the presence of symptoms of depression, anxiety, psychosis, or of severe conduct problems, the manner in which the adolescent perceives her or his environment, how the adolescent responds to stressful situations, the adolescent's self-concept, whether the young person is emotionally over- or undercontrolled, and how the adolescent relates to others.

Diagnostic Suggestions: Although it is not possible to identify specific diagnoses based on an MMPI-A profile, possible diagnoses can be suggested for follow-up based on an adolescent's test results.

Treatment Recommendations: In the final part of the interpretation, recommendations for treatment (if indicated) may be offered. These may include identification of specific treatment needs, possible impediments to successful treatment, and suggested treatment modalities.

As indicated, all of the scales and indexes described in the interpretive guidelines may serve as sources of information for the five parts of the interpretation just described. The following case example provides an annotated MMPI-A profile interpretation in which the specific profile sources for each interpretive statement are provided. A typical MMPI-A report would not include the actual sources that are mentioned here for illustrative purposes. In each section, following the annotated interpretation, we provide a distilled paragraph in the form of a typical MMPI-A interpretation.

CASE EXAMPLE

"William" is a 15-year-old adolescent male who was referred for a psychological evaluation after his parents became concerned with his deteriorating school performance and increasingly undisciplined and unruly behavior. William had received failing grades in nearly all of his freshman year classes, although he had been an average to above-average student in junior high school. He had become involved with a group of friends who were uninvolved in school activities and his parents were uncertain as to how he was spending his time with them. Recently, William was arrested for curfew violation although no formal charges were filed against him. He agreed to undergo this evaluation after his parents threatened to ground him for the remainder of the school year if he refused to participate.

William is his parents' only child. His father is a school teacher and his mother a homemaker. As part of this evaluation, he was administered a battery of tests that included the MMPI-A, the WISC-III, and the Wide Range Achievement Test–3. Scores on the latter instruments indicated that he had an average level of intelligence, with no outstanding strengths or weaknesses, and that his academic achievement level was consistent with his age and intelligence. His MMPI-A scores on the test's validity, clinical, content, supplementary, and Harris-Lingoes scales appear in Figure 16.1. Scores on the Content Component scales, and responses to critical items have yet to be incorporated into the standard scoring software.

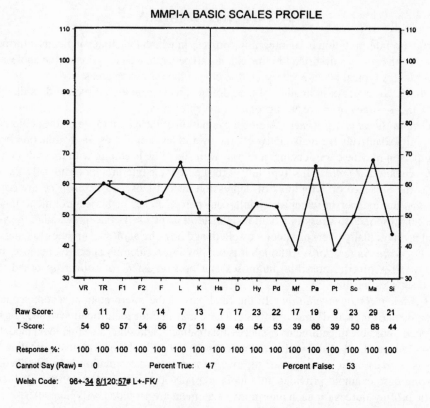

MMPI-A BASIC SCALES PROFILE

	VR	TR	F1	F2	F	L	K	Hs	D	Hy	Pd	Mf	Pa	Pt	Sc	Ma	Si
Raw Score:	6	11	7	7	14	7	13	7	17	23	22	17	19	9	23	29	21
T-Score:	54	60	57	54	56	67	51	49	46	54	53	39	66	39	50	68	44
Response %:	100	100	100	100	100	100	100	100	100	100	100	100	100	100	100	100	100

Cannot Say (Raw) =   0   Percent True: 47   Percent False: 53

Welsh Code: 96+-34 8/120:57# L+-FK/

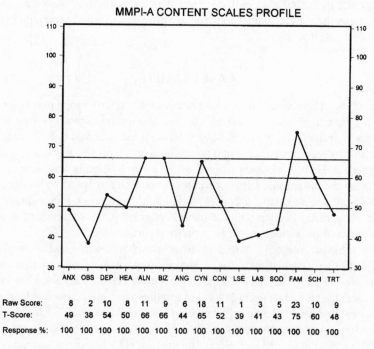

MMPI-A CONTENT SCALES PROFILE

	ANX	OBS	DEP	HEA	ALN	BIZ	ANG	CYN	CON	LSE	LAS	SOD	FAM	SCH	TRT
Raw Score:	8	2	10	8	11	9	6	18	11	1	3	5	23	10	9
T-Score:	49	38	54	50	66	66	44	65	52	39	41	43	75	60	48
Response %:	100	100	100	100	100	100	100	100	100	100	100	100	100	100	100

Figure 16.1. MMPI-A case example: William.

SUPPLEMENTARY SCORE REPORT

	Raw Score	T-Score	Resp %
MacAndrew Alcoholism-Revised (MAC-R)	27	63	100
Alcohol/Drug Problem Acknowledgment (ACK)	2	42	100
Alcohol/Drug Problem Proneness (PRO)	21	60	100
Immaturity Scale (IMM)	13	49	100
Anxiety (A)	11	45	100
Repression (R)	8	38	100

Depression Subscales (Harris-Lingoes)

Subjective Depression (D1)	7	46	100
Psychomotor Retardation (D2)	2	36	100
Physical Malfunctioning (D3)	3	48	100
Mental Dullness (D4)	4	52	100
Brooding (D5)	2	46	100

Hysteria Subscales (Harris-Lingoes)

Denial of Social Anxiety (Hyl)	3	49	100
Need for Affection (Hy2)	6	54	100
Lassitude-Malaise (Hy3)	2	42	100
Somatic Complaints (Hy4)	5	53	100
Inhibition of Aggression (Hy5)	5	66	100

Psychopathic Deviate Subscales (Harris-Lingoes)

Familial Discord (Pd1)	5	59	100
Authority Problems (Pd2)	4	54	100
Social Imperturbability (Pd3)	3	48	100
Social Alienation (Pd4)	6	55	100
Self-Alienation (Pd5)	3	45	100

Paranoia Subscales (Harris-Lingoes)

Persecutory Ideas (Pa1)	10	71	100
Poignancy (Pa2)	4	55	100
Naivete (Pa3)	4	50	100

Schizophrenia Subscales (Harris-Lingoes)

Social Alienation (Sc1)	10	62	100
Emotional Alienation (Sc2)	1	43	100
Lack of Ego Mastery, Cognitive (Sc3)	4	55	100
Lack of Ego Mastery, Conative (Sc4)	2	42	100
Lack of Ego Mastery, Defective Inhibition (Sc5)	0	33	100
Bizarre Sensory Experiences (Sc6)	8	59	100

Hypomania Subscales (Harris-Lingoes)

Amorality (Ma1)	5	66	100
Psychomotor Acceleration (Ma2)	7	52	100
Imperturbability (Ma3)	5	62	100
Ego Inflation (Ma4)	7	64	100

Social Introversion Subscales (Ben-Porath, Hostetler, Butcher, & Graham)

Shyness/Self-Consciousness (Si1)	4	43	100
Social Avoidance (Si2)	2	47	100
Alienation—Self and Others (Si3)	6	45	100

Uniform T scores are used for Hs, D, Hy, Pd, Pa, Pt, Sc, Ma, and the Content Scales; all other MMPI-A scales use linear T scores.

Figure 16.1. Continued

MMPI-A Interpretation

William's MMPI-A interpretation follows the outline listed above and includes information on the sources for the various interpretive statements. In each of the following sections, we first provide a detailed analysis of the implications of scale elevations and then indicate how this information might be integrated into actual interpretive statements.

Profile Validity

William produced a valid and interpretable MMPI-A profile. However, some of his scores on the validity scales raise cause for concern. He responded to all 478 of the test's items, an indication of cooperation with and investment in the assessment. His score on the VRIN scale (54) is well within normal limits, indicating that William responded relevantly and coherently to the test items and ruling out the possibility of random responding. This too can be viewed as an indication of cooperation with the assessment process. He produced a slightly elevated score on TRIN in the "true" direction, however this level of elevation on the TRIN scale is not sufficient to raise concerns about the validity of the resulting test profile. It does indicate a tendency to answer some of the test items "true" in an inconsistent manner. This level of elevation on TRIN is sometimes found in adolescents who experience difficulties responding to some of the "double negatives" embedded in the MMPI-A.

William's scores on the F scales are well within normal limits as is his score on K. However, he produced an elevated T-score of 67 on L. This indicates that he approached the test in a somewhat guarded and defensive manner and denied minor faults and shortcomings that most adolescents acknowledge readily. He sought to present himself as free of any bad habits or negative behavioral tendencies. His defensive response pattern was rather naïve and unsophisticated. Because of William's defensive test-taking attitude, it is possible that some areas of dysfunction may be missed or underestimated by his MMPI-A profile. Nonetheless, there is sufficient elevation on some of the MMPI-A scores, indicating that William's defensiveness was not pervasive and may be limited to one or more particularly sensitive areas of difficulty.

An interpretive statement based on this information might read as follows:

William produced a valid MMPI-A profile, although he tended to be somewhat guarded and defensive in responding to the test items. He denied minor faults and shortcomings that most adolescents acknowledge readily in an effort to appear free of any problems. Because of this test-taking approach, some of his difficulties may be missed or underestimated by the resultant test scores.

General Level of Adjustment

Williams's MMPI-A scores indicate that he is experiencing some adjustment difficulties at this time. However, these do not appear to be overwhelming him. Rather, it appears that he is having difficulties in some particular areas of his life. His within-normal-limits scores on the F scales and generally moderate scores on the MMPI-A Clinical and Content scales indicate that William likely believes that he is able to handle his problems on his own. However, the specific scales on which William produced elevated scores, particularly Clinical scales 6 and 9 and the Content scales Adolescent Alienation and Adolescent Bizarre Mentation, suggest the possibility of pronounced dysfunction that may include psychotic symptomatology.

An interpretive statement based on this information might read as follows:

William is experiencing some adjustment difficulties at this time. However, he does not feel overwhelmed by his problems. There are, however, indications in his MMPI-A profile that he may be manifesting early signs of significant dysfunction.

Symptoms and Traits

William's elevated score on Clinical Scale 9 indicates that he is likely to have substantial acting out problems, he may be experiencing significant behavioral and academic problems at school, and that he may be involved with alcohol or drug use. He likely is resentful of authority figures is prone to act out impulsively. He may be viewed by others as extraverted and outgoing, but he tends to be self-centered and has an unrealistically positive self-appraisal. His scores on the Harris-Lingoes subscales for Scale 9 do not identify any of these interpretive statements as requiring emphasis or de-emphasis.

William's elevated score on Scale 6 indicates that he tends to be guarded, evasive, and suspicious of others and very sensitive to perceived criticism or rejection. He tends to blame others for his difficulties and likely presents as being moody and unpredictable. Adolescents who produce elevations on this scale often have academic and behavior problems in school. Examination of William's scores on the Harris-Lingoes subscales for Scale 6 indicates that his elevated score on this scale was driven particularly by an endorsement of items reflective of persecutory beliefs. William sees his environment as threatening and not supportive.

William's elevated sore on the Content scale Adolescent Family Problems indicates that he reports experiencing substantial dysfunction in his family life. He believes that his parents find excessive fault in him and reports the presence of significant discord among members of his family. He does not believe that he can count on members of his family in times of trouble and believes that his parents often punish him without cause. Parents of adolescents who produce elevations on this scale often disapprove of their peers.

William's elevated score on the Adolescent Alienation content scale indicates that he reports experiencing emotional distance from others. He believes that no one, including his parents, cares about what happens to him and that his peers do not have a high opinion of him. William likely has difficulties self-disclosing and feels awkward in situations where he has to talk in front of a group.

His elevated score on the Content scale Adolescent Bizarre Mentation indicates that William reported having rather strange thoughts and experiences. He may feel that there is something wrong with his mind and that others are plotting against him. He may have had some bizarre sensory experiences and other symptoms suggestive of psychosis. However, it is also possible that some of the experiences reflected in this score may be a product of drug use, particularly hallucinogenic drugs.

William's elevated score on Adolescent Cynicism indicates that he has misanthropic beliefs. He believes that others are out to get him and will use unfair means to take advantage of him. He his likely to look for hidden motives if someone does something kind for him.

William's elevated score on Adolescent School Problems indicates that he reports having significant academic and behavioral problems in school. He is likely uninvolved in school activities and may be a member of a fringe group.

William's scores on the MacAndrew Alcoholism and Alcohol/Drug Problem Prognoses scales are both moderately elevated, indicating that he has personality characteristics and behavioral tendencies that place him at significant risk for developing substance abuse problems. His below-average score on the Alcohol/Drug Problem Acknowledgement scale indicates that he denies problems with substance abuse at this time.

Interpretive statements based on this information might read as follows:
William does not report experiencing any significant problems with anxiety or depression at this time. However, his MMPI-A scores indicate that he likely has significant acting out problems and that these may be most pronounced in the school setting and in his family relationships. He is prone toward acting out impulsively and may be influenced by negative peers. He tends to be very guarded and suspicious of the motives of others and may be showing early signs of thought disturbance. Conversely, some of the unusual experiences he reports may be the outcome of drug use. William perceives his environment as hostile and threatening. He believes that his family life is very dysfunctional and that he cannot turn to his parents for support or understanding. He feels emotionally distant from and has difficulties trusting others. Emotionally, William tends to be undercontrolled. He presents as having an unrealistically high self-appraisal. William may make an initially positive impression on others, but, he has difficulty forming warm and close relationships with others.

Diagnostic Suggestions

Williams elevations on Scales 9, Adolescent Family Problems, and Adolescent School problems indicate the possibility of conduct or oppositional disorder diagnoses. His elevated scores on Scale 6, Adolescent Alienation, Adolescent Bizarre Mentation, and Adolescent Cynicism point to the possibility of a psychotic disorder characterized by paranoid thinking. However, drug use may also account for some of these elevations. It is possible that he is manifesting early signs of a paranoid personality disorder. Finally, his scores on MAC-R and PRO indicate that William possesses personality characteristics, such as sensation seeking, and behavioral proclivities, such as becoming a member of a negative peer group, that place him at increased risk for developing a substance use disorder.

An interpretive statement based on this information might read as follows:
William's MMPI-A profile indicates a likely diagnosis of conduct or oppositional disorder and a possible diagnosis of a paranoid thought or personality disorder. His scores on the test also indicate that William is at significant risk for developing a substance use disorder.

Treatment Recommendations

William's MMPI-A profile indicates the presence of significant behavioral dysfunction that may be alleviated with proper intervention. Possible treatment needs include intervention for his disordered conduct and possible substance abuse. A behavioral approach may be most beneficial in confronting these areas of need. Family intervention also seems indicated based on William's highly elevated score on the Content scale Adolescent Family Problems. In light of the possibility that William may be showing early signs of a thought disturbance, a follow-up evaluation might be recommended to focus more specifically on this issue and determine whether there is a need for psychotropic medication. The absence of elevation on the Adolescent Negative Treatment Indicators scale indicates that William did not report any beliefs or attitudes that might interfere with the success of any treatment he might receive.

An interpretive statement based on this information might read as follows:
William's MMPI-A profile indicates that he may benefit from behavioral intervention targeted at his acting out behaviors and possible substance abuse and that the possibility of enrolling his family in family therapy should be explored as well. A follow-up evaluation to determine whether William is showing early signs of a thought disturbance is recommended. Should

such signs be identified, a referral to explore the possibility of psychotropic treatment would be indicated.

SUMMARY

The MMPI-A offers clinicians the most comprehensive, empirically validated instrument for assessing adolescent personality and psychopathology. Its considerable continuity with the original version of the instrument (in the form of the Validity and Clinical scales) indicates that clinicians may continue to rely on a relatively large body of literature regarding adolescent MMPI interpretation compiled more than 50 years prior to publication of the new adolescent version of the instrument. The new scales make the test more contemporary in addressing current adolescent-specific clinical concerns such as drug use, family difficulties, eating disorder, school problems, and alienation. An emerging body of literature on the MMPI-A indicates that the test provides valid and reliable information regarding a host of clinically relevant characteristics and behaviors.

SUGGESTED READINGS

Archer, R. P. (1997). *MMPI-A: Assessing adolescent psychopathology* (2nd ed.). Hillsdale, NJ: Lawrence Erlbaum Associates.

Ben-Porath, Y. S., & Davis, D. L. (1997). *Case studies for interpreting the MMPI-A*. Minneapolis, MN: University of Minnesota Press.

Butcher, J. N., & Williams, C. L. (1992) *Essentials of MMPI-2 and MMPI-A interpretation*. Minneapolis, MN: University of Minnesota Press.

Butcher, J. N., Williams, C. L., Graham, J. R., Archer, R. P., Tellegen, A., Ben-Porath, Y. S., & Kaemmer, B. (1992). *Minnesota Multiphasic Personality Inventory-Adolescent (MMPI-A): Manual for administration, scoring, and interpretation*. Minneapolis: University of Minnesota Press.

Forbey, J. D., & Ben-Porath, Y. S. (1998). *A critical item set for the MMPI-A*. Minneapolis, MN: University of Minnesota Press.

Graham, J. R. (1993). *MMPI-2: Assessing personality and psychopathology* (2nd ed.). New York: Oxford University Press.

Hathaway, S. R., & Monachesi, E. D. (1963). *Adolescent personality and behavior: MMPI patterns of normal, delinquent, dropout, and other outcomes*. Minneapolis: University of Minnesota Press.

Marks, P. A., Seeman, W., and Haller, D. L. (1974). *The actuarial use of the MMPI with adolescents and adults*. Baltimore: Williams & Wilkins.

Williams, C. L., Butcher, J. N., Ben-Porath, Y. S., & Graham, J. R. (1992). *MMPI-A Content Scales: Assessing psychopathology in adolescents*. Minneapolis: University of Minnesota Press.

APPENDIX A
HARRIS-LINGOES AND SI SUB-SCALES

Scale 2 (Depression, D)
        D1 – Subjective Depression
        D2 – Psychomotor Retardation
        D3 – Physical malfunctioning
        D4 – Mental Dullness
        D5 – Brooding

Scale 3 (Hysteria, Hy)
        Hy1 – Denial of Social Anxiety
        Hy2 – Need for Affection
        Hy3 – Lassitude-Malaise
        Hy4 – Somatic Complaints
        Hy5 – Inhibition of Aggression

Scale 4 (Psychopathic Deviate, Pd)
        Pd1 – Familial Discord
        Pd2 – Authority Problems
        Pd3 – Social Imperturbability
        Pd4 – Social Alienation
        Pd5 – Self-Alienation

Scale 6 (Paranoia, Pa)
        Pa1 – Persecutory Ideas
        Pa2 – Poignancy
        Pa3 – Naivete

Scale 8 (Schizophrenia, Sc)
        Sc1 – Social Alienation
        Sc2 – Emotional Alienation
        Sc3 – Lack of Ego Mastery – Cognitive
        Sc4 – Lack of Ego Mastery – Conative
        Sc5 – Lack of Ego Mastery – Defective Inhibition
        Sc6 – Bizarre Sensory Experiences

Scale 9 (Hypomania, Ma)
        Ma1 – Amorality
        Ma2 – Psychomotor Acceleration
        Ma3 – Imperturbability

Scale 0 (Social Introversion, Si)
        Si1 – Shyness/Self-Consciousness
        Si2 – Social Avoidance
        Si3 – Alienation – Self and Others

APPENDIX B
MMPI-A CONTENT COMPONENT SCALES*

Adolescent depression (A-dep)
    A-dep1 – Dysphoria
    A-dep2 – Self-Depreciation
    A-dep3 – Lack of Drive
    A-dep4 – Suicidal Ideation
Adolescent Health Concerns (A-hea)
    A-hea1 – Gastrointestinal Complaints
    A-hea2 – Neurological Symptoms
    A-hea3 – General Health Concerns
Adolescent Alienation (A-aln)
    A-aln1 – Misunderstood
    A-aln2 – Social Isolation
    A-aln3 – Interpersonal Skepticism
Adolescent Bizarre Mentation (A-biz)
    A-biz1 – Psychotic symptomatology
    A-biz2 – Paranoid Ideation
Adolescent Anger (A-ang)
    A-ang1 – Explosive Behavior
    A-ang2 – Irritability
Adolescent Cynicism (A-cyn)
    A-cyn1 – Misanthropic Beliefs
    A-cyn2 – Interpersonal Suspiciousness
Adolescent Conduct Problems (A-con)
    A-con1 – Acting-Out Behaviors
    A-con2 – Antisocial Attitudes
    A-con3 – Negative peer Group Influences
Adolescent Low Self-Esteem (A-lse)
    A-lse1 – Self-Doubt
    A-lse2 – Interpersonal Submissiveness
Adolescent Low Aspirations (A-las)
    A-las1 – Low Achievement Orientation
    A-las2 – Lack of Initiative
Adolescent Social Discomfort (A-sod)
    A-sod1 – Introversion
    A-sod2 – Shyness
Adolescent Family Problems (A-fam)
    A-fam1 – Familial Discord
    A-fam2 – Familial Alienation
Adolescent School Problems (A-sch)
    A-sch1 – School Conduct Problems
    A-sch2 – Negative Attitudes
Adolescent Negative Treatment Indicators (A-trt)
    A-trt1 – Low Motivation
    A-trt2 – Inability to Disclose

Source: Sherwood, N.E., Ben-Porath, Y.S., & Williams, C.L. (1997). *The MMPI-A Content Component Scales: Development, Psychometric Characteristics, and Clinical Application.* Minneapolis, MN: University of Minnesota Press.

APPENDIX C
MMPI-A CRITICAL ITEM GROUPS

Aggression (303, 453, 465)
Anxiety (36, 163, 173, 297, 309, 353)
Cognitive Problems (141, 158, 288)
Conduct Problems (224, 249, 345, 354, 440, 445, 460)
Depression/Suicidal Ideation (62, 71, 88, 177, 242, 283, 399)
Eating Problems (30, 108)
Family Problems (365, 366, 405)
Hallucinatory Experiences (92, 278, 299, 433, 439)
Paranoid Ideation (95, 132, 136, 155, 294, 315, 332, 337, 428)
School Problems (33, 80, 101, 380, 389)
Self-Denigration (90, 219, 230, 321, 392)
Sexual Concerns (31, 59, 159, 251)
Somatic Complaints (113, 138, 165, 169, 172, 175, 214, 231, 275)
Substance Use/Abuse (144, 161, 247, 342, 429, 431, 458, 467, 474)
Unusual Thinking (22, 250, 291, 296, 417)

Note: Numbers in parentheses are MMPI-A item numbers.
Source: Forbey, J.D., & Ben-Porath, Y.S. (1998). *A critical item set for the MMPI-A*. Minneapolis, MN: University of Minnesota Press.

17

Self-Directed Search

Colby Sandoval Srsic, Antonella P. Stimac,
and W. Bruce Walsh

INTRODUCTION

The Self-Directed Search (SDS) is a self-administered, self-scored, and self-interpreted vocational interest assessment tool. The design of the SDS enables it to be used with or without guidance from a counselor to help an individual examine vocational or educational environments which may be complementary to his or her interests and personality. Since the SDS simulates the work that a counselor and client might do over the course of a few sessions, it can be used by people who do not want or do not have access to a counselor. The design and use of the SDS also enables counselors to increase the number of individuals they can reach and allows more time for addressing concerns which require direct intervention. This chapter covers the theory and rationale that are the backbone of the SDS as well as its construction and development, administration and scoring, and interpretive guidelines. A case example will also illustrate the general use of the SDS.

A brief overview of the theory and rationale behind the SDS is presented in this section; however, readers are advised to examine the suggested readings at the end of this chapter for a more detailed and expansive look at the underlying theory. Throughout the introductory section of this chapter, various words have been highlighted to emphasize their importance. Beginning practitioners should familiarize themselves with these terms, as well as the general theory underlying the SDS, because such familiarity will help to ensure accurate understanding, explanation, administration, and interpretation of the SDS.

Assumption One

The SDS was developed based on Holland's theory of vocational behavior, which rests on seven main assumptions. The first main assumption is that an individual can be classified

Colby Sandoval Srsic, Antonella P. Stimac, and W. Bruce Walsh • Department of Psychology, Ohio State University, Columbus, Ohio 43210

Understanding Psychological Assessment, edited by Dorfman and Hersen. Kluwer Academic/Plenum Publishers, New York, 2001.

based on the resemblance of her or his personality to six pure or model personality types, namely: Realistic (R), Investigative (I), Artistic (A), Social (S), Enterprising (E), and Conventional (C). Opportunities created by parents, in addition to parental attitudes, biology, and social learning are hypothesized to differentially contribute to development of preferences, competencies, interests, and values in growing individuals. These, in turn, are expected to ultimately lead to development of various personality types, each with interests and competencies in particular areas.

For example, Artistic personality types tend to be nonconforming, expressive, and imaginative and have interests in artistic activities such as those involving the manipulation of physical or verbal materials. Such interests are likely to result in artistic competencies in the realm of art, literature, or music. In contrast, Conventional types tend to be more conforming, orderly, and practical, and tend to prefer conventional activities involving systematic data manipulation (i.e., filing, reproducing, and organizing materials). Such interests are likely to result in conventional competencies with clerical or business systems.

The six model personality types also tend to show disinterest or even aversion towards particular activities. For example, Artistic types tend to be averse to systematic or ordered activities resulting in deficits in clerical or business-related competencies. Conventional types tend to be averse to unsystematic or ambiguous activities and tend to show deficits in artistic competencies.

According to Holland's theory of vocational behavior, the six personality types can be arranged on a hexagonal model (see Figure 17.1). This model assumes that the relative placing of each type suggests the relationships between types. More explicitly, those types that are closer to each other on the hexagon share greater resemblance in terms of interests and competencies, while those that are farther from each other share less resemblance.

Assumption Two

A second main assumption is that most vocational or educational environments can also be classified based on a resemblance to six model environment types, namely: Realistic (R), Investigative (I), Artistic (A), Social (S), Enterprising (E), and Conventional (C). Environments are defined based on the personality types of the people who dominate the environments as well as on the experiences and reinforcements provided by the environment. For example, an Artistic environment contains a majority of Artistic types and typically emphasizes artistic experiences (i.e., creating art forms). Artistic environments generally reinforce unconventional, individualistic world views and artistic values.

The rationale behind defining an environment in terms of the R, I, A, S, E and C types is based in part upon the assumption that vocational stereotypes are fairly reliable (e.g., carpenters tend to be handy). In addition, people found within particular vocations are assumed to have similar personalities and interests (e.g., nuclear physicists tend to have similar personality traits and interests). Such similarities between people in particular vocational or educational environments are assumed to help create a characteristic R, I, A, S, E or C environment-type.

As with the personality types, R, I, A, S, E and C environment-types can also be arranged in the same hexagonal pattern (see Figure 17.1), where the relative distance between types is an index of the similarity between types. Again, those types that are closer to each other on the hexagon share greater resemblance (e.g., Realistic and Investigative) while those farther from each other share less resemblance (e.g., Realistic and Social).

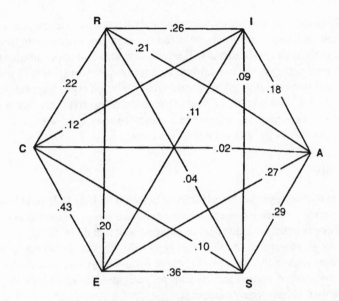

Figure 17.1. A hexagonal model for interpreting inter- and intraclass relationships. Correlations are between summary scale scores for the females [n = 1,600] in the 1994 normative sample. (Reproduced with permission from Holland, Frtizseche, & Powell, 1997.)

Assumption Three

A third main assumption is that people tend to seek environments which are compatible with their needs, values, and general personality traits. Conversely, to some extent, environments tend to seek people who are compatible with the environments. For example, Conventional personality types tend to seek Conventional environments and vice versa, while Investigative personality types tend to seek Investigative environments and vice versa.

Assumption Four

Educational and vocational behavior is predictably influenced by the interaction between an individual and his or her environment. For example, a good match between an individual's personality and her or his environment is expected to be associated with positive outcomes such as stability, achievement, success and personal adjustment. In contrast, a mismatch between a person and his or her environment (e.g., an Investigative person in an Enterprising environment) will be less likely to result in positive outcomes and is expected to be associated with attempts by the individual to: (a) change the environment to obtain a better fit; (b) change herself or himself to better fit the environment; or (d) leave the environment.

Assumption Five

The degree of congruence (or agreement) between an individual and his or her environment can be represented by the hexagonal model. For example, an Investigative person working in an Investigative environment represents a perfectly congruent person-environment match while an Investigative person working in an Enterprising environment (opposite on the hexagon) represents an incongruent person-environment match. Positive outcomes, such as stability, achievement, and satisfaction, are expected to result from person-environment congruence because a congruent environment will provide rewards and opportunities familiar to and needed by that personality type. In addition, a congruent environment will most likely reinforce abilities and personal dispositions associated with that type. Importantly, a congruent environment will also enable an individual to avoid the respective activities and ideas that he or she does not value or enjoy. Incongruence is therefore associated with greater likelihood of dissatisfaction, poor work performance, and job change.

Assumption Six

The degree of consistency (the relatedness between R, I, A, S, E and C types that represent a given individual or environment) can be indicated based on the hexagonal model (see Figure 17.1). For example, an individual or environment that most closely resembles a Realistic followed by an Investigative (adjacent) type is highly consistent compared to an individual or environment which most closely resembles a Realistic followed by a Social (opposite) type. The degree of consistency within an individual or environment is expected to moderate vocational behavior and outcomes.

Assumption Seven

Finally, a seventh assumption of Holland's theory of vocational behavior is that differentiation modifies predictions about behavior and outcomes of interactions between people and environments. Differentiation is the degree to which a person can be defined in terms of his or her similarity to a single R, I, A, S, E or C personality type (highly differentiated) versus to many personality types (undifferentiated). The concept of differentiation holds similarly for environments, as an environment may be clearly dominated by one of the R, I, A, S, E or C personality types (highly differentiated), or it may be comprised of a more even distribution of personality types (undifferentiated). A well-defined individual or environment is expected to clearly exhibit the characteristics of the model R, I, A, S, E or C type making that individual or environment more predictable than if poorly defined.

Holland's theory of vocational behavior has proven itself to be a useful way to categorize individuals and environments and derive and test hypotheses regarding interactions between the two. Empirical studies lend support to the existence of the six model personality and environment types, as well as to the hexagonal model arrangement thus making Holland's theory useful in practical settings (e.g., with the SDS).

The SDS

Specifically, the SDS consists of an assessment booklet and a classification booklet which aid a person in determining his or her personality type(s) and exploring the environments which may be most compatible with his or her personality. This tool can be very beneficial for many individuals in terms of providing a structured way for them to increase self-knowledge. The SDS also provides an avenue for individuals to organize information so that they can gain a more concrete sense of how their skills and interests fit into the world of work.

TEST CONSTRUCTION AND DEVELOPMENT

The SDS exists in a variety of forms which are designed to be used with various populations. The SDS Regular Form (Form-R) is the most commonly used and therefore will be elaborated upon in this chapter. Other forms of the SDS and the populations they are designed to help are described in brief at the end of this section.

Construction of the SDS

The SDS Form-R is designed for use with high school and college students, as well as with adults. The SDS assessment booklet for Form-R consists of a total of 228 items and is made up of eight main sections. These sections include Occupational Daydreams, Activities (6 scales; 11 items per scale), Competencies (6 scales; 11 items per scale), Occupations (6 scales, 14 items per scale), Self-Estimates (12 total ratings), How to Organize Your Answers, What Your Summary Code Means, Some Next Steps, and Some Useful Books. The following is an elaboration on the eight sections of the SDS, Form-R.

The Sections of the SDS

Occupational Daydreams

This is the first section of the SDS Form-R. An individual is instructed to list his or her vocational aspirations and their accompanying three-letter environment-codes (found in the Occupations Finder or the Alphabetized Occupations Finder). This section was included because research suggests that a person's vocational aspirations are often better predictors of future academic and career environments than objective assessment tools.

Activities

The Activities section is the second main section of the SDS and is designed to assess whether a person likes, dislikes, or is indifferent to particular R, I, A, S, E and C activities. Individuals respond "like" if they feel they would like to do a given activity or "dislike" if they are indifferent or would dislike doing a given activity. Sample items to which individuals respond "like" or "dislike" include "work on a scientific project" which represents an Investigative activity, and "learn strategies for business success" which represents an Enterprising activity.

Competencies

The Competencies section is the third main section and is designed to measure the degree to which a person feels competent in completing particular R, I, A, S, E and C tasks and activities. Individuals respond "yes" to activities on which they feel they can do well, and "no" to those they have never performed or feel they would perform poorly. For example, an individual is asked to respond "yes" or "no" to "I can play a musical instrument," which represents an Artistic competency, and to "I am a good public speaker," which represents an Enterprising competency.

Occupations

The Occupations section is the fourth main section of the SDS and is designed to assess an individual's feelings and attitudes regarding particular R, I, A, S, E and C occupations. Individuals respond "Yes" if they have an interest in the occupation or "No" if they dislike the occupation or find it uninteresting. Examples of occupations include Electrician (Realistic), Sociologist (Social), and Bank Teller (Conventional).

Self-Estimates

The Self-Estimates section is the fifth main section and enables individuals to rate themselves (as compared to other persons in the same age group) as high, average, or low on R, I, A, S, E and C abilities and skills. Two ratings for each of the six types yield 12 total ratings.

How to Organize Your Answers

This section guides an individual through tallying up the responses to the R, I, A, S, E and C Activities, Competencies, Occupations, and Self-Estimates and calculating (using simple addition) a three-letter summary person-code. As mentioned earlier, the summary person-code generally represents three of the R, I, A, S, E and C types which an individual most closely resembles. The letters are rank-ordered so that the first letter represents the personality type with which the individual shares the greatest resemblance. The second and third letters represent the second and third types most closely resembled, respectively. Occasionally, ties between letters occur, in which case an individual is instructed to include both tied letters in the summary person-code.

What Your Summary Code Means

This section is designed to help guide individuals though a search for occupations which are potentially complementary to their personality type (as represented by the three-letter summary person-code). Space is provided in the SDS for writing down the results of this search and further instructions are given as to how to proceed in the event of ties between personality types.

Some Next Steps

This section provides a number of useful steps to follow for further career exploration. For example, an individual is offered ideas on how to proceed if his or her summary person-code does not support an actual or anticipated job choice. Individuals are instructed to use the Occupations Finder to investigate the amount of education or training that is required for the occupations listed in the previous section to help determine how feasible certain occupations might be for a particular individual. Additional steps suggest consideration of one's health or physical limitations and further exploration of occupations through the use of other sources such as counselors, employment services, and individuals employed in the occupations(s) of interest. The final steps discuss the use of the SDS as a tool to aid in career exploration and address how summary person-codes may potentially be influenced by gender because males and females may respond differently.

Some Useful Books

This is the final section in which individuals can find a list of nontechnical resources which may further assist them in their vocational exploration.

Development of the SDS

Revisions to 1971 and 1985 versions of the SDS Form-R have resulted in the 1994 version. Revisions have included improvements in item content (adding new items, revising or deleting old items, attempting to remove sex bias in items) and revisions in the instructions to increase user friendliness, as well as the likelihood of an individual completing the assessment process.

The Occupations Finder has also been revised over time. Revisions include the addition of new occupations and deletion of occupations which are fast becoming obsolete. Revisions have resulted in the 1994 version which contains 1,335 occupations and each occupation's three-letter environment-code.

Reliability and Validity

A substantial amount of reliability data is reported in the *SDS Technical Manual.* Internal consistency reliability coefficients (KR-20) for the Activities, Competencies, Occupations and Summary Scales range from moderate (.70s) to high (.90s) for male and female high school and college students, as well as for adults. More specifically, the SDS Technical Manual reports internal consistency coefficients (KR-20) for female (n = 716) and male (n = 399) college students as follows: .72 to .83 for females and .74 to .84 for males on the Competencies Scales; .82 to .92 for females and .84 to .90 for males on the Occupation Scales; .90 to .93 for females and .90 to .92 for males on the Summary Scales. In addition, a sample of 45 females and 22 males ranging in age from 14 to 48 yielded test-retest correlations (over 4–12 week periods) of .76 to .89 for the Summary Scales indicating adequate stability over time. Though intercorrelations among Summary (R, I, A, S, E, C) Scales for female and male college students do not support a perfect hexagonal structure, they are generally supportive of Holland's hexagonal model and approximate it closely enough to support the model's practical use.

The *SDS Technical Manual* also reports a substantial amount of validity data to support the SDS. The manual reports results of research which suggest that the SDS has stable and adequate construct, concurrent, and predictive validity.

Available Forms

The SDS Form-R exists in a number of different translations including English Canadian, French Canadian, Spanish, Vietnamese, and Braille. In addition, the research supporting Holland's theory, as well as the cost-effectiveness and efficiency of the SDS, have encouraged the development of other forms of the SDS designed for use by people with varying degrees of education and life experience. For example, the SDS Form Easy (Form-E) is designed to be used by high school students and adults with limited educational backgrounds or reading skills. Form-E has fewer items than Form-R, and the directions have been rewritten using words commonly known by most fourth graders. In addition, Form-E exists in English Canadian and Spanish translations. The Career Planning Form (Form-CP) is designed to be used by adults and professionals in transit and individuals in organizational settings. Form-CP differs from Form-R mainly in that it does not contain the Daydreams and Self-Estimates sections and some items have been replaced with others more appropriate for organizational work settings. Finally, the SDS Career Explorer was developed specifically for use with middle school and junior high school students. The Career Explorer was developed by generating new items, as well as by pooling items from other pre-existing SDS forms. It is at an easier reading level than the SDS Form-R.

In short, the SDS in its many forms is a cost effective, efficient, valid and reliable tool which adolescents and adults can use during the course of educational and vocational exploration. The following sections will elaborate on the administration and scoring of the SDS Form-R and then present interpretive guidelines and a case example.

ADMINISTRATION AND SCORING

Administration

Administration of the SDS is rather simple given that it is self-administered, self-scored and self-interpreted; however, it is still important that administration be supervised by an individual who has adequate familiarity with interest inventories, Holland's theory, the SDS, and general occupational information. The SDS takes an average of 40–50 minutes to complete, and it can be given individually or in groups. It is generally recommended that group size be limited to no more than 25 people to insure that adequate attention can be given.

In working through the SDS assessment booklet, an individual can obtain a three-letter person-code. This code represents the three personality types which most closely resemble the individual's personality. The summary person-code and permutations of that code can be used to explore work or educational environments by matching the summary person-code to similar three-letter environment-codes found in several sources, such as The Occupations Finder, The Educational Opportunities Finder, and The Dictionary of Holland Occupational Codes. For example, an individual having an RIA summary person-code most closely resembles a Realistic personality type followed by an Investigative and Artistic personality type, respectively. Using The Occupations Finder, this individual could generate a list of occupations that are coded RIA as well as occupations coded RAI, IRA, IAR, ARI, and AIR because they are all permutations of RIA.

The SDS is frequently used with people outside of a formal career counseling context, but there are still many advantages to having an administrator facilitate the process. For example, individuals can greatly benefit from an explanation as to the rationale for taking the SDS. Administrators should explain that the SDS can be used to help individuals better understand vocational problems, generate educational and vocational possibilities, narrow the focus if there are too many possibilities, stimulate interest in future career plans, and increase general self-knowledge. Administrators need to stress that the SDS is not a "crystal ball" which will tell someone exactly what he or she should be, but rather it is an instrument that is used to stimulate self-reflection and assist an individual in taking an active role in career planning. Results from the SDS can help individuals make better-informed career decisions by drawing from an increased awareness and understanding of self, as well as the world of work.

Another role of the administrator is to select the appropriate form of the SDS. The SDS is appropriate for use with individuals who are 12 years of age or older, and there are a variety of versions from which to choose. The only significant limitation to the SDS is that it should not be used with people who are illiterate, severely mentally ill, or who have extremely complex decision-making problems.

Scoring

The SDS is scored by hand, which means results are produced more quickly and economically than with other career assessment instruments that require computer scoring. To score the SDS, individuals simply follow the directions provided. This involves transposing the scores from each section to the summary page and then summing each column vertically. The three highest types (R, I, A, S, E, or C) make up an individual's summary person-code (e.g., SEC).

Because computational errors are common, it is important for administrators to double-check the scoring. If the SDS is being administered to a group, one can simply have individuals trade with a neighbor and check the other person's computations.

It is not uncommon for individuals to have tied scores, and in this situation they should consider themselves to have several summary person-codes. For example, if an individual's highest three scores are A (32), S (32), and E (16), he or she should consider his or her summary person-code to be both ASE and SAE.

Once individuals know their summary person-code, the administrator should help them examine the degree of congruence between their summary person-codes and the codes for their current education/occupation environment. Also, it is helpful to examine the degree of congruence between an individual's summary person-code and the codes for his or her educational and occupational aspirations or daydreams. There are several ways to calculate congruence, including the Hexagon Model index, the Zener-Schnuelle index, and the Iachan index. However, for the purposes of this chapter, only two methods will be discussed in detail: the First Letter or Dominant Score Index and the C Index. Instructions for calculating other methods can be found in the *SDS Professional User's Guide*.

The simplest and most commonly used method is called the Dominant Score or First Letter index. This method involves looking at the first letter (or highest score) of an individual's summary person-code and comparing it to the first letter of an occupation or education environment-code. For example, if a woman's summary person-code is ISA and she is majoring in pre-optometry (ISR), she is said to be congruent because the first letter of her summary person-code (I) is the same as the first letter of her chosen environment-code (I). However, if this same person decided to major in architecture (AIR), she is said to be incongruent because the first letter of her summary person-code (I) does not match the first letter of her chosen environment-code (A). This method is a good one to select because, according to Holland's theory, the first letter is the type that should be given the most weight. Furthermore, studies have shown that the first type is often the most descriptive, reliable, and stable type.

The C index is a relatively new method which has received a great deal of attention in recent literature. The major advantage of this method over the First Letter index is that it uses all three of the types that make up an individual's summary person-code, and it also takes into consideration a type's position on the Holland hexagon (see Figure 17.1). This method is calculated according to the following formula: $C = 3 (Xi) + 2 (Xi) + (Xi)$ where Xi is determined by the match of the person-code relative to the environment code on the Holland hexagon.

Determining Xi
Xi = 3   if person-code is identical to environment-code
Xi= 2   if person-code is adjacent to environment-code
Xi =1   if person-code is not identical, not adjacent, and not opposite to environment-code
Xi = 0   if person-code is opposite of environment-code

For example, a woman with a summary person-code SAE, who is majoring in an SIA environment, would receive a "C" score of 3 (3) + 2 (2) + 1 = 14 because, as exemplified in Figure 17.1, the first letter of her summary person-code and the first letter of her environment-code are identical, the second letter of her summary person-code and the second letter of her environment-code are adjacent, and the third letter of her summary person-code and the third letter of her environment-code are not identical, adjacent or opposite one another on the hexagon. Scores on the "C" index can range from 0–18 with higher scores reflecting higher levels of congruence. Unfortunately, there are no strict guidelines in terms of cut offs that clearly delineate the degree of congruence. Therefore, as with any test, the use of clinician judgement and multiple sources is essential when interpreting the data.

In addition to calculating congruence, administrators should examine the degree of consistency of a summary person-code. Using the Holland hexagon, is it possible to determine the degree of similarity between each of the three types that make up a summary person-code. For example, an ASE summary person-code is more consistent than a SIC summary person-code because the types are closer to each other on the Holland hexagon in the former code then in the latter. In general, the closer the types are to one another on the hexagon, the greater the degree of consistency.

Lastly, administrators should check the degree of differentiation of a summary person-code. Remember that differentiation refers to the degree to which a person or environment can be defined by one single type. For example, if an individual's summary-person code is R (38), I (8), C (4), that code is said to be highly differentiated. On the other hand, an R (16), I (12), C(12) code is said to be undifferentiated because there is little numerical difference between the three scores. As with consistency, there are no numerical rules for determining how differentiated a code is, so once again administrators need to use their clinical judgement when interpreting the data.

INTERPRETATIVE GUIDELINES

In the "Some Next Steps Section" of the SDS, instructions for self-interpreting results are given. However, there are several advantages to having an administrator available to facilitate this process and help with more complicated or subtle interpretation issues that arise. This section will review steps that individuals who are taking the SDS can take to interpret their results. It also suggests how administrators can use the results of the SDS to aid in the career development process.

Determining a Summary Person-Code

There are several things an administrator needs to consider when determining an individual's summary person-code. Holland recommends use of the rule of 8, which states that if there is an 8-point or less difference between two scores, the difference could be due to measurement error and the scores should be viewed as equal. For example, if a woman's scores were S(42), R(37), I(28), she should assume that both the S and the R are her dominant or first letter code when determining congruence and she should consider SRI, as well as RSI environments. In addition, Holland recommends examining all permutations of an individual's summary person-code in order to expand occupational and educational options. Therefore, the above-mentioned individual should look for SRI, RSI, SIR, RIS, ISR, and IRS environments.

Interpreting the Summary Person-Code

Once a summary person-code has been derived, an administrator can draw several interpretations based upon the patterning of the code. Codes are not distributed evenly in the general population, meaning that some codes are more common than others. In general, highly consistent codes are common while highly inconsistent codes are rare. For example, 15.6% of female high school students can be categorized as SE, while only 2.3% receive the code CE. Individuals whose summary person-code is rather rare may have fewer congruent options and consequently have a more variable career path (e.g., changing jobs more often) than someone with a more common summary person-code. In addition, individuals with a highly consistent or common code frequently possess a clearer sense of identity than individuals with a rare code.

For example, a man with the highly inconsistent summary person-code, ISR, may be an individual who lacks a clear sense of identity and his interests might not necessarily complement each other. This man might greatly benefit from several sessions of career counseling in order to help him understand his unique code and discuss how this unusual pattern will affect his career path. He should prepare for the possibility that he may have a harder time finding a satisfying career and that his occupational choices may be more unstable than other people's. In addition, it may be helpful to explore how he can use hobbies to fulfill certain interests because of the difficultly of finding an occupation that would encompass all three of his interests.

Administrators should also be aware of the various reasons why an individual could exhibit a flat profile in which the scores are relatively similar. If an individual's scores are all high and close in number, this might indicate that the person has a wide variety of interests. In contrast, an individual whose scores are all low and close in number suggests a person who possibly lacks a strong sense of identity or has not had enough exposure to the world of work to develop strong preferences. Lastly, as with many assessment instruments, a low, flat profile may suggest that the person is struggling with depression which is consequently affecting self-perceptions related to interests and skills.

Another important thing to consider is that an individual's results on the SDS may be affected by a variety of factors such gender, race, age, past experiences, and familial influences. The "Some Next Steps" section of the SDS assessment booklet points out that women and men often receive different codes due to different life experiences and cultural expectations. "Because society often encourages men and women to aspire to different vocations, women receive more S, A, and C codes than men, while men obtain more I, R, and E codes (SDS Assessment Booklet, 1994)." This section also states that since almost all jobs can be successfully performed by members of either sex, individuals may want to stick with their original occupational daydreams when SDS results conflict. Thus, an important role of the administrator is to help an individual understand how these influences might have affected his or her summary person-code and how much weight should be given to these results.

Checking the Validity of the Summary Person-Code

Once a summary person-code has been generated, it is important to ask individuals how the code matches their perceptions of the skills, abilities, and interests. Additionally, administrators can be a source of information regarding the degree to which a summary person-code describes an individual, if the administrator has interacted with the individual enough to form an impression.

Generating Possibilities

Once an individual has generated all permutations of his or her summary person-code, the Occupations Finder can be used to identify possible occupations that are congruent with his or her summary person-code. The Occupations Finder lists 1,335 occupations, the amount of education required for each occupation, and a nine-digit Dictionary of Occupational Titles code for each. Previously mentioned additional resources include The Dictionary of Holland Occupational Codes and the Educational Opportunities Finder. The Dictionary of Holland Occupational Codes, which lists 12,860 occupations by Holland codes, can be especially useful when working with individuals who have unusual codes with few environments listed in the Occupations Finder.

Interpreting Occupational Daydreams

The daydreams section was not initially part of the SDS; however, it was later added due to its impressive predictive power. There are several advantages to finding the environment-codes that match an individual's occupational daydreams. It can help to: (a) promote self-direction and self-initiative; (b) promote self-exploration and understanding; (c) assist in predicting the type of environment in which an individual will eventually work; and (d) give information regarding the extent to which an individual's self concept is integrated. It is important to code all of an individual's daydreams and look for patterns that might emerge.

Congruence

In addition to coding occupational daydreams and finding unexplored environments, it is helpful to examine the degree of congruence between an individual's summary person-code and the environment-code for his or her occupational daydreams and current or possible occupational environments. In general, the higher the degree of congruence, the higher the chances are that an individual will seek out and remain in a particular occupational environment.

It can be extremely helpful to have individuals reflect on why particular occupational daydreams are or are not congruent with their summary person-code. For example, a woman may have several occupational daydreams in the medical profession (e.g., veterinarian, radiologist, and ophthalmologist); however, the results of the SDS indicate that she has little interest or perceived skill in investigative environments. Upon further reflection, she may realize that it is the values that these occupations have in common that are attractive rather than possessing interest or skill in these areas. For example, she might realize these occupations share an opportunity to earn a large income, a commitment to helping others, and a significant amount of prestige and power.

In addition to occupational daydreams, congruence between an individual's summary person-code and the environment-code of his or her current college major or occupation may help to explain dissatisfaction. Calculating congruence can also be a source of assurance for people who have recently entered or who are about to enter a particular environment.

In the workplace, calculating congruence can help explain personality differences or communication difficulties (e.g., comparing the summary person-code of one individual to another to find similarities and differences), or congruence can be used in addition to other sources of information when selecting an individual for a particular task or job.

Consistency

Remember, consistency refers to the degree of similarity between each of the three types that make up an individual's summary person-code. As mentioned earlier in the scoring section, determining degree of consistency requires clinician judgement; however, the general rule of thumb states that the closer the code types are on the Holland hexagon the more consistent the code. This information is useful in that it helps predict an individual's career. In general, the greater the consistency the more stable and productive his or her career should be. On the other hand, an individual with a low degree of consistency may be a person who will make frequent occupational changes and struggle in terms of productivity.

Differentiation

As stated in the introduction, differentiation is the degree to which a person or environment can be defined by one single type. Individuals or environments are said to be highly differentiated if they are very similar to a single type while the term highly undifferentiated is used to describe individuals or environments that are best described as an even distribution of types. This information is helpful when trying to predict how well an individual is suited to a particular environment. For example, if a person is highly differentiated, he or she may not be flexible enough to adjust to the multiple demands of a highly undifferentiated environment.

Thus, despite the fact that the SDS can be self-interpreted, there are several ways an administrator can facilitate the process. Administrators can help individuals determine and interpret their three-letter summary person-code, as well as aid in determining the validity of this code, especially when results may be influenced by factors such as sex, race, etc. The administrator can help individuals determine the degree of consistency and differentiation for their codes. Finally, after individuals have generated a list of possible occupations and majors, an administrator can help them interpret and determine the degree of congruence between their occupational daydreams and the new choices that were just generated.

CASE EXAMPLE

Sarah is an 18-year-old, Caucasian, female college student who is attending the state university approximately two hours from her home. She was referred for career counseling by her parents who are both professors at a local college. Currently, Sarah is staying at home with her parents during her six-week winter break from school.

During an initial interview, Sarah indicated that she greatly enjoyed college from a social standpoint. She reported that she had made several friends but that her performance in classes was poor from the beginning due to a lack of interest and preparation. Sarah stated that she was currently on academic probation and was not sure how she was going to tell her parents "she didn't feel cut out for college." Sarah reported she spoke to them about becoming a masseuse but that they felt she should explore other career options before making such a "rash decision." Sarah described herself as outgoing, loyal, and caring. She also indicated that she has a positive relationship with both of her parents.

Sarah's high school records indicate fair to marginal performance in all of her classes, with the exception of home economics and physical education in which she received A's. Sarah stated that she enjoyed these classes because they allowed her to talk and interact with people as opposed to just reading books. School records also indicate that she is of above-average intelligence and, when tested, she did not meet criteria for any learning disabilities. Sarah stated that she has very little interest in school; however, as her high school graduation approached, she decided to apply to the state university because she couldn't think of anything else to do and because that is what her parents expected of her.

An additional session was spent gathering information about Sarah's previous work history and work values. Sarah reported that she loved working with children as a camp counselor after her sophomore year in high school; however, the pay was minimal. During the summers after her junior and senior years in high school, she worked in the mortgage department at a local bank. She reported that her father had to pull a few strings to get her a job that paid so well; however, Sarah stated she was miserable and counted down the days until school began. When asked what was the worst part of the job, Sarah replied sitting behind a desk all day in a room all by herself. When asked what characteristics make up her ideal job, Sarah said this would be a job that let her meet new people and contribute to society by helping others. Sarah also stated that she did not want a job where she would be required to work more then 40 hours a week because she values her leisure time which she spends with her friends or two dogs.

Sarah completed the Self-Directed Search and her summary-person code is reported below.

Activities (pp. 4–5)	4	7	5	10	4	3
Competencies (pp. 6–7)	4	4	0	9	9	4
Occupations (p. 8)	9	1	3	9	4	1
Self-Estimates (p. 9)	2	2	2	7	8	2
	3	4	3	7	8	3
Total Scores	22	18	13	42	33	13
	R	I	A	S	E	C

Sarah's summary person-code is SER because these are her three highest scores. She reported being little surprised by the first two codes, given her outgoing nature and the fact that both her parents are business professors. However, Sarah was concerned that the third code, Realistic, did not adequately describe her. Upon further discussion, it was revealed that she associated the Realistic type with traditionally male occupations and was concerned that she did not possess the physical strength to succeed in these masculine activities. Sarah reported she thought of construction worker or police officer when she thought of Realistic occupations and that she didn't have much interest in these areas.

Following this revelation, a session was spent helping Sarah become aware of other Realistic occupations that were not traditionally masculine such as occupational therapist, child care worker, picture framer, and floral designer. Time was also spent exploring Sarah's gender stereotypes in relation to occupational choices and what it meant to Sarah to be labeled "Realistic." The goal of this session was to help Sarah expand her occupational choices as much as possible.

Following this session, Sarah listed all possible permutations of her summary person-code (RSE, RES, ERS, ESR, SRE, and SER). She used the Occupations Finder to identify several occupations she would like to explore including cook, automobile mechanic, child day-care worker, occupational therapist, apartment manager, airplane pilot, and animal trainer. Also, using the dominant or first-letter index, Sarah looked at the congruence between her summary person-code and her occupational daydreams. She found several congruent occupations including masseuse, social worker, and film director. After reviewing her list of possible occupations, Sarah eliminated social worker, film director, and occupational therapist because of the educational requirements. Sarah indicated that at this time she is not interested in returning to college but that she would like to keep these occupations in mind for the future. When asked which occupations she would most like to explore further, she reported child day-care worker, animal trainer, and masseuse. Sarah agreed to set up informal interviews with people already working in these areas in order to gain more information regarding how she could begin to pursue these occupations.

Time was spent discussing the fact that Sarah's code is rather consistent, meaning that she should have many choices which are congruent with her summary person-code and that she would likely have a stable and productive occupational history. The consistency of her type also indicates that her skill and interest areas compliment each other quite well and that her identity is rather solidified.

Sarah's summary person-code also appears moderately differentiated in that there is a rather large distance between her first two codes (S and E) and her third code (R). This indicates that Sarah seems to possess a clear sense of her interests and skills. Sarah was advised to perhaps weigh the first two codes more heavily than the third when making an occupational choice due to the degree of differentiation of her summary person-code. Sarah was also briefed on the possibility that her third code could change over time given the fact that it is a relatively low score and its proximity to the scores of the other three types that did not make up her summary person-code.

The last session was spent facilitating a dialogue between Sarah and her parents. They reported disappointment in her unwillingness to return to college; however, they stated that they would support her decision since she seemed to be working towards specific occupational goals. Sarah agreed that the SDS facilitated her career development by validating her previous interest in becoming a masseuse and giving her some additional options which she had not previously considered.

SUMMARY

The purpose of this chapter was to familiarize the reader with the seven main assumptions of Holland's theory of vocational behavior and how they can be applied in a concrete way using the SDS to increase self-knowledge and generate a list of possible college majors and occupations.

The SDS is an instrument which assesses skills and interests and identifies similarity between an individual and six person-types. The major advantage of the SDS is that individuals need relatively little, if any, assistance with administration, scoring, and interpretation. In addition to efficiency, it is cost effective, valid, reliable, and comes in various forms allowing it to be used with a wide range of individuals.

Once an individual has competed the SDS, there are three major factors to consider when interpreting the results. Congruence generally refers to the degree of similarity between individuals and environments. Consistency refers to the degree of similarity between each of the three types that make up either an individual's summary person-code or a college major or occupation's environment-code. Finally, differentiation refers to the degree to which a person or environment can be defined by one single type.

As with any inventory, the results of the SDS must be interpreted in a context which takes into consideration various sources of information. The major point to pass on to individuals is that the SDS cannot give someone the magic key but rather it is a helpful tool that can help increase self-knowledge and begin to guide an individual through the career decision-making process.

Below are several sources that provide further detail about Holland's theory of vocational behavior and the SDS. Additionally, several sources are listed which are recommended to be used adjunctly in the administration and interpretation of the SDS. These sources have been mentioned throughout this chapter. Finally, we recommend that administrators should take the SDS themselves to obtain experiential familiarity in addition to using the didactic information provided. This will allow for a deeper level of comfort and understanding of the instrument.

SUGGESTED READINGS

Gottfredson, G. D., & Holland, J. L. (1996). *Dictionary of Holland occupational codes (3rd ed.)*. Odessa, FL: Psychological Assessment Resources.

Holland, J. L. (1994). *The occupations finder*. Odessa, FL: Psychological Assessment Resources.

Holland, J. L. (1997). *Making vocational choices: A theory of vocational personalities and work environments (3rd ed.)*. Odessa, FL: Psychological Assessment Resources.

Holland, J. L., Fritzsche, B. A., & Powell, A. B. (1994). *The Self-Directed Search technical manual*. Odessa, FL: Psychological Assessment Resources.

Holland, J. L., Powell, A. B., & Fritzsche, B. A. (1994). *The SDS professional users guide*. Odessa, FL: Psychological Assessment Resources.

Rosen, D., Holmberg, K., & Holland, J. L. (1994). *The educational opportunities finder*. Odessa, FL: Psychological Assessment Resources.

III

Integration

18

Integrated Report Writing

William J. Burns and Bady Quintar

INTRODUCTION

A psychological report is a clinical document that has as its primary purpose to describe and interpret information gathered or discovered in the process of a psychological evaluation. The literary challenge facing the report writer is to organize, integrate, and synthesize the information gathered in the examination process and to subsequently generate a carefully planned and meaningful report which is relevant to the referral questions. Such a skill is not learned quickly. Many years of training in psychopathology, interviewing, psychometric test interpretation, case conceptualization, and report writing are necessary to learn to interpret and communicate results of a psychological evaluation in a clear, concise, and precise manner.

In the early history of clinical psychology, report writing focused almost entirely on the listing of test scores. Currently, psychological reports are less focused on test scores and more directed toward the production of a practical document which:

1. identifies a specific problem(s),
2. explains the sources and maintaining conditions of the problem(s), and
3. provides a well-conceptualized solution to the problem(s).

In modern reports, the psychological functions in question (such as intelligence, affect, social skills, memory, perception) are described in such a way that the referral questions are answered. Today's reports are "action oriented." That is, they serve as a prescription for actions, such as psychotherapy, occupational choice, instructional programs, or forms of intervention. Since report writers must be keenly aware of the needs, concerns, and expectations of the report consumer, modern reports are written from the reader's point of view. In fact, the value of the report is measured by:

William J. Burns and Bady Quintar • Center for Psychological Studies, Nova Southeastern University, Fort Lauderdale, Florida 33314.

Understanding Psychological Assessment, edited by Dorfman and Hersen. Kluwer Academic/Plenum Publishers, New York, 2001.

1. the clarity and directness with which it answers the referral questions,
2. the logic with which it organizes, integrates, and describes the psychological functioning of the individual, and
3. the appropriateness of the recommendations which are offered.

In order to achieve such objectives, report writers should avoid using jargon, technical terms, abstract concepts, convoluted sentence structure, sweeping generalizations, overworked clichés, and hyperbolas. Instead, they should strive to report their conclusions in a simple, concrete, clear, and parsimonious fashion.

THE PROCESS OF CLINICAL INFERENCE

Clinical inference is the use of human judgment and reasoning to interpret data gathered from the psychological examination. In generating a series of hypotheses about assessment data, the examiner uses the principles of formal logic to draw conclusions: i.e., to arrive at a set of diagnostic statements descriptive of the person's current psychological functioning, as well as prognostic statements about the person's future functioning. Two types of reasoning are at the basis of formal logic: inductive and deductive. Induction is the process of reasoning from the particular to the general, drawing general conclusions after examining specific aspects of a case. Deduction is the process of reasoning from the general to the particular, in which the conclusion is drawn that a particular case is a verified example of a known general principle or premise. It is the former, inductive logic, that is used most often in the formation of hypotheses about the meaning of the findings of a psychological evaluation.

Inductive Inference

Psychological examiners gather a wide variety of data from which they attempt to make general conclusions or inferences about the examinee. An example of inductive reasoning is found in the process of arriving at a diagnosis in the *Diagnostic and Statistical Manual* (DSM) of the American Psychiatric Association. Many behavioral criteria must be met by each DSM disorder to verify the accuracy of applying that diagnosis to a specific client. The process of inductive reasoning is a type of logic in which the examiner uses particular data (test responses, behavior observations, background information from interviews and records) to make general conclusions. Specific aspects of the test findings, observations, interview data, and records are combined to provide support for a specific hypothesis or inference about personality and behavioral style. The examiner is aware that the information available is partial and that it is only one tiny sample of all of the behaviors in that person's life. Therefore, the examiner makes the assumption that the limited sample of data obtained in the assessment is representative of the person's typical way of behaving, thinking, and feeling. Examiners attempt to assess the validity of this assumption of representativeness through use of response-set or validity scales, as well as through their own subjective estimation of the representativeness of the data collected. For this reason, a psychological report should inform the reader about the examiner's estimation of the representativeness of the findings.

Biases in the Reasoning Process

Inductive reasoning is the inferential structure by which the report writer maintains logical accuracy in hypothesis formation and maintains logical sequencing of evidence that leads to conclusions about assessment data. But the series of judgments required to create hypotheses and integrate them into a report are complex and vulnerable to several important biases. Four specific biases in human reasoning have been identified that are known to cause erroneous judgments in clinical inference (Achenbach, 1985). The four biases are:

1. False Behavior Relationships. Experienced clinicians who have observed patient behaviors, thoughts, and emotions that appear to be commonly associated may infer correlations between these patient attributes, when in reality there is no correlation or association between these attributes in the population. For instance, a clinician may observe that children who have been sexually abused remove the clothes of dolls in play therapy. In actuality such behavior may be observed in many young children in play therapy, and is, therefore, not specifically correlated with a history of sexual abuse.

2. False Symptom/Disorder Relationships. Certain symptoms are considered by clinicians to be typical of a specific disorder. At one time it was widely believed that brain damage resulted from hyperactivity in children. Studies of the prevalence of specific symptoms in children with brain damage revealed that externalizing symptoms may be more frequent at earlier ages and internalizing more frequent at later ages of childhood. Ignoring the actual base rates of symptoms in clinical samples of patients may lead to an erroneous judgment about the probability that a patient has a specific disorder based on the presence of a certain symptom.

3. False Use of Clinical Cases. As an examiner becomes acquainted with a new patient, there frequently comes to mind vivid memories of a former patient with similar mannerisms, style of relating, and presenting complaints. It is very easy for an examiner to erroneously use these available memories of a former patient to shape clinical inferences about the new patient. Such inferences may influence a clinician to ignore differences between the two cases and to ignore similarity with other former cases that are less available in memory.

4. Failure to Use Disconfirmatory Evidence. Examiners may give excessive attention to selective aspects of their data, in order to confirm their beliefs about a specific client. Hypotheses formulated early in the evaluation process need to be confirmed or disconfirmed. Research shows that clinicians tend to favor confirmation and resist disconfirmation of hypotheses formulated earliest in an evaluation. Therefore, to avoid this bias, examiners need to weight disconfirming evidence equally with confirming evidence, especially in the case of early-formulated hypotheses.

REPORT FORMAT OUTLINE

The following is a traditional order of headings for a psychological report. This format will be used to label the sources of information in the case examples presented below.

Format for a Psychological Report
   1. Identifying Data

Name: Age:
Date of Birth: Years of Education:
Marital Status: Occupation:
Date of Examination: Address:

   2. Referral Questions Referral questions must be clearly stated, since they determine what questions will be asked in the interview, what tests will be administered, and what findings will be emphasized in the report. It is the purpose of a report to answer the referral questions.

3. **List of Evaluation Procedures**
4. **Behavioral Observations** An accurate description and interpretation of the patient's behavior, attitudes, and conversation during the evaluation sessions is necessary to provide evidence for hypotheses formulated in the test findings and history.
5. **Background History** Medical and school records are often necessary to obtain objective information about history. Self-reported history given during an interview is valuable because it indicates the patient's perceptions of the history, which is often more important for understanding the patient's problems than the factual events. The interview should include early developmental and medical history, as well as more recent experiences. Relationships with parents, as well as peer relationships, should be included. School and occupational history are important to include.
6. **Test Findings and Interpretations**
7. **Summary and Conclusions**
8. **Diagnostic Impressions (DSM-IV)**
9. **Recommendations**
10. **Signature and Title of the Examiner**

THE APPLICATION OF CLINICAL INFERENCE

The conclusions at the end of the report represent the end product of a chain of clinical inferences arrived at by inspecting, analyzing, and integrating information gathered from a variety of sources into a cohesive, plausible, and meaningful set of interrelated hypotheses. The sources of information include: referral questions, behavioral observations, background information, clinical interviews, and test data.

The Referral Question

Prior to the selection of an appropriate, well-balanced test battery, the examiner should consider carefully the referral questions. Issues addressed in the referral question determine the tests to be given, observations to be made, and the person or persons to be interviewed, as well as what collateral information is needed to answer the referral questions. Additionally, the battery designed to answer referral questions may need to be changed during the assessment to account for unforeseen aspects of the case. Psychologists who do not design their evaluation to answer the referral questions tend to scatter their attention to too many irrelevant issues. It is a false assumption that a greater multiplicity of tests increases the likelihood of obtaining the most relevant information. Such a scattered approach to testing, in addition to being time consuming, expensive, and unnecessary, tends to yield redundant and superfluous information.

Behavioral Observations

After reviewing the referral questions and selecting a well-balanced and planned battery of tests, examiners turn their attention to the examinee's behavior during the course of the evaluation. To augment the information gleaned from test findings and to improve their clinical inferences, examiners are encouraged to keep a verbatim record of the examinees' verbal asides and behaviors during the course of the evaluation. Detailed descriptions should be made of any unusual behaviors or statements. Observations gathered during the course of testing, verbal asides, and responses to test stimuli offer a rich pool of behaviors from which examiners draw inferences. These descriptions of the client's behaviors will be integrated with the clinical inferences made from test results. Their value lies in their objectivity. States of mind inferred from test data are less objective than behavioral observations, and will, therefore, need to be verified through integration with the behavioral observations.

Background Information

Knowledge of background information is crucial to the understanding of the examinee' levels of functioning and past achievements. Background information should include the following: developmental history, family constellation, familial interactions, school and medical history, social growth, activities, and interests. Knowledge of historical background is an essential link to an understanding of a person's present behaviors. Inferences drawn from background information are based on the assumptions that an individual's behavior tends to be rather consistent and that the best predictor of a person's future course of action is past behavior.

Interview and Test Data

Self-reported information obtained from a clinical interview, from projective measures, and actuarial tests, and information gleaned from behavioral assessments provide the basis for the final aspects of clinical inference. Not all data gathered in the assessment process should be included in the report. It is the dual purpose of the integration phase of inference not only to select those aspects of the data that have provided solutions to the referral questions, but also to bypass data that is redundant or otherwise not contributory. The report writer must strike a balance between under- and overinclusiveness of information. There must be a deliberate effort to bypass any information that will distract from the main focus of the report (no matter how interesting or useful for other reasons). On the other hand, relevant information should not be bypassed merely for the sake of brevity. One method for maintaining such a balance between reports that are overinclusive and reports that are underinclusive is to have an inference plan.

STAGES OF CLINICAL INFERENCE

The inference plan suggested here is to proceed through three stages of inference, beginning with very specific hypotheses about test responses, interview data, background information, and behavior observations. This process ends with an integration of these hypotheses in a well conceptualized report.

1. Stage One: Hypotheses Based on Raw Data. The first step in the inferential process is to create a number of independent hypotheses which interpret each component of the raw data derived from the evaluation. Since these hypotheses are each derived separately from the analysis of each source of raw data, each of these hypotheses may "suggest" a different aspect of the character structure of the examinee and her or his typical ways of behaving.

2. Stage Two: Integration of Raw Data Hypotheses. Following formulation of a wide range of hypotheses in the first stage of inference, the psychologist attempts to integrate the information in these raw data hypotheses. From these integrations, the examiner postulates second stage or integrated hypotheses, which link and synthesize the personality characteristics of the examinee with the various ego functions which work synergistically to crystallize these characteristics into his or her personality structure. It is this second stage of inference which produces integrated statements about the essential characteristics of the examinee's level of day-to-day functioning.

3. *Stage Three: The Final Synthesis.* The third and final level of inference is achieved by synthesizing the integrated hypotheses of level two and postulating diagnostic statements that best describe the person and his overall level of functioning.

ADULT CASE #1: A PSYCHODYNAMIC APPROACH

A Brief Example of the Application of the Three Levels of Inference

Brian, a 27-year-old college student was referred for psychological testing by his psychiatrist. Brian had been very distressed by his inability to concentrate on his studies. When he tried to study, he had unwanted (ego-dystonic) thoughts of sexually molesting his neighbor's nine-year-old daughter who frequently played in the street by his home. To interrupt these unwanted thoughts, Brian developed a ritual of leaving his studies, jogging around the block, returning to his room, and putting on his headset to play loud music.

During the psychological testing, Brian was compliant but restless. He was often dissatisfied with his answers because he believed that they were not precise or detailed enough to convey his ideas clearly and completely. Indeed, his responses were far more detailed than expected, and his attempts to be precise resulted in an increase in pedantic and indecisive responses. Furthermore, when presented with affectively charged material, he responded in a highly intellectualized sterile fashion. His MMPI-2 codetype was 7-9, and he had an elevated Obsessive Content Scale (OBS). On the Rorschach, the constellation for the obsessive style index was positive, and his EB ratio indicated an ambitent problem-solving style.

The *first stage of inference* in the case of Brian was to hypothesize on the basis of the referral complaints that he had obsessive-compulsive problems (inability to concentrate, instrusive ruminations, and ritualistic behaviors). On the basis of behavioral observations, it was hypothesized that he was anxious (restless, indecisive) and preoccupied with orderliness. His MMPI-2 codetype and Rorschach Inkblot Test positive constellation Obsessive Style Index (OBS) each supported a hypothesis of an obsessive-compulsive disorder. On the basis of the EB ratio of the Rorschach, a hypothesis was formulated that Brian is a person who is indecisive in his problem-solving style.

In the second stage of inference, an integration of the separate hypotheses from the interview, MMPI-2, and Rorschach offered considerable evidence for a diagnosis of obsessive-compulsive disorder (DSM 300.3). The separate hypotheses may be combined into a descriptive summary as follows: "Brian is an anxious, indecisive person who is driven by the need to be precise, complete, and punctilious." From a psychodynamic point of view, Brian's obsessive-compulsive tendencies may be conceptualized as a type of ego defense system whose purpose was to protect him against the intense feelings of anxiety which threatened his emotional adjustment. Brian apparently maintains a measure of emotional stability by resorting to intellectualization, isolation of affect, and reaction formation. His impulse to sexually molest his neighbor's daughter is being held in check in a very tentative fashion, because his style of coping is inconsistent. Therefore, he needs to begin psychotherapy as soon as possible.

The third stage of inference in the text of the psychological report is a final refinement of the integrated hypotheses of the stage two inference. A final integration of the intrapsychic conflict and the development of the disorder might be stated in the report in the following fashion: "The inner conflict between Brian's powerful impulses to be a sexual abuser and his weakened defenses has been resolved temporarily by the formation of an obsessive-compulsive orientation. His obsessive-compulsive disorder is manifested in symptoms of unwanted ruminations and compulsive rituals. This pathological adjustment has failed to provide Brian with an adequate means of coping with his inner conflicts. He is in urgent need of a psychological treatment which will address these conflicts."

ADULT CASE #2 (RZ): CONCEPTUALIZATION USING A PSYCHODYNAMIC APPROACH

The purpose of this Case #2 is to present the three stages of inference in greater detail than in Case #1. The assessment data are described in a condensed fashion to avoid wordiness, but the data are labelled according to source.

Referral Information. RZ is a 22-year-old caucasian male who referred himself because of stress and anxiety about his lack of progress in meeting the life goals which he had set for himself. He asked for a professional analysis of his decision-making difficulties and for professional guidance about how to refocus his life.

Interview and Background History. RZ is an undergraduate college student who lives with his girlfriend in a large city in the southeastern U.S. He was reared in New York, where his parents lived until he entered high school. His only sibling, an older sister, was born in the Phillipines, where his father was stationed in the military. RZ describes his father as a very private person who is insecure about trusting people, even his own children. During his childhood, RZ's father was infrequently at home because he worked long hours saving money to buy a house. RZ described his mother as more emotionally available than his father, although she worked nights in a bank and slept during the day when he was a child. Neither of his parents finished high school.

During his later childhood, his parents moved their residence several times. When he was 10 years old, his parents separated for a year. The moving and separation bothered him a great deal. He became very angry at his father for leaving the family and maintained this anger, even after his father returned to the family. During this time he had difficulty concentrating in school, and he began to fantasize about becoming a baseball player.

EZ's life became more stable when the family moved to the Southeast. He entered and graduated from the same high school. His grades improved, and he was captain of the baseball, football, and track team. During the last two years, he has been attending college but feels very unstable about his life goals. RZ summarized his life, thus far, as fitting into four distinct periods. He described the first 10 years with his family as "happy and good." The next four years after his parent's separation were described as unstable and "crumbling down." He viewed his high school years as very happy ones. He said, "After high school graduation things began to become rough again." He believes that his life after high school has brought back some of his pre-high-school feelings of instability. He said," I found myself moving around a lot trying to find out what I was going to do with my life and that is where I am at right now." He feels that the only goal that he has been able to accomplish is going to college. He regrets losing a college scholarship because he was injured and could not play football.

He regards his current girlfriend as the best friend that he has ever had, and he noted that she is always there when he needs her.

The Minnesota Multiphasic Personality Inventory. The code-type for RZ's MMPI-2 clinical scales was 2-9-8-4. The T-scores for the depression (Scale 2) and hypomania (Scale 9) scales were both 77, an elevation of more than two standard deviations above the mean. Therefore, the probability that the descriptors for these scales apply to RZ is very high. The consistency and validity were within acceptable limits.

The Rorschach Inkblot Test. RZ gave 15 responses, which made his protocol interpretable but meager. The ratio between his human movement and color responses (EB) was 2:2. The Exner Coping Deficit Index (5) was the only positive constellation, but his Suicide Constellation (7) was nearly positive.

The Wechsler Adult Intelligence Scale. EZ's Full Scale IQ on the WAIS-III was 87, nearly one standard deviation below the mean. His Verbal IQ was 95 and his Performance IQ was 81. His lowest verbal subtest scaled scores were Vocabulary (7) and Information (8). His lowest performance subtest scaled scores were Picture Completion (4) and Block Design (7).

The Thematic Apperception Test. On Card 1, RZ told a story about a little boy who was frustrated as he tried to learn to play the violin in compliance with his parents' wishes. On Card 2 he told a story about a young woman whose parents wanted her to finish her education because they did not do so. She respected what her parents said. On Card 3BM he described a little boy who wanted something and was not able to get it. He pouted and cried to get his way. When his parents refused, he did something that they did not want him to do in order to pay them back. On Card 7BM he described a father giving his son advice. RZ said that in the future they become closer because he learns to understand his father.

The Rotter Incomplete Sentences Blank. RZ completed several sentences in which there was concern about his future. Sentence #24 was: *The future* is unclear (Q) I don't know what is going to happen. He also completed several sentences in which there were signs of his current feelings of emotional instability. Sentence #6 was: *At bedtime* I cannot sleep (Q) too many things on my mind (Q) What am I going to do with myself? Several sentences describe his personal suffering when his needs are not met. Sentence #20 was: *I suffer* a lot (Q) from not doing what I want to do in life (Q) play ball.

ANALYSIS OF CASE #2 (RZ)

Presenting Problems: Stage One Inferences

Hypothesis #1: RZ's self-referral supports the hypothesis that he is motivated to seek out the cause of his problems.

Hypothesis #2: RZ's self-referral for stress and anxiety supports the hypothesis that he is feeling a moderate degree of discomfort with his present life.

Psychological Interview: Stage One Inferences

Hypothesis #1: RZ's childhood experiences have negatively impacted his life. He had a turbulent life particularly after age ten, when his parents separated. His mother and her two children became increasingly less secure and moved several times. The frequent changes of residence, school, and neighborhood during puberty and early adolescence contributed to feelings of insecurity and instability. It is possible that RZ learned during this time to view interpersonal relationships as transient, and that he learned to disengage and reengage quickly with each new neighborhood and school. The depressive feelings which he complains about and the uncertainty as to what the future holds for him are not unlike the feelings that he had as a child when the future was always uncertain.

Hypothesis #2: RZ wishes to fulfill some of his parents desires for him. His belief is that his parents, who had insufficient formal education, have emphasized schooling for both of their children. He views his parents as wishing to live their dreams through their children, rather than to find out what their children are interested in and help them realize their own dreams.

Hypothesis #3: RZ portrays a picture of a distant father who abandoned his family. Interestingly, this hypothesis may reflect only RZ's current perception of his father, rather than historical fact. Contrary to the notion that he has not felt some closeness to his father, RZ's feelings about a father come to light in a Thematic Apperception Test story in which he describes a close, friendly father who is giving guidance to his son. But that more complex aspect of his mixed feelings of love and hate for his father is not a part of the first stage of inference and will be described later on at the integration stage.

Hypothesis #4: Rodney feels very close to his mother, despite her unavailability during his childhood. His successful formation of a relationship with his girlfriend may be related to these his feelings about his mother.

Hypothesis # 5: Rodney's successes at schoolwork and athletics in high school have left him with feelings of confidence about himself. They have given him the desire to formulate realistic aspirations for himself rather than mere dreams, or much less, the dream fulfillment of his parents.

Hypothesis # 6: Rodney's main concern about himself is that he is not progressing in his lifelong goals. He is confused about the reasons why he does not meet these goals. He wants to know if he has any cognitive, emotional, or social problems which might be preventing him from meeting his goals.

Psychological Testing: Stage One Inferences

Stage one inferences for test findings are often generated, these days, from computer programs that provide scoring and interpretation of test data. Examples of such software programs are those for the WAIS-III, MMPI-2, and Rorschach. After obtaining a printed report from such a software program, however, the report writer is still faced with the task of selecting the most appropriate material for the final report. Thus, the task of stage one inference may be accomplished by generating a series of hypotheses about the same test, whether by software or by hand. Next, stage two integrated inferences are generated by combining related hypothese may within a single test or among several tests. To make more evident how stage one hypotheses lead to stage two integrations, the stage one hypotheses cited below have been selected to reflect similar themes that have been judged by the examiner to be related.

1. The Minnesota Multiphasic Personality Inventory–2. The first descriptor listed for the 2-9 codetype is "self-centered and narcissistic." Therefore, the first hypothesis suggested by the leading correlate of the 2-9 codetype for RZ is that he is self-centered and narcissistic.

2. The Rorschach Inkblot Test. When the computer software of Exner (Rorschach Interpretation Assistance Program, or RIAP) was used to generate inferences about RZ's responses, the first positive key variable (CDI > 3) directed the search strategy to the third in a sequence of clusters of structural data: self-perception. Among the structural data in this self-perception cluster were Fr + rF = 4, FD = 2, An + Xy = 1, and the Egocentricity Index $(3r + (2)/R) = .93$. The first hypothesis generated for this data by the RIAP software was "a core element in this subject's personality is a narcissistic-like tendency to overvalue personal worth." This hypothesis was selected from the software report for focus at this point because it is easily integrated with the MMPI-2 hypothesis above.

3. *Thematic Apperception Test.* On Card 3BM, RZ told a story about a little boy who wanted something and was deprived of it by his parents. He tried pouting and crying to get his desires satisfied. When his parents refuse, he does something to pay them back. The hypothesis generated by the examiner and selected for its potential for integration with the above MMPI-2 and Rorschach hypotheses was that RZ views revenge as an appropriate response when his wishes are denied (an attitude that could very well be generated by a self-centered personality).

4. *Rotter Incomplete Sentences Blank–Adult Form.* In response to Sentence Stem #20, *I suffer,* RZ wrote, "a lot from not doing what I want to do in my life." The hypothesis generated by the examiner was that RZ is reporting that he experiences ongoing emotional pain because he is not able to do the things that he wants. Similarly to patients with a narcissistic personality disorder, RZ experiences painful affect when his dreams go unfulfilled

Presenting Complaints: Stage Two Inferences

An integration of the two hypotheses from stage one might be to conclude that RZ's motivation to purpose professional help is at least partially influenced by his current degree of emotional discomfort.

Psychological Interview: Stage Two Inferences

A very helpful procedure during the integration phase is to label each content sentence with the hypothesis number and the source of data. Such an approach facilitates the rapid identification of the source of statements, enabling the report writer to retrieve and revise inferences. An example of this approach follows.

Integration #1: RZ interprets the emotional distance between himself and his father as a form of developmental deprivation that has had a destabilizing effect on his life similar to the instability which RZ experienced during the many times that the family was socially uprooted to move residences (Interview, Hypotheses # 1 and 3).

Integration #2: The negative impact of paternal distance and family moves has been to partially retard RZ's social and emotional development and to reduce his confidence in his ability to determine his own future (Interview, Hypotheses # 1, 3 and 6).

Integration #3: On the other hand, RZ has perceived his mother's emotional closeness as a positive force in his life, which has helped him to mature in his relationship with women, and to partially counterbalance the negative impact of his father's emotional distance (Interview, Hypotheses #3 and 4).

Integration #4: His success in high school academics and athletics helped to build some of the social and emotional confidence which had developed slowly in childhood (Interview, Hypotheses #1 and 5).

Integration #5: RZ feels a strong need to fulfill his parents' unmet need for achievement, as though such an accomplishment will substitute for his ambivalence about planning his own future (Interview, Hypotheses #2, 5 & 6).

These five integrated statements combine, relate, and interpret the six hypotheses from the interview in a second stage of inference. Notice that the statements include:

1. Clear labeling of RZ's perceptions and interpretations as self-report data, e.g., RZ "*interprets* the emotional distance between himself. . . ."
2. Using abstract but understandable terminology to categorize the relationships between life events, e.g., "Social-emotional development."
3. Making inferences about relationships between events without using absolute or global terminology, e.g., "*partially* counterbalanced the negative . . . , *helped to build* social-emotional*.*"

Since these hypotheses and integrations have been generated only from the interview, they await confirmations from the other assessment data. Use of the label (interview) may seem unnecessary at this point, when the integrations are all within a single source of data. However, integrations also need to be made between interview hypotheses and the hypotheses from other sources of data. An example of such an intersource hypothesis makes use of a potential hypothesis from the TAT data cited above and an interview hypothesis. This intersource hypothesis may be stated as follows:: Although RZ portrays a picture of his father as an emotionally distant man who abandoned his family (interview, Hypothesis #3), this perception may be motivated by his unresolved anger at his father for leaving the family (interview). In his projective stories (TAT), he describes a father who is close, friendly, and wise. The final integration, then, is that RZ has mixed feelings about his father, which include both love and hate, both hope and disappointment, and both fantasy and reality.

Psychological Testing: Stage Two Inference

The stage one hypotheses for data from each of the psychological tests above have been selected for integration by the examiner because of their similar content. They have all inferred a self-centeredness in RZ. The examiner must go beyond the specific focus of each test inference and fit the single hypotheses to a model of personality. In this case, the conceptual model of choice might be DSM-IV, Axis II, Narcissistic Personality Disorder (Cluster B, 301.81). DSM-IV describes Narcissistic Personality Disorder as a "pervasive pattern of grandiosity (in fantasy or behavior), a need for admiration and lack of empathy." The disorder begins in early adulthood. The DSM-IV diagnostic conceptualization calls for verification of at least 5 of 9 criteria, such as, "is preoccupied with fantasies of unlimited success." This latter criteria was verified in RZ's continuous focus on his desire to become a famous baseball star. Sufficient criteria were verified for the Narcissistic Personality Disorder diagnosis through the use of the *Structured Clinical Interview for DSM-IV.*

Final Integration of All Findings:
The Integrated Report, Diagnostic Section

Using the DSM-IV conceptualization of findings, the integrated hypotheses may finally be related to diagnostic categories of psychopathology.

1. Narcissistic Personality Disorder, DSM-IV 301.81, Axis II was confirmed.
2. Although RZ was not found to meet DSM critieria for Avoidant Personality Disorder, findings described him as lonely, lacking in family support, angry at perceived family pressure to achieve, fearing failure, feeling socially alienated, and having superficial social relationships (interview).
3. Although DSM-IV diagnosis of Dysthymic Disorder was not confirmed because RZ does not report a consistent depressed mood, he does report signs of depression. EZ

said that he has insomnia (Incomplete Sentences), poor self-esteem, and concentration deficits (interview), as one would find in Dysthymic Disorder. RZ's MMPI-2 codetype 2-9 often is interpreted to represent depression masked by agitation. RZ's suicide constellation on the Rorschach was nearly positive, and he endorsed one critical item on the MMPI-2 which acknowledged thoughts of self-harm.

4. A significant discrepancy between RZ's Verbal IQ of 94 and his Performance IQ score of 80 on the WAIS-III raised the suspicion that he has difficulty with new learning, especially when task materials are visual-spatial. Since diagnosis cannot be either confirmed or disconfirmed in this case, a referral to a neuropsychologist for further assessment is advised.

Final Integration of All Findings: Dynamic Section

To integrate RZ's test and interview hypotheses into a description of his personality makeup, it is necessary to use a conceptual model. For the case of RZ, a psychodynamic model was chosen. A dynamic point of view includes the examinee's own interpretation of the facts, as well as the examiner's diagnostic point of view. For instance, we might say in the report, "RZ's perception of his father as an emotionally distant man (Hypothesis #3, interview) is the result of deprivation of physical and emotional contact with his father as a child. This deprivation has also contributed to the development in adulthood of a narcissistic personality disorder. RZ has added his own emotional alienation to his feeling of emotional deprivation by his father."

It is traditional in a dynamic conceptualization to describe the coping mechanisms by which the examinee tries to adjust to his psychopathology. For instance, we might include all of the following:

1. "RZ uses rationalization to cope with his feelings of self-doubt, especially when he is unable to assert his will (TAT, Card 3BM). He states that he has 'learned that you don't get everything that you want.'"
2. "In the face of conflict, RZ's first instinct is to walk away and avoid, but with the encouragement of others he is able to resolve conflicts (TAT, Card 4). He switches between isolation/constriction of anger and hostile outbursts of anger towards his family."
3. "RZ's preoccupation with decisions about the future keeps him from anxiety about current issues." (Interview)
4. "He presents as an anxious-agitated individual, while internally he is more depressed." (MMPI-2 2-9)

It is also traditional in a dynamic conceptualization to hypothesize about the source of the anxiety and depression that underly RZ's emotional discomfort. For instance, we might say in the report, "RZ's unresolved bid for autonomy, as described in his projective story themes, and his unresolved feelings of abandonment by his father both point to very early sources of emotional conflict."

Final Integration of All Findings: Conclusions

After presenting an integrated description of EZ's personality, conclusions must be offered to answer the referral questions. As a self-referral, RZ asked why it was that he was not able to make progress in his life goals and why he felt anxious and depressed. In answer to these diagnostic questions, the report conclusions might include the following:

"RZ's perception that his father failed to recognize, nurture, and allow his self-identity to develop may be an accurate perception of one of the sources of his problems, but his problems are not due in their entirety to his father's emotional distance. The main source of his current inner conflicts are unresolved developmental issues from early childhood. EZ's perceptions provide him with only partial insight the origins of his problems. By hindsight, he feels a need to have his father help him to attain an autonomous self and to learn to assert his will. To avoid the feelings associated with this loss of developmental progress, RZ has learned to rationalize and to swallow his feelings. He has adjusted to these feelings in a more permanent fashion by overcompensating and overvaluing his self, as a narcissistic personality disorder. His symptoms of depression and anxiety are signs of the inner turmoil which he experiences. His problems with object relations and progress in a career are further negative effects of his inner turmoil."

Final Integration of All Findings: Recommendations

Recommendations for treatment, further assessment, and consultation by other professionals should be listed after the conclusions in the form of specific, planned, defined statements. In the case of RZ, one recommendation will be to obtain a neuropsychological evaluation. It is the responsibility of the examiner to recommend a specific neuropsychologist, and if possible, to oversee the scheduling of an appointment. If such scheduling is accomplished before the publication of the report, the time and place of the neuropsychological assessment may be listed in the recommendations. Another recommendation for RZ will be to schedule an appointment with a psychotherapist to begin a course of psychological treatment for his disorder. Again, it is the responsibility of the examiner to facilitate the referral to a psychotherapist and, if possible, to list the time and place of the first appointment.

PSYCHOLOGICAL ASSESSMENT OF CHILDREN AND ADOLESCENTS

Full Assessment Battery for Children and Adolescents

Although brief screening methods are often used out of expedience due to constraints on time and money, use of a comprehensive battery of psychological tests in the assessment of children has an important advantage. Unlike adults, children and adolescents are limited in their ability to adequately describe the context in which their problems occur. They are likely to have inadequate memories for the circumstances in which events occur, and they may not recall events in sufficient detail to enlighten an examiner about the subtle aspects of their problems. Furthermore, children and adolescents may not have matured sufficiently in their ability to conceptualize their problems to understand the relationship between their daily life events and these problems. A thorough battery of psychological tests may compensate for some of this inadequacy. Through the use of multiple informants and multiple test strategies, a psychological examiner can make accurate estimates of the details of the child or adolescent's problems.

The Components of a Full Battery for Children and Adolescents

A thorough battery of tests for children and adolescents typically includes assessment approaches which gather information using all of the following five components.

1. *History.* The history of the child or adolescent's medical, developmental, psychiatric, social, and school progress should be gathered from reliable sources.

2. *Abilities.* Several subtypes of abilities should be assessed within major content areas. Sufficient subtypes of content should be assessed to detect subtle aspects of the problems that have been stated in the referral question. For instance, a referral question about cognitive abilities would call for the assessment of such subtype categories as intelligence, memory, attention, concentration, concept formation, and achievement. A referral question about emotional adjustment might call for use of such subtype categories of content as behavior, personality, peer relationships, self-concept and emotional stability.

3. *Surroundings.* An evaluation of the child or adolescent's behavior in each of the settings of their current life should be carried out. For instance, visits to the home to observe the interaction of family members and to the school to observe classroom behavior might be essential components of an evaluation which had a referral question about socially inappropriate behaviors.

4. *Sources.* It is essential to make use of information from each of the adults who is with the child or adolescent during a significant part of each day. The mother, father, teacher, coach, employer, and caretaker may each contribute unique and important information concerning the problem.

5. *Instruments.* The use of a wide range of assessment instrument types, such as psychometric tests (achievement, IQ), projective techniques (Rorschach, TAT), behavior assessment (fear inventories, reinforcement history), self-report inventories (self-concept scales), and rating scales (Child Behavior Checklist) each offer a different perspective on the problems of the child or adolescent.

A well-planned selection of instruments for use in the full assessment battery is the first step toward the writing of a well-informed report. After each of the five aspects of assessment have been completed, the findings must be analyzed for use in the report.

Integration of Evaluation Information

A thorough battery of tests, which contains information about multiple areas of psychological content, obtained from various settings and sources through the use of many psychological techniques, offers the evaluator an interpretative challenge. The most valuable psychological reports are those which are able to organize such a vast array of information into clear statements which answer the referral questions and provide a rationale for the recommendations at the end of the report. The following case study of an adolescent offers an application and adaptation of the method of integrated report writing suggested earlier in this chapter for adult full battery cases.

A CHILD CASE (#3, S.K.)

Sarah is a 14-year-old female, who was referred by her case worker for evaluation of her psychological adjustment. She had recently been placed in a residential treatment facility, after unsuccessful foster placement. She had been removed from parental custody a year earlier due to parental neglect and physical abuse. The foster parents had reported oppositional-defiant behavior, unexplained outbursts of anger, and suicidal threats.

Referral. Two referral questions were formulated in consultation with the referring social worker. The first referral question focused on Sarah's current psychological status. Specifically, does she meet criteria for a psychological disorder, and what is the risk of suicide? The second referral question was concerned with Sarah's intervention setting. Is the current residential treatment facility an appropriate placement for her during the coming year, and should any changes be made in her treatment in the residential setting?

Assessment Instruments. To gather information concerning the first referral question about Sarah's current psychological status, the following assessment techniques were used:

- The Kiddie-Schedule for Affective Disorders and Schizophrenia in School-Age Children 6–18 Years–Present Conditions (K-SADS-P).
- The Minnesota Multiphasic Personality Inventory–Adolescent (MMPI-A).
- The Beck Hopelessness Scale (BHS).
- The Rorschach Inkblot Test (RIT).
- The Thematic Apperception Test (TAT).

Although, in reality, all assessment devices were used for both referral questions, two subsets of tests are listed here to provide a demonstration of their use in the analysis of the case. The following set of instruments were used in this case to gather information concerning the second referral question regarding intervention.

- The Wechsler Intelligence Scale for Children–Third Edition (WISC-III).
- The Wide Range Achievement Test–Third Edition (WRAT-III).
- The Rotter Incomplete Sentences Blank (RISB).
- The Child Behavior Checklist (CBCL).
- Unstructured Interview.

REFERRAL QUESTION #1: PSYCHOLOGICAL STATUS

1. First Stage of Inference: Hypothesis Formation

Similarly to the approach suggested for the intepetation of adult findings, analysis of child assessment data may be accomplished in three stages. The first stage is that of hypothesis formation.

K-SADS-P. Using the child as informant, criteria were met for DSM-IV diagnoses of Major Depression and Post Traumatic Stress Disorder. During the K-SADS-P interview, Sarah was alert, cooperative, and coherent in her responses. Although she was slightly overtalkative in elaborating her responses, the examiner considered the interview to be consistent and accurate. Therefore, the first hypothesis is that Sarah has comorbid affective and stress disorders, which are impairing her social and school functioning (Kiddie-Global Assessment Scale). Sarah reports that her feelings of depression are intense and that she becomes irritated and cranky with others. It is her opinion that the abuse which she experienced as a child is the source of her problems. Having been abused has left her with a chronic sense of guilt and low self-esteem. She is often fatigued, has poor concentration, and avoids people because of her depressed feelings.

MMPI-A. Sarah's seventh grade reading equivalent on the WRAT-III was sufficient for her to read the items on the MMPI-A. The protocol was complete and showed item consistency. Although the K scale and TRIN were within normal limits, the L scale was elevated, indicating some defensiveness about minor personal flaws. On the other hand, a mild elevation of the

F scale indicated an endorsement of a wide variety of symptoms. Therefore, the clinical scales were judged to be interpretable. The most elevated clinical scale was 6 (Pa), with the Harris-Lingoes subscale Pa1 (persecutory ideas) most elevated. These findings support a second hypothesis about Sarah's emotional adjustment. She feels misunderstood and different from others. She is interpersonally sensitive, and her efforts to be liked and appreciated go unacknowledged. Sarah reported that she becomes so angry at her peers that she drives them away.

2. The Second Stage of Inference: Hypothesis Integration (Referral Question #1)

Clinical Scale 2 (D) on the MMPI-A was also found to be elevated. This finding provides further evidence for Hypothesis #1 concerning presence of an affective disorder. An elevation on Scale 2 indicates a high likelihood that Sarah's adjustment is similar to that of patients with major depression. Furthermore, elevated Harris-Lingoes subscales of D1 (subjective depression) and D5 (brooding) indicate that Sarah endorsed items concerning nervousness, worry, brooding, dysphoria, and feelings of inadequacy. Taken together, these two pieces of information offer good evidence that Sarah is depressed and possibly suicidal.

Beck Hopelessness Scale. On the BHS, Sarah endorsed 14 of 20 items in the pessimistic direction. She endorsed such statements as, "All I can see ahead of me is unpleasantness." This was consistent with items endorsed on the MMPI-A, such as "The future seems hopeless to me." On the MMPI-A, Sarah's endorsement of the suicidal ideation item "I sometimes think about killing myself" is consistent with her report that she has suicidal thoughts. It appears that much suicidal ideation is intermittent, since she failed to endorse the MMPI-A item "Most of the time I wish I were dead." Taken together, loss of hope reflected in the BHS and the suicidal ideation endorsed on the MMPI-A help to qualify Hypothesis #1 about an affective disorder. There is a genuine suicide risk. Sarah's social worker needs to be alerted to the risk in order that precautions may be taken at the residential setting.

The Rorschach Test. None of the constellations were positive, but an elevated Lambda indicated an overly constricted manner of processing information. In other words, Sarah does not allow herself to think about all of the connotations of what she sees. This places her at risk for acting before she thinks and for acting in unconventional ways. It is known that patients with PTSD report experiencing loss of control over their thinking. Taken together with Sarah's self-report about feeling misunderstood, guilty, and depressed, there is support for inference that she is experiencing PTSD. Her opinion that the abuse is the source of much of her problems also provides evidence for this hypothesis.

TAT. Sarah told TAT stories which contained themes about sad and lonely children, stories about happy, popular, abused children, and suicidal children. Her last TAT story was an actual description of her own abuse and foster placement. The story themes all seem to fit Sarah's life either in reality or in her fantasies about how good life could be. There seems to be a side to Sarah's that has some hope, even if in a very polyannish way. She experiences her sadness and the heavy weight of her abuse history, while at the same time nourishing a hope for a better life. This hopeful side of Sarah will be to her advantage in benefitting from psychological treatment.

3. The Third Stage of Inference: Report Writing (Referral Question #1)

Sarah's comorbid major depressive disorder and post-traumatic stress disorder are the emotional sequelae of a history of abuse and foster placement. These disorders are a barometer of just how much Sarah's history has impacted her ability to adjust. In other words, the internal suffering of this adolescent is manifested in her diagnoses. She attests that her episodes of depression, as well as those times without depression, are both accompanied by the vivid memories of abuse and loss of her family. Her emotional disturbance is significant, but well focused in its historical origin. The evidence from the K-SADS-P, MMPI-A, BHS, Rorschach and TAT converges to tell the story of social alienation, sadness, aloneness, and hopelessness that result from an abuse history. The answer to referral question #1 is clear. Sarah's diagnoses of major depression and PTSD call for intensive treatment.

REFERRAL QUESTION #2: AN APPROPRIATE TREATMENT SETTING

Similarly as with the three stages of inference listed above for referral question #1, the report writer should progress through the three stages of inference for referral question #2. In this sample case, the hypotheses generated by findings from the WISC-III, WRAT-III, RISB, CBCL, and interview should be used in an integration phase and finally a report-writing phase. In Sarah's case, a Full Scale IQ of 88 and reading achievement standard score of 93 did not present evidence of a learning disability. Rather, her significantly low WISC-III subtest scores in arithmetic and vocabulary made it evident that her abuse history and foster placement had impaired her ability to benefit from traditional education. The most plausible hypothesis is that Sarah is in need of remedial education placement because she must make up for her past history, rather than because her brain is unable to learn. Her adequate reading ability attests to her ability to learn. On the RISB, she described her preoccupation with her social condition (The happiest time is when I am with my brother . . . I have trouble going to sleep) and how her preoccupations have gradually impacted her learning (In the lower grades I did better in school...I can't remember well . . . I failed seventh grade . . . Reading is easy for me because I like it"). The answer to referral question #2 is that residential placement is the best alternative for Sarah as the present time. She needs a setting that can provide her with remedial education, intensive psychotherapy, and a supportive milieu. If her current setting is able to provide these three interventions, then it is appropriate.

The final written report for Sarah can be a very brief summary of these findings in which the two referral questions are answered. What a reader wants to see in the report are:

1. the best answer to the referral questions,
2. the weight of evidence to support the hypotheses about the examinee,
3. the logic used to infer the hypotheses.

In the above sample case of Sarah, these three components have been prepared for the final report through the use of a three-stage process. The reader never sees the lengthy process that is involved in the first two stages of report writing. It is because the first two stages are there, however, that the final report may be brief and to the point.

APPENDIX I.
THE LANGUAGE OF A PSYCHOLOGICAL REPORT

Writing Styles to be Avoided.

1) *The Overuse of Generalized Statements.* Generalized statements that apply to the majority of people, but do not describe a characteristic that is specific to the examinee, are often irrelevant and useless verbiage in a report. An example of such an irrelevant statement would be to say that "people who respond in an aggressive fashion are likely to isolate themselves from interpersonal situations." A specific application of such characteristics to an examinee would be "This person's story themes on a projective test suggests that he feels so uncomfortable in and around people that he uses aggression to avoid interpersonal situations."

2) *The Use of Technical Psychological Jargon.* Textbooks of psychological testing are filled with abstract technical words which are meaningful to psychologists. Words and phrases such as Freedom from Distractibility Factor, visual-spatial synthesis, hypochondriasis, and hysterical features are examples of such jargon. Such psychological jargon should not appear in a written report, since it tends to mystify rather than clarify, even for educated readers, the issues under consideration. An example of the use of such jargon in a sentence would be "this patient's ego functions are so taxed by id impulse derivatives on the one hand and superego injunctions on the other that he is rendered helpless to make decisions." A more parsimonious jargon-free statement of the same content might be "the intensity of this patient's conflicts interfere with his ability to be decisive".

3) *Excessive Use of Superlative Adjectives.* Superlative adjectives, such as in overwhelming anxiety, the most incapacitating anger, and extreme tension, exaggerate the emotional state of the examinee and reduce the credibility of the report. Patients with overwhelming anxiety would not be able to sit through four hours of testing, and patients with incapacitating anger would not be able to adjust outside a mental hospital.

4) *Conclusions Based on a Single Test Item.* When making a generalization about an examinee, it is important to justify such a generalization by linking it to basic and, whenever possible, concrete data either from the test responses or behavior during the course of testing. Thus, the statement that the patient has a poor self-concept becomes increasingly convincing if it is enriched with critical incidents which led to that conclusion. For instance, the patient's repeated self-descriptive statements "I feel so stupid," and "I am doing so poorly on these tests" provide evidence of self-concept. Also, responses on psychometric tests may provide evidence of insufficient self-esteem.

5) *The Use of Too Many Examples to Justify Inferences.* Avoid filling the report with too many examples to justify the inferences made. Examples should be used to illustrate and clarify the issue in question, but too many may distract. Some psychologists believe it is not necessary to give many examples to support their clinical inferences, while others assume that a conclusion is definitely fortified when it is followed by a few relevant examples.

SUGGESTED READINGS

Achenbach, T. M. (1985). *Assessment and taxonomy of child and adolescent psychopathology.* Newbury Park, CA: Sage.

Groth-Marnat, G. (1997). *Handbook of Psychological Assessment* (3rd ed.). New York: John Wiley & Sons, Inc.

Kamphaus, R. W. & Frick, P. J. (1996). *Clinical assessment of child and adolescent personality and behavior.* Boston: Allyn and Bacon.

Sattler, J. M. (1988). *Assessment of children* (3rd ed.). San Diego: Jerome M. Sattler, Publisher.

Tallent, N. (1993). *Psychological Report Writing* (4th ed.). Englewood Cliffs, NJ: Prentice Hall.

About the Editors

William I. Dorfman (Ph.D., Ohio State University) is Professor of Psychology and Associate Director of Clinical Training in the Center for Psychological Studies, Nova Southeastern University, Fort Lauderdale, Florida. He is formerly Executive Director of Nova University's Community Mental Health Center and Chief Psychologist of its APA-approved Internship in Clinical Psychology. Dr. Dorfman is active in the education and training of professional psychologists; has published his work in professional journals and books; and has presented papers at scientific meetings in the areas of personality assessment, psychopathology, clinical interviewing, and the evaluation of trainees' attitudes toward managed health care systems and brief therapy. He has made numerous radio and television appearances discussing mental health issues, including the Oprah Winfrey Show, and is a licensed psychologist in Florida, Virginia, and California and a member of the National Register of Health Service Providers in Psychology. Dr. Dorfman has been awarded a Diplomate in Clinical Psychology by the American Board of Professional Psychology.

Michel Hersen (Ph.D., State University of New York at Buffalo) is Professor and Dean, School of Professional Psychology, Pacific University, Forest Grove, Oregon. He is Past President of the Association for Advancement of Behavior Therapy. He has written 4 books, coauthored and/or coedited 144 books, and has published more than 220 scientific journal articles; he is coeditor of several psychological journals and is coeditor, with Alan S. Bellack, of the recently published 11-volume work *Comprehensive Clinical Psychology*. Dr. Hersen has been the recipient of numerous grants from the National Institute of Mental Health, and Department of Education, the National Institute of Disabilities and Rehabilitation Research, and the March of Dimes Birth Defects Foundation. He is a Diplomate of the American Board of Professional Psychology, Distinguished Practitioner, Member of the National Academy of Practice in Psychology, and recipient of the Distinguished Career Achievement Award in 1996 from the American Board of Medical Psychotherapists and Psychodiagnosticians. Dr. Hersen has written and edited numerous articles, chapters, and books on clinical assessment.

Author Index

Subject Index